THE MANAGEMENT OF HEMANGIOMAS AND VASCULAR MALFORMATIONS OF HEAD AND NECK

THE MANAGEMENT OF HEMANGIOMAS AND VASCULAR MALFORMATIONS OF HEAD AND NECK

Editor

KS Goleria

MB FRCS (Ed) DLO (Lond) DORL (Bom)

Plastic, Reconstructive and Craniofacial Surgeon
201, Doctor House, Dr G Deshmukh Marg
Mumbai, Maharashtra, India

Foreword

Ian T Jackson

JAYPEE BROTHERS MEDICAL PUBLISHERS (P) LTD

New Delhi • Panama City • London

Jaypee Brothers Medical Publishers (P) Ltd.

Headquarter

Jaypee Brothers Medical Publishers (P) Ltd
4838/24, Ansari Road, Daryaganj
New Delhi 110 002, India
Phone: +91-11-43574357
Fax: +91-11-43574314
Email: jaypee@jaypeebrothers.com

Overseas Offices

J.P. Medical Ltd.,
83 Victoria Street London
SW1H 0HW (UK)
Phone: +44-2031708910
Fax: +02-03-0086180
Email: info@jpmedpub.com

Jaypee-Highlights Medical Publishers Inc.
City of Knowledge, Bld. 237, Clayton
Panama City, Panama
Phone: 507-317-0160
Fax: +50-73-010499
Email: cservice@jphmedical.com

Website: www.jaypeebrothers.com
Website: www.jaypeedigital.com

Inquiries for bulk sales may be solicited at: jaypee@jaypeebrothers.com

The Management of Hemangiomas and Vascular Malformations of Head and Neck

First Edition: **2012**

ISBN 978-93-5025-125-6

Printed at: Ajanta Offset & Packagings Ltd., New Delhi

Dedicated to

The memory of

My mother, Smt Bhagwati Devi,
the inspiration to pursue the medical profession and
an example of the power of compassion and love.

My father, Th Birbal Singh,
an ever living example of the value of discipline,
honesty, dedication and hard work.

My wife, Dr Pushpa Devi,
an embodiment
of understanding and sacrifice
my support and strength.

Contributors

Anil Pandurang Karapurkar
MS (Gen Surgery) MS (Neurosurgery)
Senior Consultant
Endovascular Neurosergery
Sir Harkisandas Nurrotumdas Hospital
Mumbai, Maharashtra, India

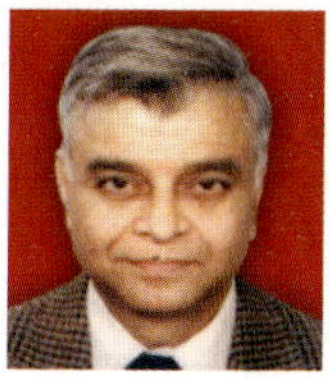

Shrinivas B Desai
MBBS MD (Radiology)
Head of the Department of Imaging
Jaslok Hospital and Research Centre
Mumbai, Maharashtra, India

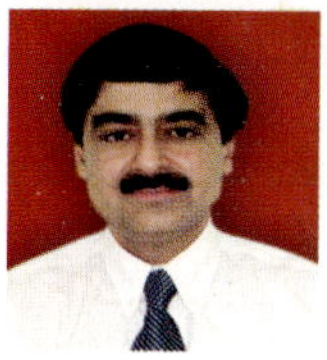

KS Goleria
MB FRCS (Ed) DLO (Lond) DORL (Bom)
Plastic, Reconstructive and Craniofacial Surgeon
Mumbai, Maharashtra, India

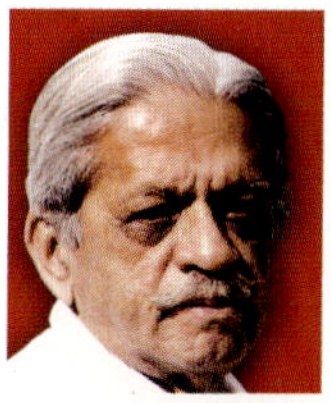

Shrirang G Pandit
MS MCh (Plastic Surgery)
Pandit Clinic
Pune, Maharashtra, India

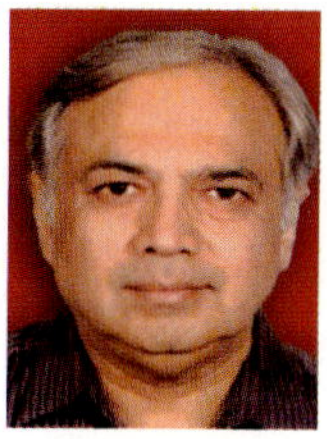

Nirmala Subramanian
MS (Gen Surgery) MCh (Plastic Surgery)
Senior Consultant Plastic Surgery
Apollo Hospital
Chennai, Tamil Nadu, India

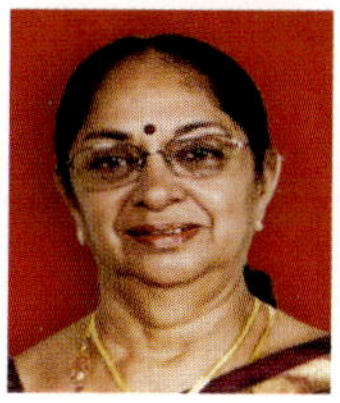

Foreword

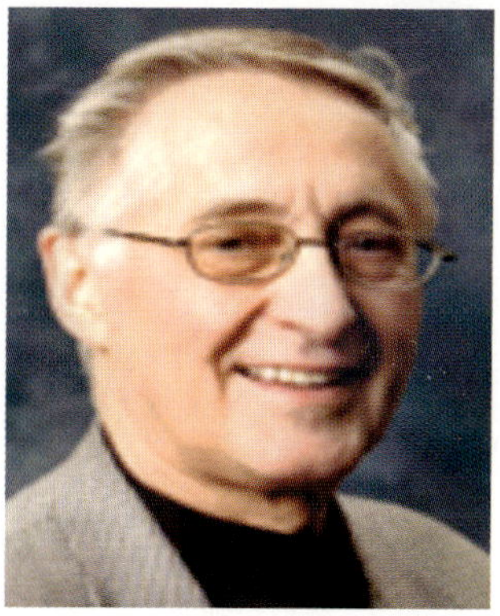

KS Goleria has been a leader of Indian plastic surgery for more than fifty years. He has pioneered many new developments in craniofacial surgery, microsurgery, cleft lip and palate surgery and now the management of hemangiomas and vascular malformations. It is not always appreciated by those from other countries that India has an incredibly large population. It is always embarrassing when presenting one's experience on 50 cases of a somewhat rare condition only to find that several of the Indian surgeons have treated many times that number, and may even present a new and excellent technique, KS Goleria is one of those individuals.

I am so pleased to have been invited to write this foreword. Dr Goleria is my friend, we have shared ideas and I have learned a great deal from him.

As with his surgery, he has considered this subject most carefully and has presented it in a logical and comprehensive manner. This is absolutely necessary since many of the presentations on this subject have been confusing and have led to poor management of these difficult problems.

The Management of Hemangiomas and Vascular Malformations of Head and Neck consists of 10 Chapters, six of which have been written by Dr Goleria. The remaining chapters are contributed by specialists in radiology, ophthalmology, laser therapy, and neurosurgery. This is truly a comprehensive cover of the field. Having known Dr Goleria over a long period of time, having operated with him, and having discussed many difficult cases with him. He has produced what I would have expected from him—a book that will be of great help to those working in this challenging field.

What I find extremely gratifying is to see the textbook coming from an Indian plastic surgeon. It is not always appreciated in the West just how much experience our Indian colleagues have. Dr Goleria is one of the fathers of Indian plastic surgery and as such is highly respected in this field. On many occasions, I have discussed problems with him and he has always been able to draw from his vast experience, and to give advice on even the most obscure conditions. We have operated together—this is where one finds the measure of the man—he is a master.

For those who are interested in this subject, this is a book, which is essential to have. It will be the book you reach for when that seemingly impossible problem turns up. If you are in the field of vascular anomalies or you plan to plunge into this, Dr Goleria's words of wisdom will be of inestimable value to you.

Ian T Jackson
MD FRCS FACS FRACS
Director
Institute for Craniofacial and Reconstructive Surgery
Southfield, Michigan
United States of America

PREFACE

The term 'hemangioma', as still commonly used, neither leads us to a specific entity, nor to a specific therapy. The term itself originates from three Greek words—the prefix *Hem* from *aima* which means blood, the middle *angio* from *aggeion* which means vessel and the suffix *oma* denoting a tumor. The terminology seems to have evolved from 'angioma' to 'hemangioma'. However, because of wide general usage both the terms *oma* and tumor came to be identified with multiplication of cellular entities and not organized entities.

Logically and to prevent confusion, the term hemangioma has come to be restricted to entities with endothelial hyperplasia and mainly to the benign, self-resolving entity, now generally referred to as the *capillary hemangioma of infancy* (CHI) or the *infantile hemangioma* (IH). All other lesions which involved the growth and conglomeration of various vascular channels, capillaries, lymphatics, venules, veins, arteries and their various combinations, but without endothelial proliferations are grouped under the term *Vascular Malformation*.

Some of these combinations are referred to as syndromes, named after the identifier of the entity. There are a number of other syndromes, where other structures participate with one or more segments of this conglomeration.

Each of the constituents of this group of lesions has a distinctive biological behavior and therefore, needs a distinctive therapeutic response. The terminological and the therapeutic confusion is aggravated by lesions having more than one component of this group in varying proportions and combinations.

Apart from plastic surgeons, a number of medical and surgical disciplines handle the management of these vascular anomalies. Their approach to the problems often differs, as does the terminology they use. This compartmentalization prevents the interdisciplinary spread of relevant experience in a common terminology. It has also generated a plethora of nomenclature creating enormous confusion of nomenclature, listed in the appendix after the last chapter, with no claim to its completeness.

This confusion in terminology lead Mulliken to pointedly remark that: "Words have been stumbling blocks on the road to an understanding of vascular anomalies." To overcome this confusion, he has developed a classification 'based on endothelial characteristics' of these lesions. This has considerably ended the terminological confusion and has found wide acceptance.

In the time frame that followed the publication of this classification, the diagnostic and therapeutic advances have been phenomenal, emphasizing a need to take full cognizance of the biological behavior of the involved channels. This was easily achieved by taking into account not only the flow rate (low or high) but also the vessel size (small or large) into their nomenclature and classification. The result is 'A Management Oriented Classification' into four groups detailed in Chapter 1. Each of these groups has distinctive biological characteristics, and a specific approach to evaluation, investigation and management.

The evolution of the classification is briefly dealt with in the first chapter. The specifics of assessment and management are elaborated in the chapter dedicated to each group. Even though this classification is presented in relation to the management of lesions of the head and neck, it is lesion and not region specific. The management—in addition—is influenced by the location of the lesion—particularly so—in the head and neck.

The cranium and the orbit significantly influence our approach to the management. Dr Anil Karapurkar, a Neurosurgeon dedicated to Interventional Radiology and Dr Nirmala Subramanian, a Plastic Surgeon dedicated to Oculoplastic Surgery have gladly contributed their vast experience to the handling of these lesions in the closed confines of their chosen specialties.

The progress in the art and science of imaging has brought precision to the understanding of the anatomical limits and the biological nature of these vascular lesions. In addition, Interventional Radiology has become an important therapeutic tool. It is but appropriate to acknowledge the cooperation and help that we have received from Dr Shrinivas Desai, and his dynamic team, at the Department of Imaging of the Jaslok Hospital and Research Center. Dr Desai has contributed a chapter entitled *Imaging for the Management of Hemangiomas and Vascular Malformations.*

The Lasers and Radiofrequency have emerged as important tools in the management of these lesions. Dr Shrirang G Pandit has dealt with this aspect of the management in the chapter entitled *Lasers in Hemangiomas and Vascular Malformations*.

The *steal phenomenon* occurring in the arteriovenous malformations, had been noticed by Virchow over a century and a half ago. Yet, it was inadequately treated almost till the advent of interventional radiology. It poses formidable management problems and challenges—ablative and reconstructive. The concluding chapter deals with this phenomenon.

Deformity is a feature, common to all hemangiomas and vascular malformations of head and neck.

The genesis of the deformity may lie in the lesion itself—its existence, growth and sometimes involution.

Deformity may also be an expression of the secondary skeletal deformities, which may occur with the passage of time, either as skeletal hypertrophy and overgrowth or as skeletal atropy. An iatrogenic deformity associated with therapeutic interventions often needs to be treated.

'Timely and effective intervention minimizes deformity' is a thought that under-runs this text, based as it is on the biological behavior of the lesion. 'Wait, till the child grows' is as bad a decision as 'rushing in where the angels fear to tread'.

KS Goleria

Acknowledgments

I owe the inspiration to write this book to my friend Dr HG Doctor who persuaded me to share my experience of over fifty years. During this period, India has grown from a country with poor infrastructure and poor resources, to a country with islands of excellence and a plethora of problems whose experience is worth sharing with the world, not always very advanced.

The management of these lesions requires a team effort at various levels and in multiple disciplines.

Each of the contributors, to the four invited chapters, have created areas of excellence in their respective fields. I am grateful to them for having readily accepted my invitation, in spite of their extremely busy schedules. It is an old adage which says, 'If you want something done, give it to the person who is busy'. I had followed this adage and it did prove itself. They have done an admirable job.

The contribution of the Department of Imaging and Interventional Radiology at the Jaslok Hospital, led by Dr Shrinivas Desai and the Department at the GS Medical College and King Edward Memorial Hospital led by Professor Uday Limaye, to the management of these lesions, was a part of the team work deserving recognition and acknowledgment.

The postoperative results are again, an expression of team work. I must acknowledge the contributions of our Anesthetists, Intensivists, Residents, the OT staff and the Nursing staff, in a number of locations.

For the help in editing and organizing the illustrations, I acknowledge the help of Mr Pravin Chavan, Department of Medical Photography, Jaslok Hospital and Research Center, Mumbai.

Individual contributions from some friends have been acknowledged in the text.

I acknowledge the help, cooperation and patient understanding of M/s Jaypee Brothers Medical Publishers (P) Ltd, New Delhi, India and their staff.

The help that I received from my Secretary, Mrs Audrey Sequeira in retrieving, integrating and organizing the data with dedication and devotion deserves a special recognition.

Contents

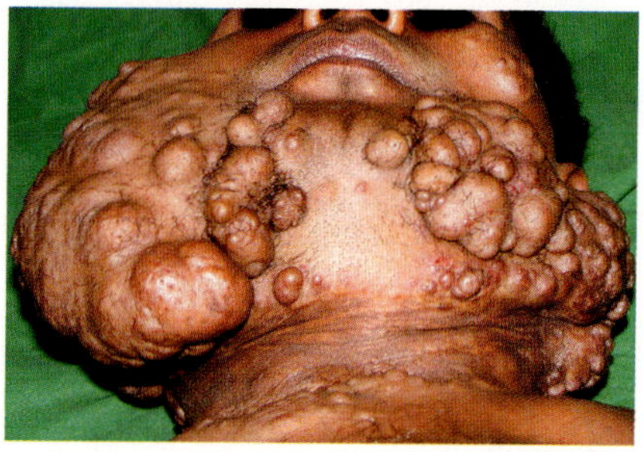

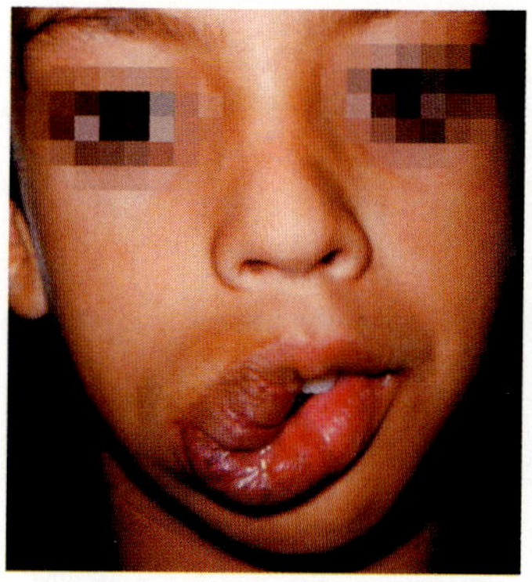

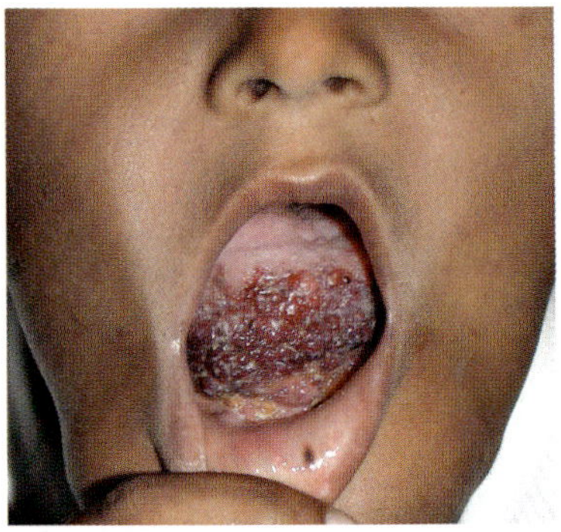

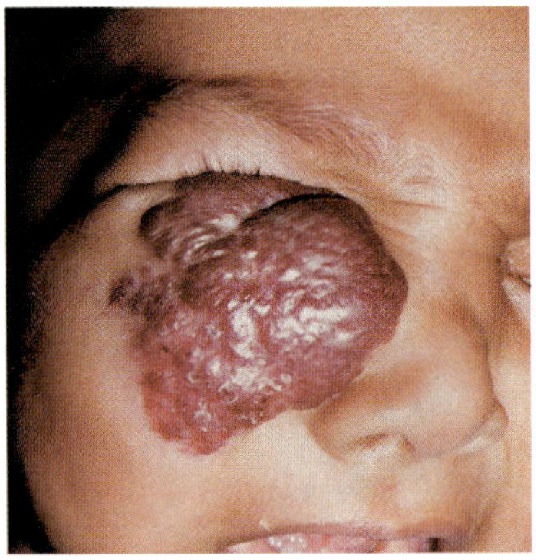

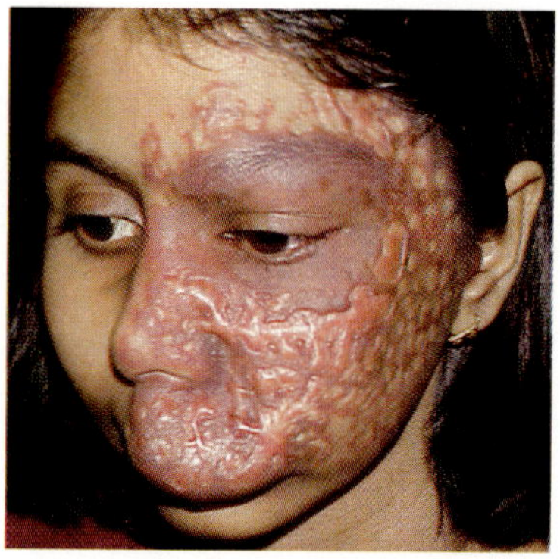

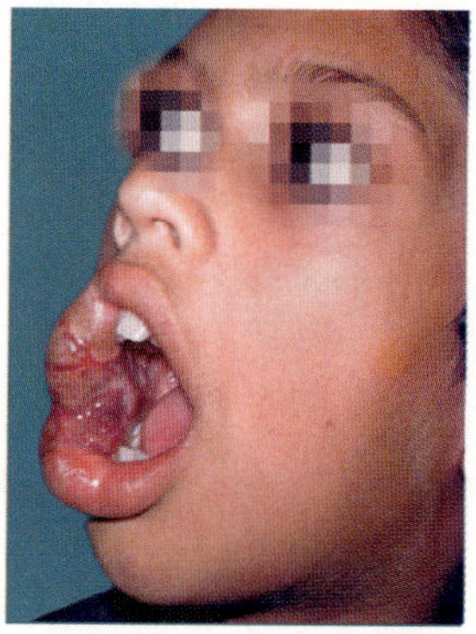

1

HEMANGIOMAS AND VASCULAR MALFORMATIONS—A MANAGEMENT ORIENTED CLASSIFICATION

KS Goleria

Hemangiomas and vascular malformations are a group of lesions, governed by the biological behavior of the constituents and modulated by their anatomical location. The Biological behavior is common to a specific biological unit, but its expression is conditioned by the local anatomy. The therapeutic perceptions too have varied and evolved over the years. An evolution of the classification is natural.

In medical parlance, the generic term 'Hemangioma' has been used loosely. If the purpose of a name is to articulate an identity, the term has singularly failed in that objective. In common usage, it covers a variety of vascular anomalies. The use of this omnibus term alone, merely creates confusion in perception, not infrequently resulting in a faulty approach to the management.

THE FIRST BIOLOGICAL CLASSIFICATION (1863)

The first Biological Classification found expression in 1863, in Rudolph Virchow's three volume treatize on Blood Vessels. Virchow is regarded as the father of cellular pathology. His study of the vascular malformations of the head (including the intra-cranial ones) is incredible. He roughly classified them as:

- Angioma Simplex—implying capillary or strawberry hemangiomas.
- Angioma Cavernosum—implying subcutaneous hemangiomas and venous malformations.
- Angioma Racemoseum—implying racemose (cirsoid) aneurisms or arteriovenous malformations.

To Virchow's student Wagner goes the credit of identifying the lymphangiomas as a distinct entity.

Virchow's terminology and grouping persisted well into the 20th century but gradually lost its relevance because of a sustained explosion in the nomenclature of these lesions (see in the Appendix).

Finally, order was restored by the Biological Classification put forward by Mulliken and Glowacki (1982).

MULLIKEN AND GLOWACKI'S BIOLOGICAL CLASSIFICATION (1982)

Mulliken and Glowacki confined the use of the term Hemangioma to lesions characterized by increased endothelial turnover and endothelial proliferation. The other lesions were grouped as Vascular Malformations. The Tables 1.1 and 1.2 below are essentially based on their work.

The First Group (Table 1.1) are the hemangiomas represented by the Capillary Hemangioma of Infancy and its variants, the congenital hemangiomas—RICH (the Rapidly Involuting Congenital Hemangioma) which rapidly involutes, NICH (the Non-Involuting Congenital Hemangioma) which does not involute and the phenomenon of Hemangiomatosis.

It is logical to add the malignant lesions with these characteristic viz. hemangio-endothelioma (Angiosarcoma) and hemangiopericytoma, to this group, even though the management of the first and sometimes of the second, falls in the realm of Oncosurgery.

Conventionally, added to this group is *Pyogenic granuloma*, rarely more than 6 to 8 mm. in diameter, which appears to be acquired in childhood, but sometimes even later. To begin with it is sessile but later may become pedunculated. Its histological characteristics are those of a hemangioma (the Congenital Hemangioma of Infancy). It is associated with frequent bleeds. A cautery ablation is curative.

The second group (Table 1.2) is concerned with the vascular malformations. These have been classified by them on the basis of the identity of the channel and the intensity of the flow. In addition, the classification takes cognizance of the combinations and establishes their identity by the initials of the combining entities.

Mulliken and Glowacki's classification takes into account the biological structure of the involved channels and has been a great step forward in sorting the terminological confusion that prevailed earlier.

However, a number of other classifications followed three of these need a special mention.

TABLE 1.1
Biologic Classification—Hemangiomas
(Based on the work of Mulliken JB and Glowacki J (1982) Characterized by Increased Endothelial Proliferation and Endothelial Turnover)

Benign	*Malignant*
Hemangioma of infancy or Capillary hemangioma or Strawberry nevus Rapidly Involuting Congenital Hemangioma (RICH) Noninvoluting Congenital Hemangioma (NICH) Pyogenic granuloma	Hemangioendothelioma (angiosarcoma) Hemangiopericytoma

TABLE 1.2
Biologic Classification—Vascular Malformations
(Based on the work of Mulliken JB and Glowacki J [1982])

Low flow	*High flow*
Capillary malformation (CM) Lymphatic malformation (LM) Venous malformation (VM)	Arterial malformation (AM) (multiple arteriovenous fistulae)
COMBINATIONS	
Capillary-venous malformation (CVM) Lymphatico-venous malformation (LVM) Capillary lymphatic malformation (CLM) Capillary lymphatico venous malformation (CLVM)	Arteriovenous malformation (AVM)

(Syndromic lesions are characterized by a variety of combinations)

THE HAMBURG CLASSIFICATION (1988–1989)

Under the inspiration and leadership of Prof Stefan Belov of Bulgaria, 'The Hamburg Classification (1988 and 1989) was proposed in an international consensus document, by the International Society for the Study of Vascular Anomalies (ISSVA). In this classification, vascular anomalies were divided into groups on anatomical, pathological and embryological criteria into vascular tumors or hemangiomas and vascular malformations or angiodysplasias.

Each of these was subdivided into slow-flow or fast-flow entitles.

Five types of these malformations were further identified, as dominantly arterial, venous, lymphatic, with arteriovenous shunts and combined forms. Each of these, were sub-divided into truncular and extratruncular forms.

The classification as borrowed from BB Lee, et al is given in the Table 1.3. As mentioned earlier, classification in Table 1.3 is essentially based on anatomical, pathological and embryological criteria.

THE IAN JACKSON CLASSIFICATION (1993)

Concerned by the plethora of nomenclature confusing the scene of hemangiomas and vascular malformation and to ensure that the participating teams functioned at the same wavelength, Jackson, et al (1993) found the old classifications to be 'descriptive, extensive and too complicated. They evolved a simple classification of these lesions, incorporating the blood flow as an important factor both in diagnosis and management. This was a simple, easy to use clinical classification and grouped these vascular lesions (Table 1.4).

THE ORBITAL SOCIETY'S CLASSIFICATION

J Rootman in 1999, propounded a very similar hypothesis, on the basis of which, a very similar classification was adopted by the Orbital Society. The only tangible difference was that the group III of the Jackson's classification dealing with lymphatic malformation (lymphovenous malformation) was labeled as 'No Flow' group.

TABLE 1.3
The Hamburg Classification

A. Hamburg Classification* of congenital vascular malformations (CVMs)—types;
   Predominantly arterial defects
   Predominantly venous defects
   Predominantly arteriovenous (AV) shunting defects
   Predominantly lymphatic defects
   Combined vascular defects
B. Hamburg Classification of CVMs§ forms—embryological subtypes
   Extratruncular forms
   Infiltrating, diffuse
   Limited, localized
   Truncular forms
   Aplasia or obstruction
   Hypoplasia, aplasia, hyperplasia
   Stenosis, membrane, congenital spur
   Dilation
   Localized (aneurysm)
   Diffuse (ectasia)

* Based on the consensus on Congenital Vascular Malformations (CVM) through the International Workshop in Hamburg, Germany, 1988, and subsequently modified—Capillary Malformations was not included earlier.

§ Developmental arrest at the different stages of embryonic life, earlier stage—extratruncular form; later stage—truncular form.
Both forms may exist together; may be combined with other various malformations (e.g. capillary, arterial, arteriovenous shunting, venous, hemolymphatic, and/or lymphatic); and/or may exist with hemangioma.

TABLE 1.4
The Jackson Classification

i. Hemangioma
ii. Vascular Malformations
   a. Low flow lesion (venous malformation)
   b. High flow lesion (arteriovenous malformation)
iii. Lymphatic Malformation (lymphovenous malformation).

THE BIOLOGICAL BEHAVIOR OF THE VARIOUS CHANNELS

The last two decades have been a witness to a phenomenal increase in the therapeutic potential of treating these lesions and the selection of the treatment plan depends on the tissue response to the therapeutic modalities. Therefore, a look at the biological behavior of the various channels involved, becomes necessary.

The Hemangiomas

The Hemangiomas, which have a small channel high flow system, lined by endothelium which is vigorously proliferative to begin with and totally involuting thereafter. The spontaneous total involution is a significant and preponderant biological characteristic of this group.

The Vascular Malformations

The Small Channel Group

The small channel group is composed of the lymphatics, the capillaries and the venules. All the three are lined by a single layer of endothelium, histologically indistinguishable from each other and characterized by a low flow. They are distinguished from each other only by their contents.

The other common characteristic is incessant growth. However, the pattern of growth and its aggressiveness differ between the channels. The microcystic lymphatic malformations are the most dominating and aggressive. In the mixed channels, which are not uncommon, they impart to the whole lesion their aggressiveness. They do not respect tissue planes, grow round important structures and continue to grow at least till puberty and frequently longer. Aggressive recurrences are not uncommon, specially in the younger age groups. This observation of the combinations is applicable to lymphatics, capillaries, and venules in decreasing order of aggressiveness. Venules often conglomerate and are seen in the conglomeration as veins with all the characteristics of that channel including phleboliths. The incessant growth in the capillaries usually expresses itself, as hypertrophy and hyperplasia of the vessel walls, and of the adjacent soft and hard tissues—both the integument and the bone.

These malformations exert gentle, but persistent compressive pressure, which can obstruct low pressure physiological channels in the head and neck.

Specific characteristics can be attributed to each of the small channels:

- Over a period of time, lymphatic malformations, which are the commonest, distort, weaken and demineralize the skeleton.
- Capillary malformations often increase bone formation as well as, induce skin hypertrophy and hyperkeratinization.
- Formations of pure venules are uncommon. However, the venules which represent the initiation of the return flow are a part of many of these malformations.
- The behavior of small channels is usually dictated by the predominant channel.

The Large Channel Group

The large channels on the other hand belong to two distinctive groups.

- The large low flow channels are the venous malformations (VMs). They have and maintain a distinctive identity in the tissues and grow over a period of time by displacing other structures. They are (unless clotted) soft, compressible and non-pulsatile and their appearance may show significant change, associated with a change of posture. The low flow channels have pockets of sluggish flow, wherein are generated the tell-tale phleboliths.
- The large high flow channels are the arterial (AMs) and the arteriovenous malformations (AVMs). They are warm and pulsatile to touch. Frequently, particularly in the more superficial lesions, a reddish pink hue overrides the natural skin color. Small superficial lesions and larger deep lesions present as a bulge associated with these characteristics. An important biological and radiological

characteristic is the presence of multiple 'niduses' *(or nidi)*, which essentially are arteriovenous fistulae.

Local tissue hypertrophy is common. Recurrence after ablation is attributed to a nidus escaping the knife.

WHY A MANAGEMENT ORIENTED CLASSIFICATION?

Under the heading of 'Hemangiomas and Vascular malformations' we are confronted by a multitude of lesions and a formidable list of diagnosis (see Appendix), based on a variety of considerations, e.g. the name of the primary observer the location of the lesion, the components of the lesion — both vascular and nonvascular, etc.

However, this group of lesions owe their identity to the presence of various channels. Each channel has a distinctive biological behavior. The constituent channels decide the lesions biological behavior.

This in turn is significantly conditioned by a their location in the vascular tree, the rate of flow and the size of the channels. These parameters are relevant to the management. A classification based on channel size and the flow intensity is therefore relevant and has the advantage that:

i. The investigative modalities to specifically identify each of these channels are well identified.
ii. The therapeutic response of each channel to a therapeutic modality is distinctive. It is usually possible to clinically suspect the diagnosis, confirm it by specific investigations and initiate the appropriate therapeutic measures.

A classification based on the channel size and the flow intensity is therefore relevant.

This grouping is clinically possible. In each group, the confirmation of the diagnosis is possible by a specific investigation, thereby avoiding unnecessary exposure to radiation, controlling the costs and facilitating an appropriate therapeutic plan.

Presented in Table 1.5 is a management oriented classification which is based on these criteria. The evaluation and management of each of these is group oriented, as

TABLE 1.5
Hemangiomas and Vascular Malformations—A Management Oriented Classification
(Based on the biological behavior of the participating vascular channels)

Capillary Hemangiomas of Infancy (CHIs) (spontaneously involuting lesion) *Characterized by* A Small Channel High Flow System,
Capillary, Lymphatic, Venules Combinations (CLVCs) *Characterized by* Small Channel Low Flow Vascular Malformations
Venous Malformations (VMs) *Characterized by* Large Channel Low Flow Vascular Malformations
Arterial and arteriovenous malformations (AVMs) *Characterized by* Large Channel High Flow Vascular Malformations

are the modern developments in investigation like, ultrasonography, CT scan, MRI and DSA and in therapy like lasers, radio frequency, embolization, etc. Therefore, this classification is user friendly.

SUMMARY

The 'hemangiomas' and their management have puzzled the surgical mind for almost two centuries. Virchow organized his vast experience in the cranial and intracranial 'hemangiomas' and gave the first biological classification of these lesions to the world. It is obvious that his primary concern was for, what we identify today, as the large channel lesions.

It was Virchows student Wagner, who first identified the Lymphangiomas. Over the years, the other small channels, the combinations of various channels, their varying locations and their varying tissue associations came into the picture. Virchow's classification which held sway over the 19th century faded away in the 20th, lost in a flood of nomenclature.

We owe it to Mulliken, et al who over a quarter of a century ago, gave us their biological classification and restored order to a chaotic field and nomenclature.

This quarter of a century in its turn, has been a witness to an unparalleled growth in technology, both diagnostic and therapeutic, characterized by accuracy and precision. This technology has changed the way we look at and treat the 'hemangiomas and Vascular Malformations' and has led to this 'management oriented classification'.

The consequences of their presence and the approach to their management are further modulated by their location.

BIBLIOGRAPHY

1. Haris GJ. Vascular Malformation a concensus statement on terminology and its clinical implications Am. J Ophthalmology 1999;127:453-55.
2. Jackson IT, Carreno Raphel, Potparic Zoran, Hussain Karim. Hemangiomas, Vascular Malformations, and Lymphovenous Malformations: Classification and methods of Treatment. Plastic and Reconstructive Surgery 1993;91:1216-30.
3. Lee BB, J Laredo, TS Lee, S Huh, R Neville. Terminology and classification of congenital vascular malformations. Phlebology, Royal Society of Medicine Press 2007;22:249-52.
4. Loose DA. Surgical treatment of vascular malformation (arterial, venous, lymphatic, arteriovenous and combined) Vasomed 2001;13:96-105.
5. Mulliken JB. Glowacki J. Hemangiomas and vascular malformations in infants and children: a classification based on endothelial characteristics, Plast and Reconstr Surg 1982;69:412.
6. Rootman J. Vascular malformations of the overt hemodynamic concepts. Orbit 2003;22:103-20.
7. Virchow R. Angiome. In Die krankhaften Geschwiilste. Vol. 3. Berlin, August Hirschwald 1863;306-425.

2

IMAGING FOR THE MANAGEMENT OF HEMANGIOMAS AND VASCULAR MALFORMATIONS

Shrinivas Desai

Modern imaging techniques can readily differentiate and confirm the hemangiomas and vascular malformations into the four clinically identifiable and management oriented groups as indicated below:

CHIs
Capillary Hemangiomas of Infancy
(Small Channel High Flow System)

CLVCs
Capillary, Lymphatic, Venule Combinations
(Small Channel Low Flow Vascular Malformations)

VMs
Venous Malformations
(Large Channel Low Flow Vascular Malformations)

AVMs
Arterial and Arteriovenous Malformations
(Large Channel High Flow Vascular Malformations)

ROLE OF RADIOLOGICAL INVESTIGATIONS

Appropriate imaging helps in delineation of the lesions and in depicting the involvement of adjacent vital structures (e.g. neurovascular bundles, respiratory or alimentary passages, etc.) and helps in determining the depth of the invasion.

This information provides the guidelines for supportive investigations, helps in elucidating the treatment plan and guiding the management.

Radiological imaging, before and after pharmacological therapy is a tool to monitor the therapeutic response.

Long-term prognosis can be suitably explained to the patients with the aid of images.

INITIAL WORK-UP

Sonography and Doppler

The initial evaluation is usually done with sonography and Doppler which are useful in examining soft-tissue masses that are suggestive of hemangiomas or vascular malformations.

Vessel density as depicted on Doppler, has been used in differentiating other types of masses from vascular malformations and is helpful in differentiating low from high-flow systems.

Delineation of lesions in terms of depth of invasion and involvement of underlying structures by ultrasound is somewhat inadequate as the high frequency probes have limited penetration.

The sonographic depiction of abundant low-flow vascular channels is useful in predicting potential success of percutaneous sclerosis.

CT Scan

CT is useful in depicting the delineation of the lesion and its relationship with the underlying soft tissues and bone. Osseous hyperplasia, deformity and invasion is accurately visualized and helps in surgical management.

MRI

MRI is useful in confirming the nature of lesions. Most information needed to examine the lesion is available from a combination of T1-weighted, fat-saturated T2-weighted, and gradient-echo (flow-weighted) MR images. Visualization of the lesions in all three planes can be done by using 3D sequences.

Extent and depth of invasion of the lesions is shown superlatively with MRI. We find the axial plane to be the most helpful in depicting the relationship between the lesion, neurovascular structures and tissue planes.

Gadolinium-enhanced images have been advocated as helpful in differentiating between low-flow vascular malformations such as lymphangiomas and venous malformations.

MRI does not expose the patient to radiation and has better soft tissue delineation where it scores over CT. However, for osseous involvement CT is a must.

Angiography

Angiographic studies are valuable in establishing the extent and type of vascular malformation. With the advent of CT and MRI, their primary diagnostic role is somewhat limited.

Their accurate depiction of the blood supply and drainage, and associated intraorbital or intracranial extensions, are important from a therapeutic point of view, especially in high flow lesions.

The role of angiography in the era of cross-sectional imaging facilitates therapeutic intervention.

HEMANGIOMAS (CAPILLARY HEMANGIOMAS OF INFANCY)

A Small Channel High Flow System

They are also known as "Strawberry Hemangiomas" which appear as an erythematous macule, a blanching macule, or an area of localized telangiectasia. Increased proliferation and turnover of endothelial cells, mast cells, fibroblasts, and macrophages are characteristically seen in these lesions.

We have seen hemangiomas as the most common head and neck tumors in infancy and childhood.

Hemangiomas can be evaluated on a gray scale ultrasound and color Doppler. They are seen as well-defined soft tissue masses with both arterial and venous flow. The lesions are mostly hypoechoic. However a few can be heterogeneous or hyperechoic. Vessels are distributed both centrally and peripherally. They show a high density of vessels, i.e. more than 5 per sq cm. Post-involution the hemangioma becomes isoechoic with loss of arterial and venous flow.

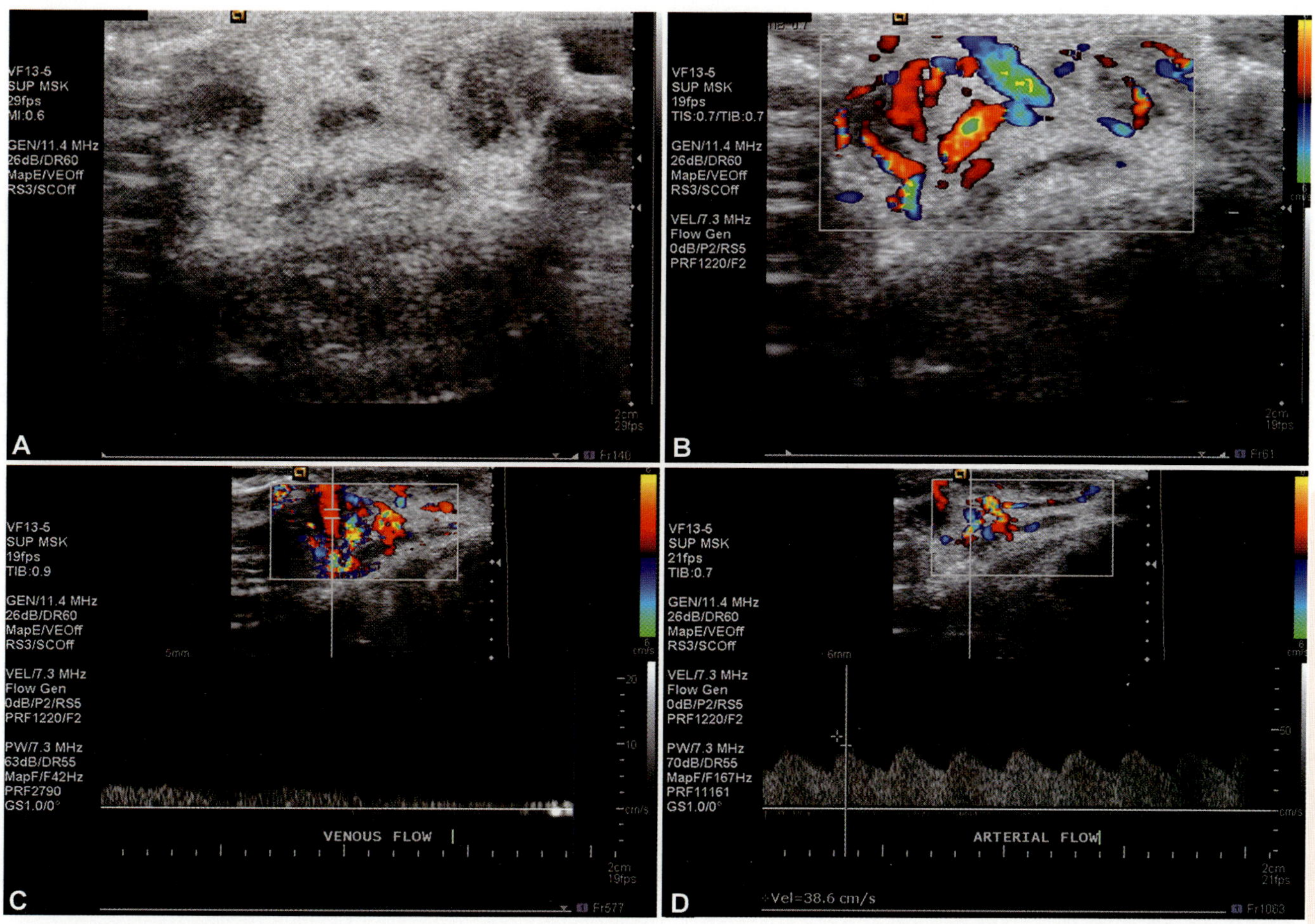

FIGURES 2.1A TO D

(A) Well-defined hyperechoic hemangioma with vascular channels; (B to D) The hemangioma shows multiple vascular channels on color Doppler with arterial and venous flow

They are well delineated on CT, where they are seen as soft tissue density lesions, isodense to the muscle with diffuse postcontrast enhancement.

MRI is extremely good at characterizing hemangiomas, which are identified as isointense to hyperintense to the muscle on T1WI and hyperintense on T2WI. Multiple flow voids are seen within the lesions, which represent central and peripheral high-flow vessels and prominent draining veins. The lesions are seen to have homogeneous enhancement on postcontrast scans.

There may be areas of hyperintensity on T1WI in the involuting period (Figs 2.2A and B), secondary to fatty replacement.

The presence of a parenchymal mass differentiates hemangioma from the other high-flow vascular anomalies such as AVM, which may exhibit reactive soft-tissue changes but no discrete mass.

Angiography

On angiography, in the arterial phase, a circumferential network of arteries are seen which give off numerous small feeding vessels. In the capillary phase, one can see an intense circumscribed tissue staining with some lobular organization. In the venous

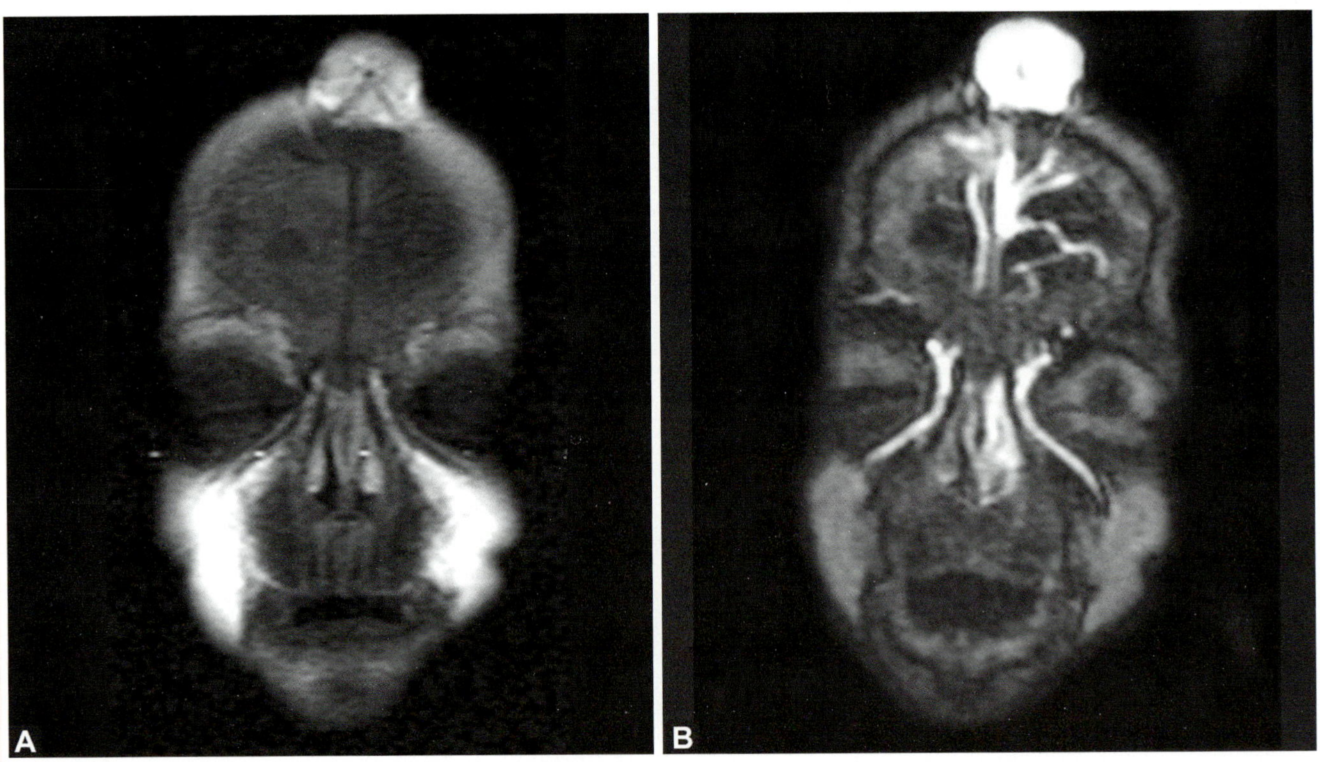

FIGURES 2.2A AND B

(A) Well-defined mass lesion in the midline scalp with prominent flow voids seen on T2W1; (B) Hemangioma in the proliferative phase indicated by the homogeneous post contrast enhancement phase, small veins drain toward, the base of the mass. The lobules are separated by linear or patchy radiolucencies.

As the hemangiomas involute there is an increase in the separating radiolucencies and reduction in the intensity of the tissue staining.

The two angiographic features that distinguish hemangiomas are: A well circumscribed mass and the presence of intense, persistent tissue staining, usually organized in a lobular pattern.

The arterial architecture also differs from that in the vascular malformations. The hemangiomas are supplied by multiple (two to four) slightly enlarged branches of normal adjacent systemic arteries. In some lesions, these proximal feeding arteries form an "equatorial" network at the periphery of the mass, sending smaller feeding arteries into the lesion at right angles to the peripheral vessels. The smaller feeding arteries are closely packed and roughly parallel. In most cases they taper in a normal fashion. Some lesions show arborization of the proximal feeding arteries, so that small branches supply individual parenchymal lobules without an equatorial vessel.

Direct arteriovenous shunting is not demonstrated angiographically.

In those hemangiomas in which venous drainage was well demonstrated, small veins appeared to drain each lobule and then to opacify large veins at the base of the mass. Additional small veins drained toward the surface of the mass, communicating with dilated but otherwise normal regional veins.

The presence of a parenchymal mass differentiates hemangiomas from the other high-flow vascular anomalies such as AVM, which may exhibit reactive soft-tissue changes but no discrete mass. The enhancement pattern and vascularity differentiates the high-flow enhancing hemangioma, from the low-flow, non-enhancing lymphatic malformation. The vascularity and early enhancement may help to differentiate hemangioma from venous malformation. However, characteristic imaging features may not be as easily observed with small hemangiomas.

Involuting hemangiomas enhance less intensely, have diminishing vascularity overtime, and have an increasing proportion of fibro-fatty matrix.

The reason for the extensive description of capillary hemangiomas of infancy is that, unlike vascular malformations they require no treatment and are self-involuting.

VASCULAR MALFORMATIONS

They are formed as a result of abnormal development of blood or lymphatic vessels rather than increased endothelial cell turnover. They are usually first spotted in late infancy or early childhood.

They are distinguished from hemangiomas by their steady increase in size corresponding with the growth of the child and with failure to involute. Sudden rapid enlargement is seen to occur due to trauma, infection or endocrine changes, normally seen at puberty and during pregnancy. They are commonly associated with skeletal changes.

The vascular malformations are subdivided into three groups:

1. CLVCs—Capillary Lymphatic Venule Combinations
2. VMs—Venous Malformations
3. AVMs—Arteriovenous Malformations.

Capillary, Lymphatic, Venules Combinations (CLVCs)

(Small Channel Low Flow Vascular Malformations)

Capillary Malformations

They are also referred to as port-wine stains, capillary hemangiomas and nevus flammeus. The lesions consist of nests of dilated capillaries whose walls lack smooth muscle and elastic fibers.

CMs, most frequently involve the head and the neck region. Of facial CMs, 45 percent are more or less restricted to 1 of the 3 areas supplied by the divisions of the fifth cranial nerve and 55 percent involve an area innervated by more than 1 division of the fifth cranial nerve, crossing the midline or occurring bilaterally.

They are seen in association with various syndromes such as:

a. Sturge-Weber syndrome where there is a capillary malformation in the distribution of the trigeminal nerve with involvement of the choroid plexus and leptomeninges.
b. Ataxia-telangiectasia (Louis-Barr syndrome), where oculocutaneous telangiectasias are associated with cerebellar ataxia.
c. Osler-Weber-Rendu syndrome —identified by hereditary hemorrhagic telangiectasia with multiple mucocutaneous and visceral vascular malformation.
d. Wyburn-Mason syndrome has facial capillary malformation and retinal or optic pathway arteriovenous malformations.
e. Cobb's syndrome has posterior thoracic capillary malformation overlying spinal cord arteriovenous malformations.

Capillary malformations are usually small in size and are not well visualized by USG.

The CT is also normal in most cases. In few instances a faint increase in density may be seen on the postcontrast scans. Hence, CT is not the ideal modality to visualize these lesions.

MRI is a better modality for detection of these lesions, which are seen on postcontrast studies as poorly delineated foci of increased signal intensity. In cases where hemorrhage has occurred within the lesion, multiple hypointense foci can be seen within the lesion on T1W1, T2W1 and SW1 representing blood products.

These lesions show multiple nests of capillary like vessels with vascular staining in the capillary phase on angiography (Figs 2.3A and B).

Thus, imaging is used not only to visualize the extent but also to diagnose associated lesions and to elucidate syndromic varieties.

Lymphatic Malformations

Lymphatic malformations are cystic masses composed of dysplastic endothelium lined lymphatic channels filled with protein rich fluid. These lesions are classified on the size of the cysts as microcystic, macrocystic, or mixed.

These lesions can be detected antenatally in a few cases during obstetric ultrasonography especially in the second and third trimesters. However, they usually present at birth or within the first few years of life. In some cases the anomalies are undetected until there is sudden enlargement as a result of hemorrhage or infection—particularly viral infections—due to large quantities of lymphatic fluid production from lymphoid follicles in the cyst wall.

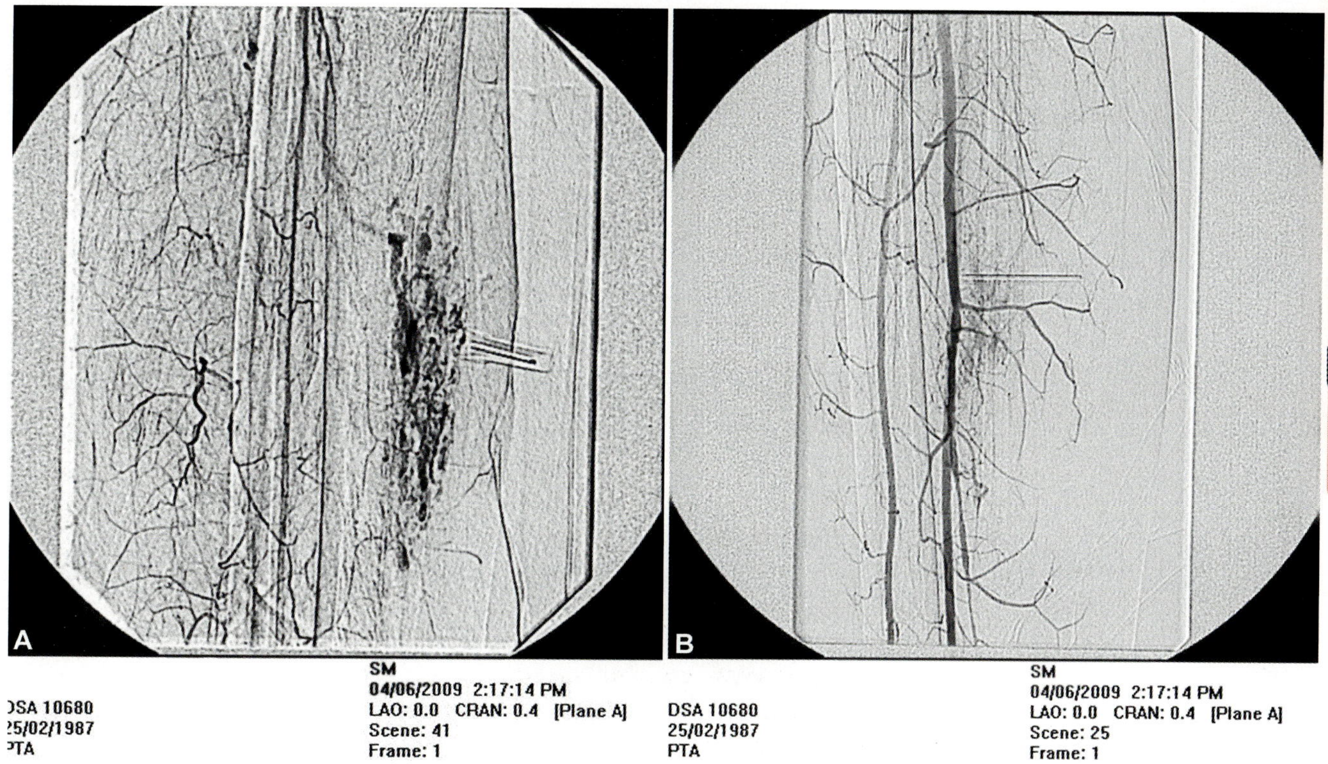

FIGURES 2.3A AND B

(A) Angiography showing small vessels filling in the capillary phase which are diagnostic of capillary malformations, (B) Postembolization, the lesion shows complete occlusion.

The most common locations for lymphatic malformations include the neck and the oral cavity (approximately 75%) and axilla (approximately 25%).

The usual mode of presentation is the presence of a mass or the mass effect causing alteration of function. These anomalies have a tendency to involve multiple fascial compartments. They are frequently associated with skeletal distortion and overgrowth. Thus, macroglossia is usually associated with an overgrowth.

Complications occur from secondary hemorrhage or infection causing sudden enlargement that may obstruct vital passages such as the airway, the esophagus, etc.

Lymphatic malformations can occur as part of generalized disorders such as Turner's syndrome (45XO), Noonan's syndrome, Trisomy 21, Trisomy 13, and Trisomy 18.

On sonography, the lesion's appearance depends on the size of the cystic space. Macrocystic LM reveals a uni- or multilocular cystic mass sometimes containing echogenic debris with intervening stroma. Microcystic LMs appear hyperechoic because of numerous interfaces.

On Doppler, arterial and venous flow is seen within the septa and the stroma corresponding to the histological presence of arteries and veins within the cyst walls and stroma. The high mean Resistive Index (RI) values and low mean peak venous velocities are suggestive of their slowly progressive behavior.

Uncomplicated malformations are seen as multiple hypodense lesions on non-contrast CT. On post-contrast scans, the cyst walls and/or septations enhance but the fluid contained within the cystic space does not enhance. If the lesions are secondarily complicated by hemorrhage, hyperdense components with fluid-fluid (blood-fluid) levels may be visualized (Fig. 2.4A).

These lesions are best characterized by MRI as hyperintense on T2W1. However, when they are complicated by hemorrhage or infection the signal intensity is variable depending on the protein content and the presence of blood products. Following the administration of contrast, the cyst walls and septations show enhancement, however, the central portion of the cyst does not enhance. Large and/or anomalous adjacent

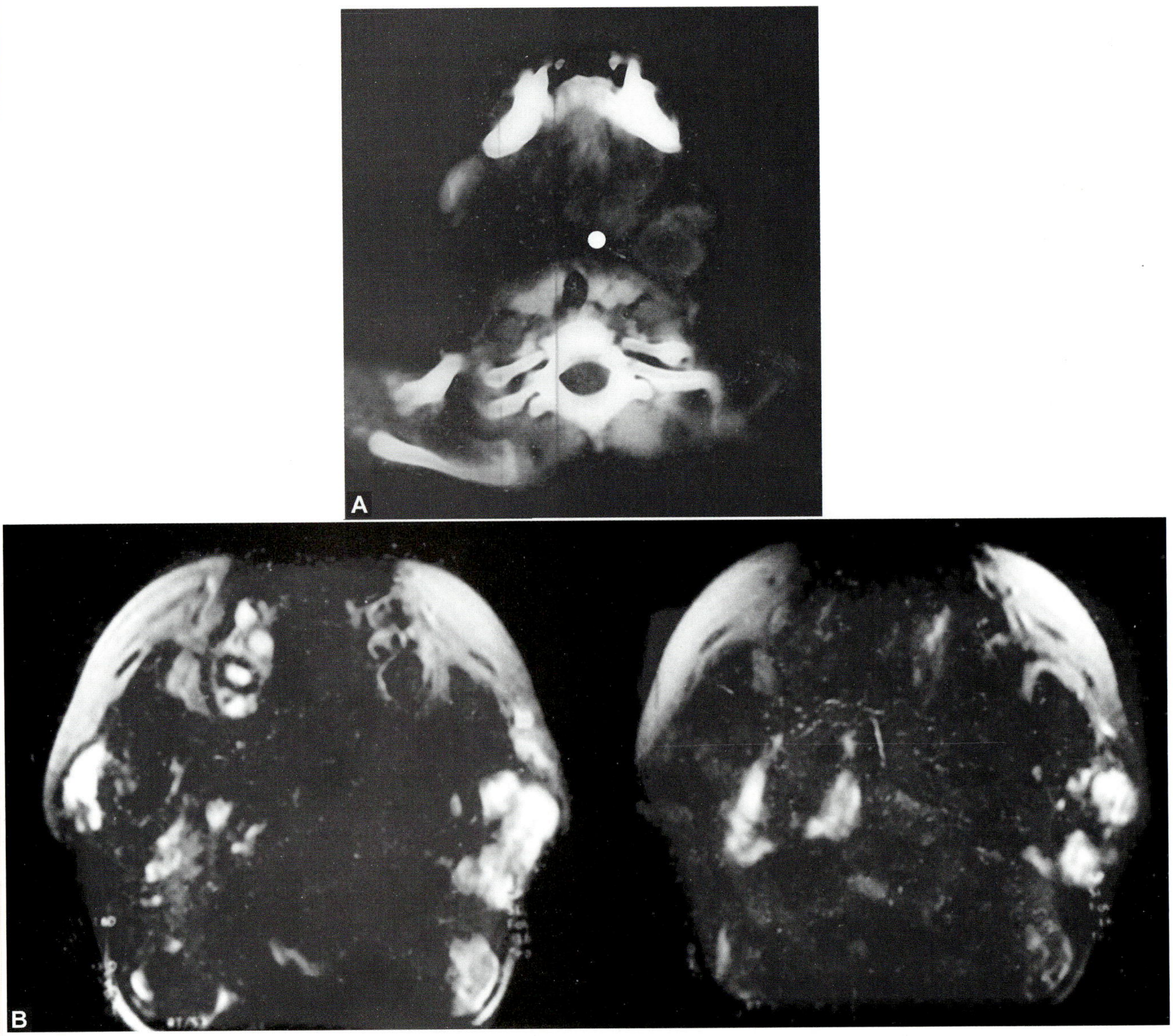

FIGURES 2.4A AND B

Macrocystic lymphangiomas: (A) Hypodense cystic lesions with peripheral enhancement on contrast enhanced CT; (B) Hyperintense lesions in the soft tissues on T2W1 venous channels are often seen, and communication between the LM and adjacent veins is frequently present (Fig. 2.4B).

In the fetus or the newborn, the differential diagnosis for multiseptated macrocystic lesions is teratoma, venous malformation or lymphatic malformation. The presence of fluid-fluid levels, lack of fluid enhancement and absence of phleboliths, differentiate lymphatic malformation from venous malformation. The absence of fat or calcification within the lesion differentiates lymphatic malformation from a teratoma.

Microcystic lesions are more difficult to differentiate from other lesions, as the cystic spaces may be so small that the lesion appears more diffusely enhancing.

Venous Malformations
(Large Channel Low Flow Vascular Malformations)

The venous malformations are dysplasias of small and large venous channels associated with a variable amount of hamartomatous stroma. They are low flow lesions that are seen as the most common vascular malformations to involve the oral cavity.

VMs are present at birth, but the age of presentation depends on size, location and interference with normal function. VM can be single or multifocal and localized or extensive.

In our experience, they are predominantly soft-tissue masses. Some lesions can infiltrate deeply along fascial planes with involvement of the underlying bone and muscle. Unlike hemangiomas, they do not show osseous invasion. The muscles they involve in the face in descending order are the masseter, trapezius and sternocleidomastoid muscles. When located in the extracranial head and neck, these malformations may enlarge in size and cause airway compromise.

Familial forms of VM include blue-rubber bleb nevus syndrome, familial multiple glomangioma and cerebral cavernous malformation.

Ultrasound and Doppler

On B-mode ultrasound and Doppler, venous malformations can either be seen as dilated vascular channels diffusely involving the subcutaneous tissues or as well-defined sponge like collection of vessels. Considering these lesions are low flow in nature, they may show venous flow within the vessels, however arterial flow is characteristically absent. The lesions show a variable vessel density.

CT Scan

Soft tissue density lesions, i.e. of muscle attenuation are visualized on non-contrast CT. The lesions show variable patterns of enhancement. On the postcontrast scan, usually in the venous phase, the lesions show heterogeneous enhancement. Delayed images show a more homogeneous pattern of enhancement. These lesions are low flow, hence the enhancement may not be sufficient on CT to enable separation of their margins from the surrounding muscle. Phleboliths which are characteristic of these lesions appear as rounded, lamellated, calcific densities on CT.

MRI

On MR imaging, the lesions are either isointense or hyperintense to muscle on T1W1 and hyperintense to muscle on T2WI. On the postcontrast scans, they show variable enhancement. On dynamic scans, early postcontrast images may show heterogeneous enhancement which is homogeneous on the delayed scans. The presence of venous lakes which are seen as discrete areas of homogeneous high signal intensity, helps to characterize these lesions. Phleboliths may be present and appear as round, low-signal-intensity lesions on MR imaging. MR venography may reveal dilated or anomalous veins in the vicinity of venous malformations.

Arteriography of venous malformations reveals either no findings, or a delayed mass associated venous or capillary blush with variable stasis, pooling or puddling. Feeding vessels are either normal or slightly enlarged and draining veins may be dilated. Direct percutaneous cannulation with contrast injection of the VM, typically shows interconnecting sinusoidal spaces and adjacent normal or dilated venous channels (Figs 2.5A and B).

AVMs

Arterial and Arteriovenous Malformations

(Large Channel High Flow Vascular Malformations)

These lesions result from abnormal blood vessel morphogenesis and arteriovenous malformations. They are high flow lesions by virtue of their arterial components. AVMs represent a direct connection between the arterial and the venous systems. Lesions tend to grow with the child but can enlarge rapidly as a result of thrombosis, infection, or hormonal stimulation.

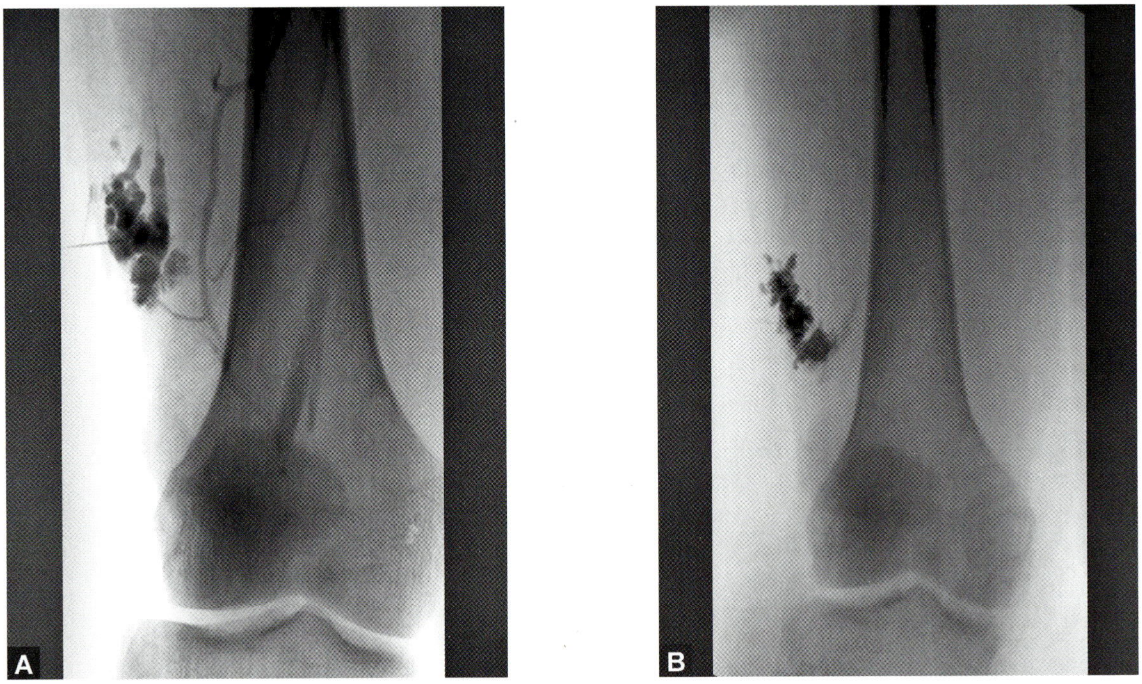

FIGURES 2.5A AND B

Direct percutaneous venography: (A) Venous malformations show larger channels than capillary malformations with prominent feeding vessels and opacification of the enlarged draining veins; (B) Postembolization there is complete outlining of the lesion by the sclerosant

Ultrasound and Doppler

Gray scale ultrasound and color Doppler shows multiple dilated tortuous vascular channels diffusely involving the subcutaneous soft tissues. The lesions show arterial and venous flow with high vessel density. They however do not show any soft tissue mass, which is the characteristic that helps us to differentiate them from hemangiomas of infancy, which are also, classified as high flow lesions during the period of growth. As these lesions show direct connection between the arterial and the venous systems, they usually show a Resistive Index that indicates low-resistance flow.

CT Scan

CT reveals multiple soft tissue density structures on the plain scans. They show intense enhancement on the postcontrast scans with multiple enhancing tortuous vessels.

MRI

On MRI, the enlarged arterial components, which are characteristically seen, appear as flow voids on T1 and T2 weighted images. They show good enhancement and appear as a cluster of vessels on the postcontrast MR angiography scans. Although, the lesions can be associated with surrounding edema or fibrofatty stroma, usually no focal discrete soft-tissue mass is found.

Angiography

On angiography, arterial malformations are characterized by rapid flow with enlarged, tortuous arteries seen in the arterial phase and enlarged tortuous draining veins in the venous phases. Parenchymal staining is unusual. Angiography and DSA (Digital Subtraction Angiography) are extremely useful for preoperative embolization of these lesions and in planning surgical intervention.

Combined High and Low Flow Lesions

Combined vascular malformations with features of both high flow and low flow lesions may be seen in few patients occasionally. These lesions can attain enormous proportions with involvement of the deep musculature and subcutaneous tissues. On MRI, these lesions demonstrate serpiginous flow voids, characteristic of arterial malformations and soft tissue infiltrating component typical of venous malformations.

Figures 2.6A to M illustrate a case study of a 'Combined High and Low lesion'. The patient shown in this figure was operated 15 years ago for this type of a lesion extensively pervading the lower face and neck. The surgery had involved the replacement of a significant part of the neck skin with a split skin graft. The patient had now come with a massive bilateral lesion of the lower face and neck. The various facets of this unusual lesion are illustrated.

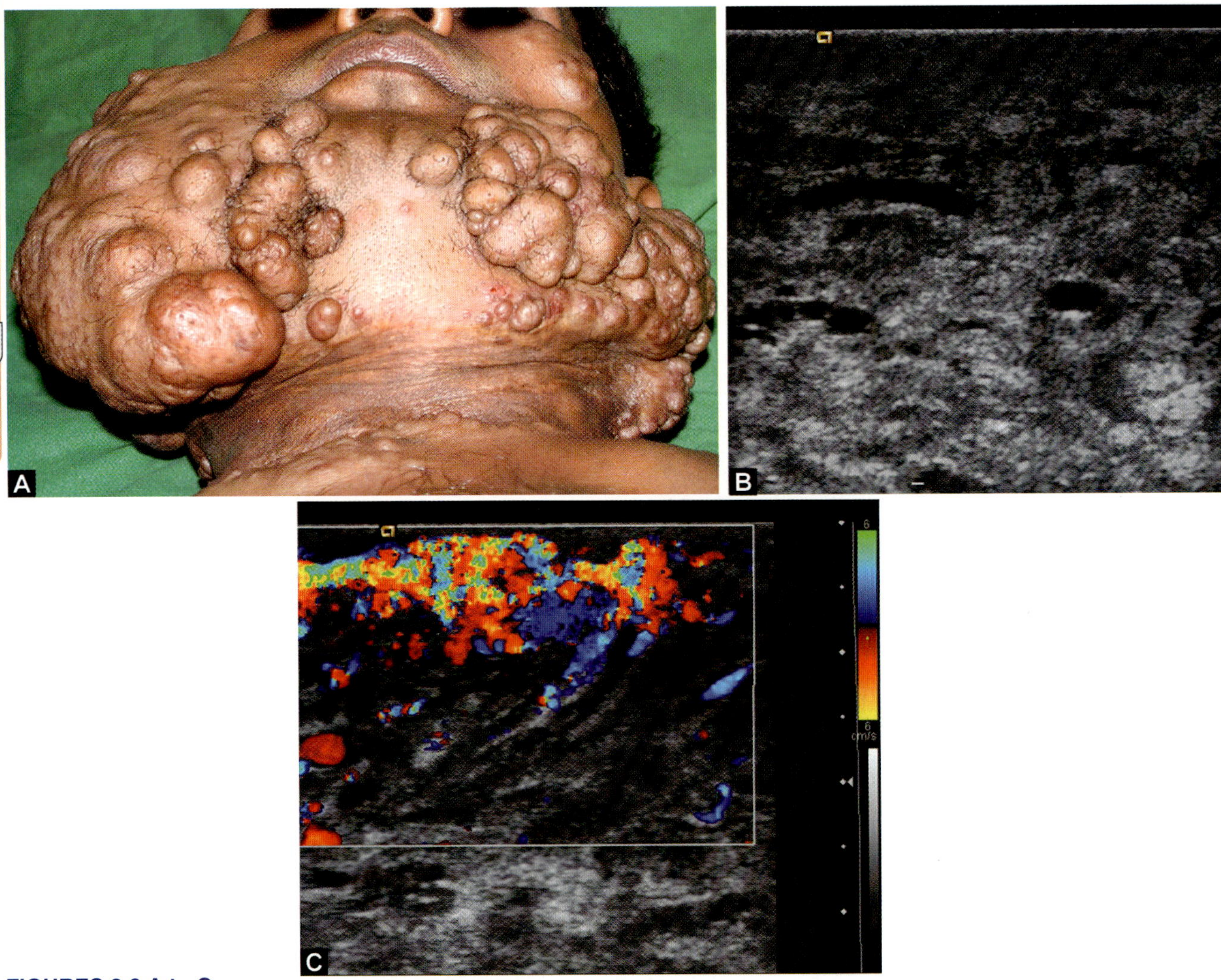

FIGURES 2.6 A to C

(A) Clinical photograph; (B) MRI shows a heterogeneous lesion with multiple hypoechoic vascular channels; (C) Abundant vascularity of superficial surface with flow in vascular channels

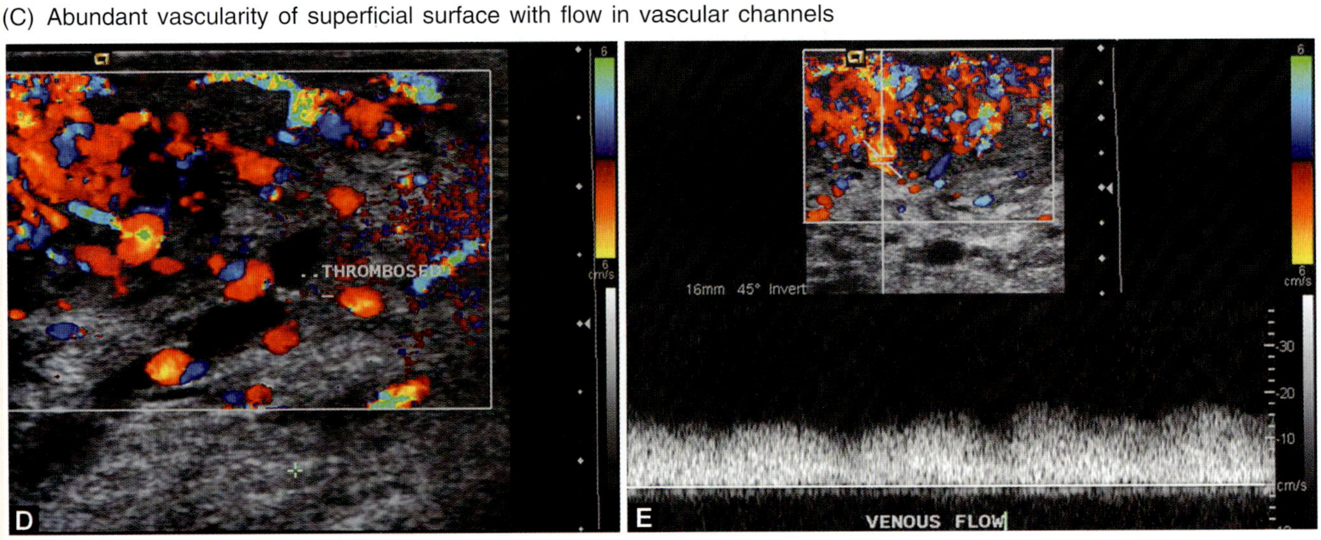

FIGURES 2.6 (D and E)

The vascular channels show both the arterial and venous components

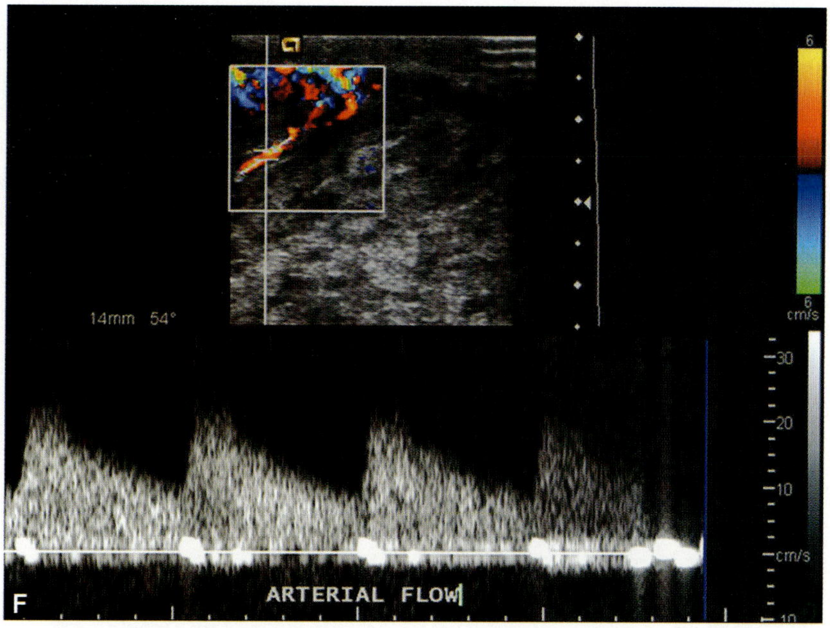

FIGURES 2.6 F

The vascular channels show both the arterial and venous components

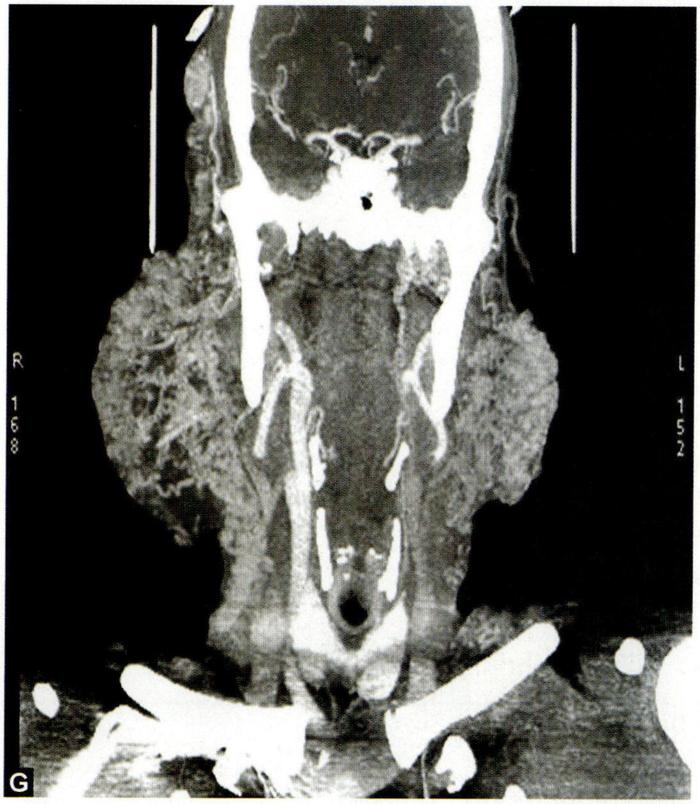

FIGURES 2.6 G

(G) Arterial phase contrast enhanced CT shows enhancement of the lesion and the prominence of the arterial components

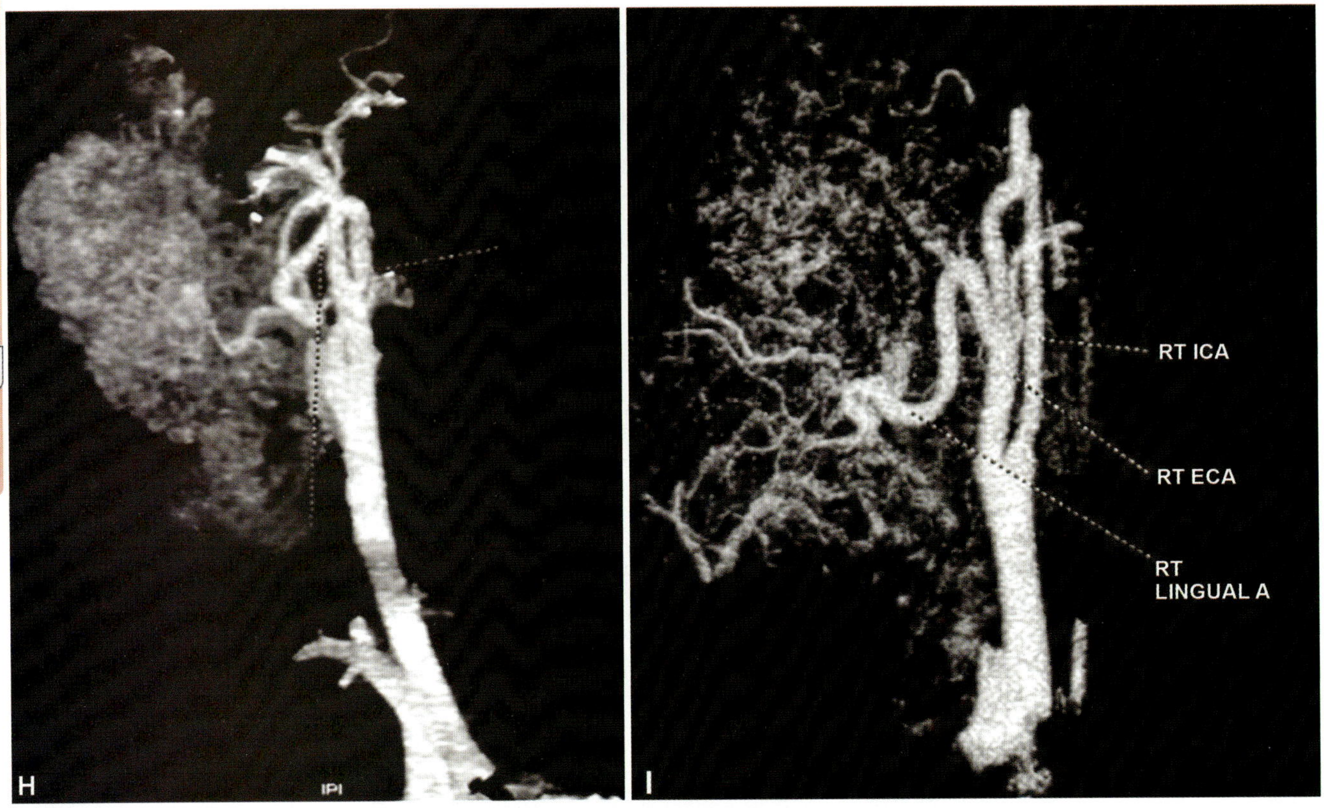

FIGURES 2.6 G to I

3D volume rendered images. *Note:* Lingual arteries supplying the lesion

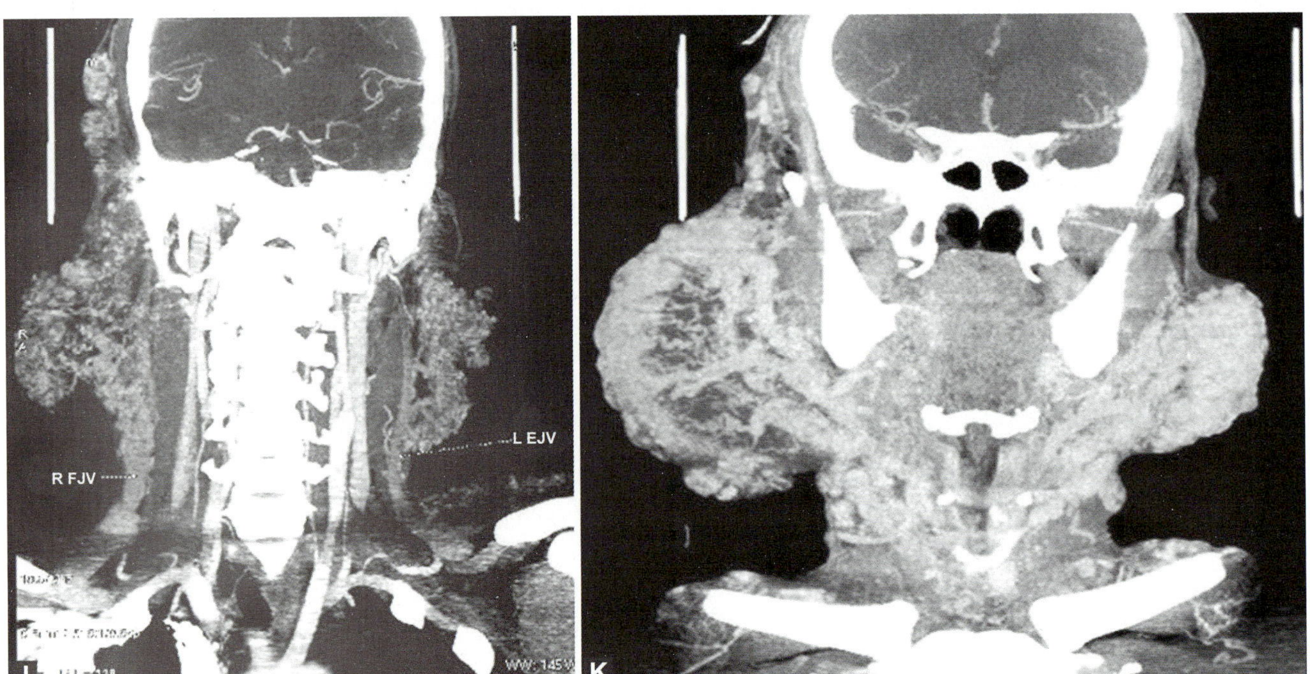

FIGURES 2.6 J and K

(J) Early draining dilated veins and consequentially dilated external jugular vein; (K) Delayed phase: Contrast filling in the matrix with persistent enhancement.

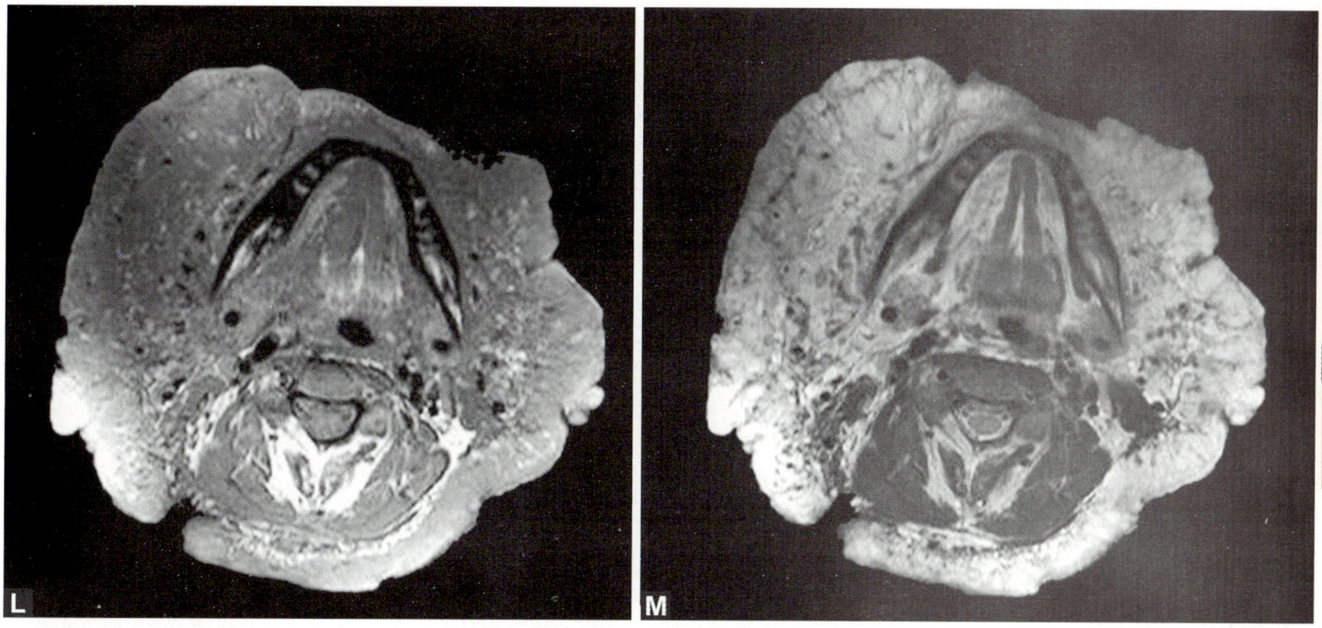

FIGURES 2.6 L and M
(L) MRI: T2W1 image—Hyperintense lesion with multiple flow voids,
(M) MRI: T1W1 image—Hypointense to Isointense lesion with multiple flow voids

Imaging Controlled Ablation

Imaging controlled RF ablation of select localized vascular malformations without surgical exploration is now a part of our management protocol. This technique is particularly useful for the ablation of deep seated localized vascular malformations. Focused MR under MRI control is used as a precision tool for this purpose.

We are already using this technology for the vascular lesions of the rest of the body. The protocol for the head and neck lesions is being developed.

CONCLUSION

It is obvious that radiological imaging plays an important role in diagnosing and delineating the lesions. Advantages of ultrasound and MRI are absence of radiation which is an important consideration as most of the patients are in the pediatric age group.

CT is a valuable tool used to visualize osseous involvement. With the advent of 64 slice CT scanners vascular anatomy is well visualized by CT angiography. Digital subtraction angiography is used mainly for therapeutic purposes and for follow-up of treated cases. The use of Imaging controlled 'Radio Freqency' (RF) is emerging as a valuable quick, precise and safe tool for the ablation of these lesions selectively.

BIBLIOGRAPHY

1. Barnes PD, Burrows PE, Hoffer FA, Mulliken JB. Hemangiomas and vascular malformations of the head and neck: MR characterization. AJNR 1994;15:193-95.

2. Cohen JM, Weinreb JC, Redman HC. Arteriovenous malformations of the extremities. Radiology 1986; 158:475-79.
3. Donnelly LF, Adams DM, Bisset GS, III. Vascular malformations and hemangiomas. AJR Am J Roentgenol 2000; 174:597-608.
4. Dubois J, Garel L, Gignon A, Laberge L, Filiatrault D, Powell J. Imaging of hemangiomas and vascular malformations in children. Acad Radiol 1998;5:390.
5. Dubois J, Patriquin HB, Garel L, et al. Soft-tissue hemangiomas in infants and children: Diagnosis using Doppler sonography. AJR 1998;171:247-52.
6. Koeller KK, Alamo L, Adair CF, Smirniotopoulos JG. Congenital cystic masses of the neck: Radiologic-pathologic correlation. Radiographics 1999;19:121-46.
7. McCormick WF. The pathology of vascular ("arteriovenous") malformations. J Neurosurg 1966;24:807-16.
8. Meyer JS, Hoffer FA, Barnes PD, Mulliken JB. Biological classification of soft-tissue vascular anomalies: MR correlation. AJR Am J Roentgenol 1991;157:559-64.
9. Murphey MD, Fairbairn KJ, Parman LM, Baxter KG, Parsa MB, Smith WS. Musculoskeletal angiomatous lesions: radiologic-pathologic correlation. RadioGraphics 1995;15:893-917.
10. Paltiel HL, Burrows PE, Mulliken JB. Color Doppler ultrasound of soft tissue vascular anomalies. Radiology 1994;193:292-95.
11. Van Rijswijk CS, van der Linden E, van der Woude H, van Baalen JM, Bloem JL. Value of dynamic contrast-enhanced MR imaging in diagnosis and classifying peripheral vascular malformations. AJR Am J Roentgenol 2002;178:1181-87.
12. Vilanova JC, Barcelo J, Smirniotopoulos JG, et al. Hemangioma from head to toe: MR imaging with pathologic correlation. Radiographics 2004;24:367-85.

CAPILLARY HEMANGIOMA OF INFANCY (CHI)

3

A SMALL CHANNEL FAST FLOW LESION

KS Goleria

NOMENCLATURE

Capillary hemangioma of infancy (CHI) is a true 'angioma', with the characteristics of a benign tumor- and essentially a small channel but fast flow lesion. It differs significantly from other small channel lesions by being a self resolving disorder (Figs 3.1A to D). It is variously known as 'Strawberry Nevus', Hemangioma, Benign Hemangio-endothelioma, etc. The multiplicity of nomenclature has added confusion to the nomenclature of the vascular lesions. The term 'capillary hemangioma of infancy (CHI)', is a fairly explicit nomenclature deserving universal adoption.

INCIDENCE AND DISTRIBUTION

CHI is the most common tumor of infancy occurring in 4 to 10 percent of white infants. The incidence in the colored population is reported at about half of this figure. I have not come across the incidence figures in the Indian or Chinese population. The incidence in India appears to be low. The few statistics available are from a couple of institutions and not comparable to the data available in the west.

The Western literature indicates that they occur most frequently in the Craniofacial region (60%) followed by the trunk (25%) and extremities (15%) (Matheys Vol 5 Pg 22 Ref 13). The lesions are reported to be 3 to 5 times more common in girls than in boys. In 80 percent, the lesions are single and in 20 percent multiple.

THE BIOLOGICAL PROGRESSION

Manifestation and Proliferation

In its commonest expression, CHI appears as a pinkish spot at about three weeks of age and grows rapidly in the first few months of life. In the earliest phase, there is proliferation of the endothelial cells forming syncytial masses with or without lumens. The increase of the vascular channels appears to be a response to endothelial proliferation and the increase in tissue volume. In lesions located under the skin, the surface is raised with increased turgescence and purple hue. The deeply located lesions show a

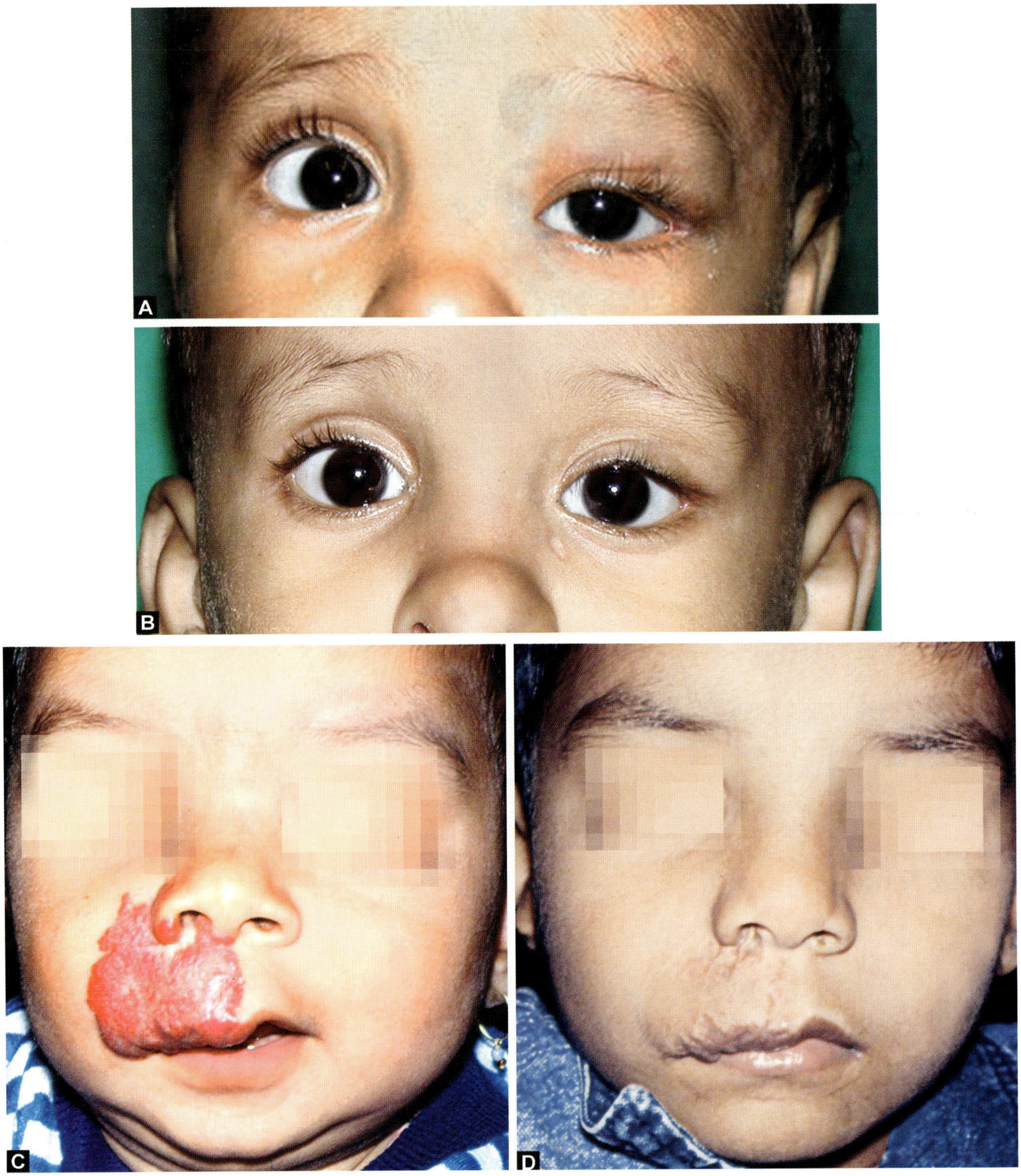

FIGURES 3.1A to D
Spontaneous involution: (A and B) CHI of left upper lid—involution without scarring (common); (C and D) CHI of right upper lip—involution with minimal scarring (occasional)

bulge and usually a purplish hue. Often both the superficial and deep lesions coexist. In the craniofacial region, they can interfere mechanically with vital functions, e.g. vision and respiration.

Involution

The onset of the phase of involution, is often heralded by a change in color from a bright crimson to a dull purple, appearance of one or more whitish patch in the central area and decrease in turgidity. The involution starts at about 9 months of age concomitantly with the ongoing proliferation, but becomes the dominant feature by 12 months of age. Spontaneous total resolution by 5 to 8 years of age is the norm even in very large lesions. The involution is usually complete. Relevant is Lister's remark, based on an observation of 93 hemangiomas (1938) — "no exception has been found to the rule that naevi which grow rapidly during the early months of life, subsequently retrogress and disappear of their own accord, on the average of about the 5th year of life". Since then biology has not changed. Spontaneous resolution was confirmed by Wallace (1953) after a study of 290 cases. As Wallace pointed out in a large number of cases it was impossible to make out the site of the lesion after the resolution was complete. Spontaneous total resolution by 5 years of age (Fig 3.1) is the norm, even in very large lesions. Occasionally, some residual lesion may still be seen. Some workers aver that involution may continue till 8 years of age — "the final degree of improvement is achieved by the time the child is 8-year-old" (Thompson and Burrows). Occasionally, taking into consideration social and psychological pressures, a small residual unresolved lesion may need a surgical intervention at the age of 5 or 6.

Both the proliferative and the involutionary phases have histologically distinctive features, and both coexist for a period of time.

Postinvolution

The period immediately after involution has been called the post-involutional phase. In the vast majority of cases, there is no trace of the lesion and the tissue looks normal. Once in a way, we come across minor scarring and deformity or small atrophic patches. I attribute these to the not so uncommon central patches of superficial ulceration, possibly related to episodes of infection, corrosive applications or minor trauma.

In the western world, where the incidence of these lesions is far more common and the care more specialized and intensive, ulceration during the proliferative phase has been attributed to the growth of the lesion surpassing epidermal elasticity and blood supply. A telangiectatic lax crepe like skin referred to as anetoderma is also described. Rarely a massive hemangioma on spontaneous resolution might leave behind a minimal hypertrophy of the skeleton which is attributed to increased vascularity.

A CASE STUDY

Figures 3.2A to L illustrate the Biological progression of a CHI which had threatened the infant's respiration. The three month old infant, with a CHI in a 'proliferative phase' and in severe respiratory distress was hospitalized to the intensive pediatric care unit of our hospital. The CHI involved the lips, both cheeks, the lower face, the floor of the mouth and front of the neck. In addition she had a typical superficial lesion on the sternum.

Case Study: Biological progression of a CHI with threat to respiration (Figures 3.2A to L)

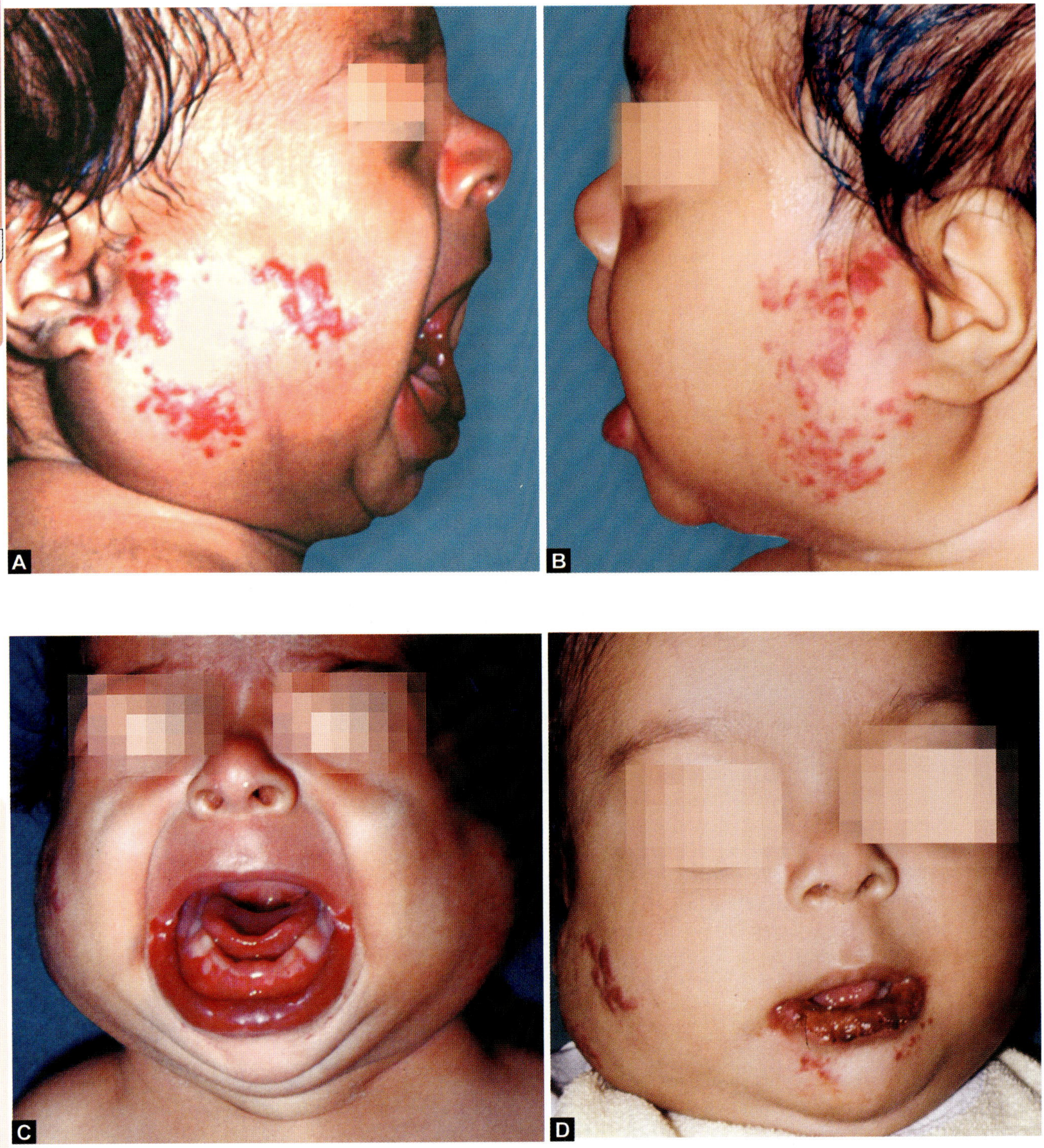

FIGURES 3.2A to D

Biological progression of a CHI with threat to respiration: (A to C) On emergency admission the child was in severe respiratory distress. The child showed immediate benefit with Oxygen therapy and the simultaneous initiation of steroid therapy relief. In 48 hours, the child had fully settled down; (D) Shows the response after 2 weeks of therapy.

Case Study: Biological progression of a CHI with threat to respiration (Contd...)

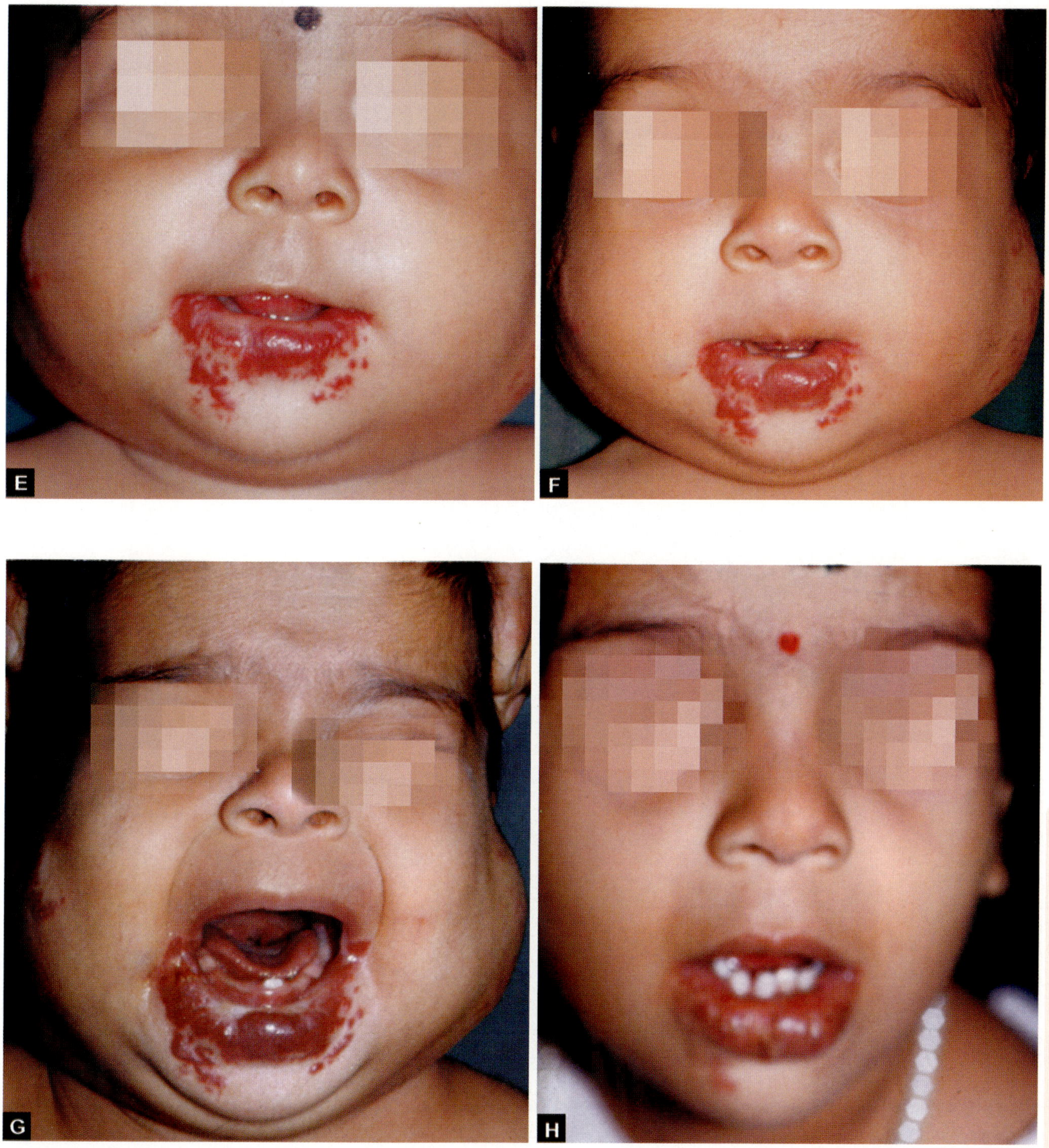

FIGURES 3.2E to H
Biological progression of a CHI with threat to respiration: (E) The response after another 4 weeks; (F) Shows a mild steroid withdrawl rebound seen 10 days later; (G) 5 months after 1st intervention (age 8 months); (H) At age of 2 years illustrates the continuing involution

Case Study: Biological progression of a CHI with threat to respiration (Contd...)

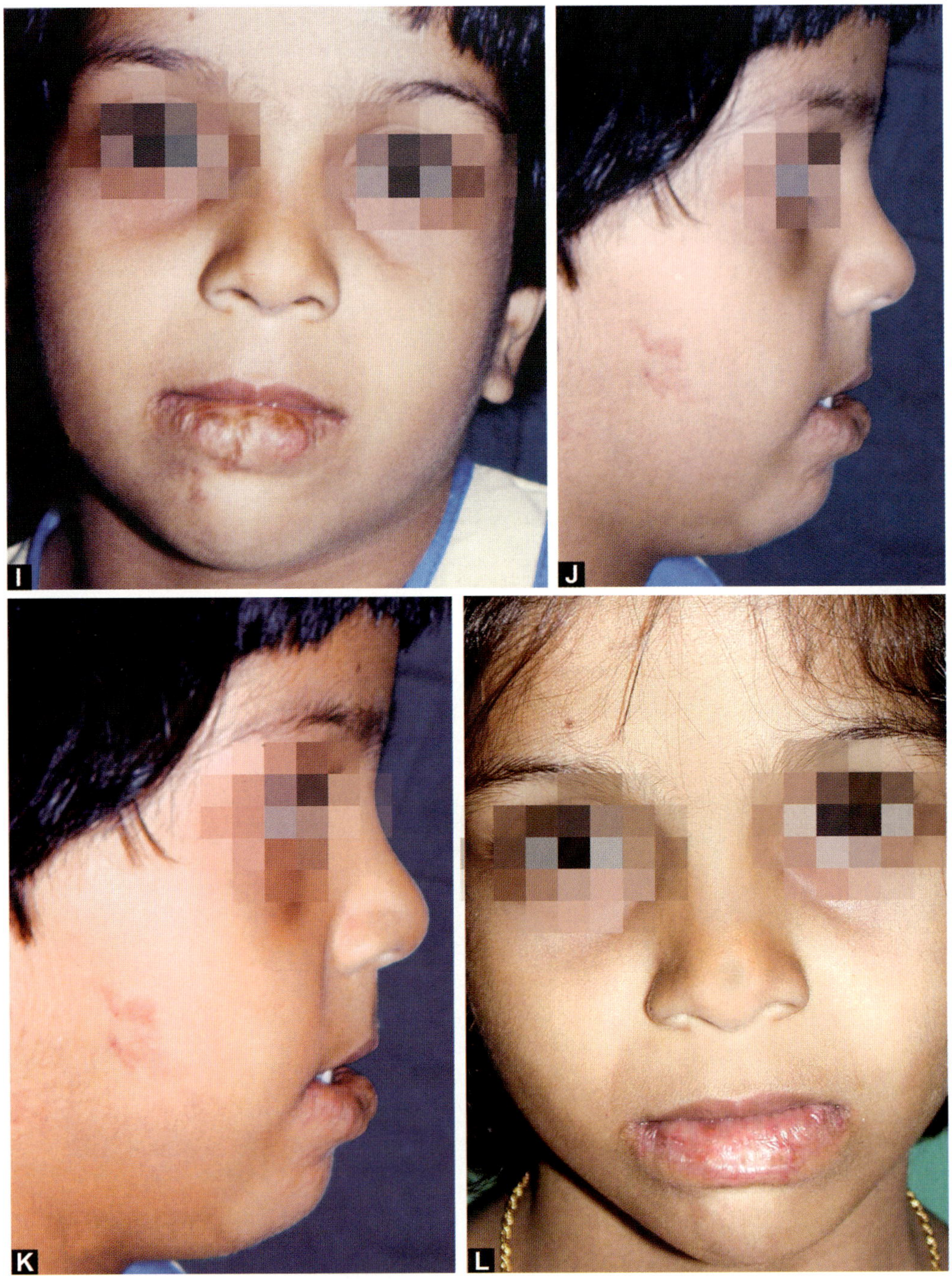

FIGURES 3.2I to L
Biological progression of a CHI with threat to respiration: (I to K) Illustrate the status at the age of 5 years; (L) Shows the patient at 10 years. Note residual scarring under lower lip border needing a small surgical intervention

FIGURES 3.2A to L
Biological progression of a CHI with threat to respiration

DIAGNOSIS

This biological history of CHI, distinguishes it from all other vascular malformations. Yet errors in diagnosis can occur and are preventable. To quote Mulliken (1990), "Two axioms help to distinguish hemangioma from vascular malformation. The first is that *'not all hemangiomas look like a strawberry'*. The skin overlying a deep hemangioma may be of normal color, a bluish tint, or (in rare instances) a pale shade with scattered telangiectasia. The corollary axiom is that *not all strawberry-like vascular lesions are hemangiomas.* A capillary cutaneous, capillary venous, lymphatico-venous or pure venous malformation look remarkably similar to a hemangioma". A careful examination does distinguish them (Figs 3.3A to D).

The biological progression, strawberry color — a bright scarlet — that gradually deepens during the first year of life and the following involution, are diagnostic of CHI (Fig. 3.3A).

Capillary vascular malformations grow persistently and have a persistent hue depending on their composition (Fig. 3.3B).

At times, a venous malformation can closely mimic a CHI, but it can be easily distinguished by its thin walls and compressibility (Fig. 3.3C).

An anterio-venous malformation (AVM) in children is bright pink in color and is pulsatile (Fig. 3.3D). Biological behavior and clinical observation usually give a good indication of the lesion's identity.

Special Investigations

Frequently, no special investigations are needed for the management of a patient with CHI. When in doubt, or when visceral hemangiomatosis is suspected, ultrasonography and MRI are useful aids, which not only confirm the diagnosis but help in defining the depth and extent when contemplating therapeutic interventions (see Chapter 2). They are particularly useful when one is suspecting a systemic multicentric involvement which disturbs circulatory balance and threatens life.

VARIANTS

Congenital Hemangiomas

They are present and fully developed at birth. They manifest as two variants — RICH (Rapidly Involuting Congenital Hemangioma) which involutes within a few months and NICH (Non Involuting Congenital Hemangioma) which does not involute. These exhibit telangiectasis and are warm to touch and need surgical excision.

Hemangiomatosis

Occasionally lesions located in organs have been reported. They are usually discovered incidentally, during an imaging procedure in the child. Since they are asymptomatic and self resolving, they are ignored.

Rarely, however, during early infancy, multiple and/or extensive visceral (particularly hepatic) or extensive cutaneous CHIs, may be associated with high output cardiac failure, hepatomegaly and anemia. These manifestations carry a high mortality and requires urgent appropriate intervention.

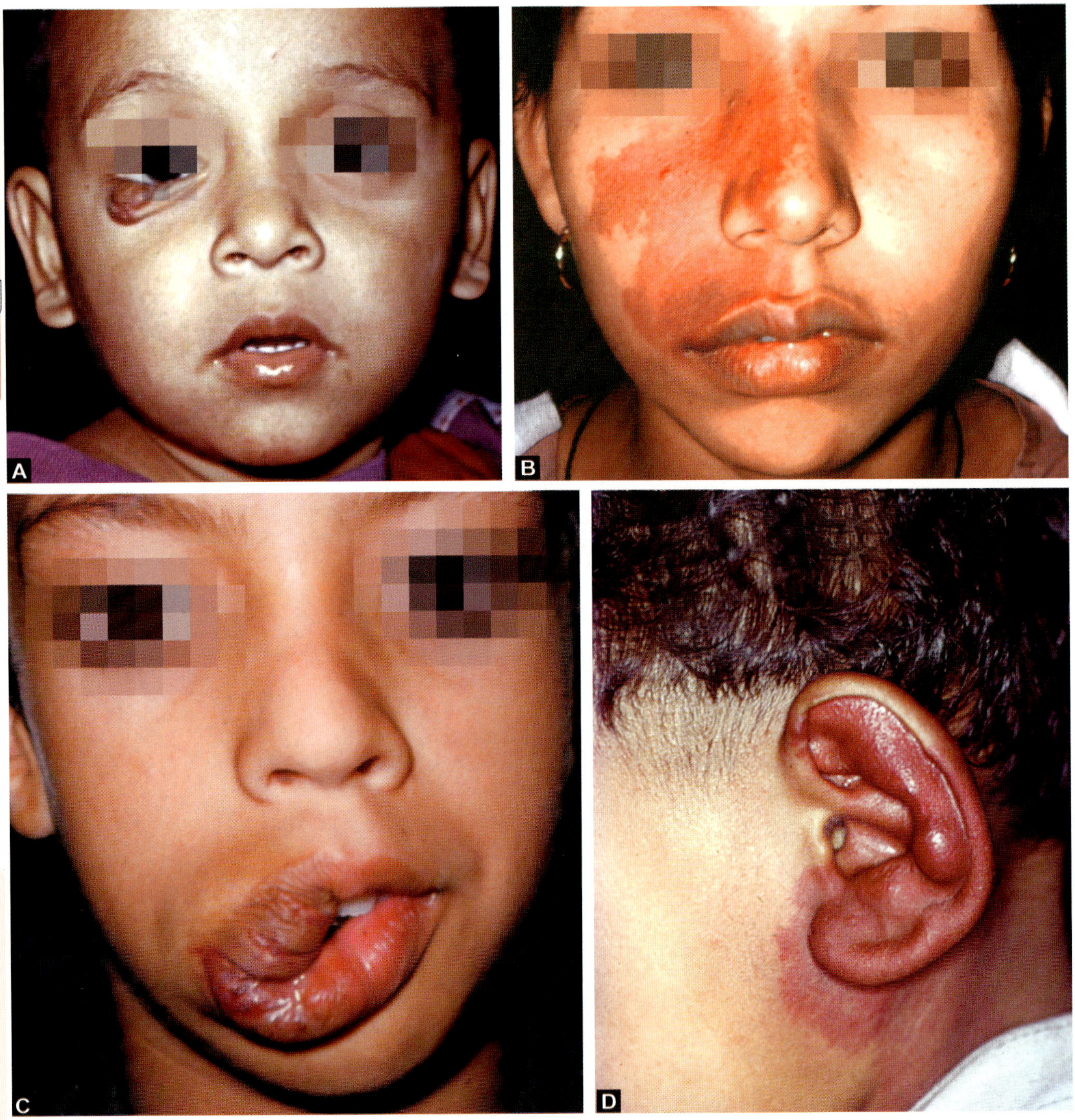

FIGURES 3.3A to D

The Main Differential Diagnosis: (A) A CHI seen at 9 months. Note early signs of involution; (B) A CM seen at the age of 22 years with significant hyper-keratinization; (C) A VM can at times strongly simulate a CHI; (D) An AVM too is bright red and growing and is strongly pulsatile

The infants having multiple small cutaneous lesions could be simultaneously having multiple visceral hemangiomas, common in liver, but could also occur in brain, GI tract, or lung. These can be confirmed by Sonography or MRI.

Intrahepatic group is more frequently seen in female babies. These may be asymptomatic, but not uncommonly, very early in life exhibit anemia, congestive cardiac failure, hepatomegaly and a bruit over the liver. Differential diagnosis of these includes malignant neoplasms and arteriovenous malformations (AVMs).

A second less common group shows no shunting but presents with massive hepatic enlargement and secondary hepatic and renal failure. Mortality rate in hepatic hemagiomas is very high (30 – 80%).

MANAGEMENT

General and Prophylactic

Spontaneous Healing

Spontaneous healing, as illustrated in the case study given above, is the distinguishing feature of CHI. In the vast majority of cases, spontaneous healing does not leave behind tell-tale marks (Figs 3.1A and B) Occasionally one encounters minimal scarring which can easily be managed (Figs 3.1C and D). Primary surgical management of these lesions is totally unjustified. Yet total inaction is neither warranted nor appropriate. Prevention and management of certain complications is important.

Urgent/early Intervention

Urgent intervention is indicated when respiratory obstruction threatens life or ulceration and bleeding pose problems. Hemangiomatosis involving multiple deep structures (particularly the liver) needs aggressive evaluation, monitoring, team-work and therapy.

Proliferative phase and interference with vital functions: Lesions on the face can sometimes interfere with vital functions. When involving the eyelids the vision can be blocked. Even when one pupil is obstructed it can lead to the suppression of vision of that eye and interfere with the development of binocular vision (detail in Chapter 5). Large lesions of the lower face and neck can interfere with the respiratory function. The most favored and time honored approach is the use of steroid therapy.

These lesions respond to heavy doses of corticosteroids during the proliferative phase. Steroids should be used only if vital function like respiration or vision are affected. Heavy doses are required. A number of regimes have been prescribed. In vogue is cortisone in the dose of 2 to 3 mg/kg/day for 2 to 3 weeks (See case study — Fig. 3.2-cited above). If there is a good response, the therapy may be continued for some more time at dosage of 1 mg/kg/day. However, it should be tapered off as early as possible.

No significant gains are seen on administration of steroids during the involutionary phase.

Lesions in and around the Orbit

Lesions in and around the orbit pose very special problems particularly related to the orbit's anatomy and likely to affect the vision. The management of lesions involving the orbit are detailed in Chapter 5.

Ulceration

The thin epithelium over the CHIs tends to desiccate and ulcerate. My experience suggests that in our country this could be due to a fear of touching these lesions resulting in an inadequate hygiene and a lack of use of emollients, resulting in desiccation and consequentially ulceration. These are prevented by local hygiene, local emollients and protected by soft clothing, particularly in winters.

Ulceration is also fairly common in the western world and occurs mainly in the early proliferative phase. It is attributed to the growth of the lesion surpassing epidermal elasticity and blood supply.

Treatment of all these ulcerations is essentially conventional: wound toilet and protection, prevention or treatment of infection as appropriate, relief of pain with the use of analgesics and surface anesthetics.

Today, ectodermal growth hormone substitutes appear to present new therapeutic opportunities (See Surface Application).

Bleeding

These lesions as mentioned earlier belong to the 'small channel high flow' system and can bleed profusely in response to trauma. Guarding them against direct trauma is essential. Balancing the needs of protection viz-a-viz the needs of personality development have to be balanced. As the involution proceeds, the bleeding tends to be less severe.

It is essential to educate the parents on the immediate control of bleeding following injury. This is best achieved by a direct gentle finger pressure applied without interruption for 10 to 15 minutes while seeking medical help.

Intralesional Steroids

Intralesional corticosteroid injections are an alternative to systemic corticosteroids. A total of 10 to 15 mg of triamcinolone acetomide (10 mg/ml) is injected into the lesion. The treatment can be repeated in every 4 to 6 weeks. This treatment modality carries the risk of embolization of the retinal artery and blindness. Therefore, intralesional corticosteroid therapy should be limited to nonperiocular CHIs. Other adverse effects include, subcutaneous fat atrophy, epidermal necrosis, and temporary dyspigmentation of the treated area. However, these are all quite uncommon.

Some authors prefer using intralesional injections of betamethasone (6–12 mg), or triamcinolone (40 mg) locally.

It needs to be emphasized that in the management of the CHI primary surgical intervention can produce unnecessary scars and deformity and should be avoided. However, it may be required to deal with the residual scarring or deformity at the end of involution.

Intralesional Sclerosant

The patient in Figures 3.4A and B presented to us at the age of 5 years with what looks like a poorly resolved CHI. The clinical history revealed that at the age of one year the child had been given an injection into the lesion locally. It probably was a sclerosent, and given the fact that this intervention occurred at a time when both the proliferative and the involuntary phases coexist, interference with the involutionary process is a logical consequence as expressed in Figure 3.4A. Surgical interventions corrected the deformity.

Surgical Intervention

Surgical intervention is essential for the management of noninvoluting congenital hemangiomas (NICH). Surgery may also be needed in the management of interference with vital functions like vision or respiration. A small lesion with recurrent bleeding, too is best removed.

Residual scarring at the end of involution usually needs a surgical intervention.

Residual lesions towards the end of the involutionary phase (5 to 6 years of age) may be treated by a surgical intervention to help managing the psychological problems.

A surgical intervention may be needed in the management of interference with vision or respiration.

Use of Lasers

Lasers are a relatively new tool in the management of CHI. The use of lasers for CHI is described in Chapter 6. Nd: Yag or Intense Pulsed Light (IPL) are the favored modalities. IPL has been successful, in treating ulcerated CHI lesions. Several studies have demonstrated the efficacy of IPL, while minimizing side effects like purpura and scarring.

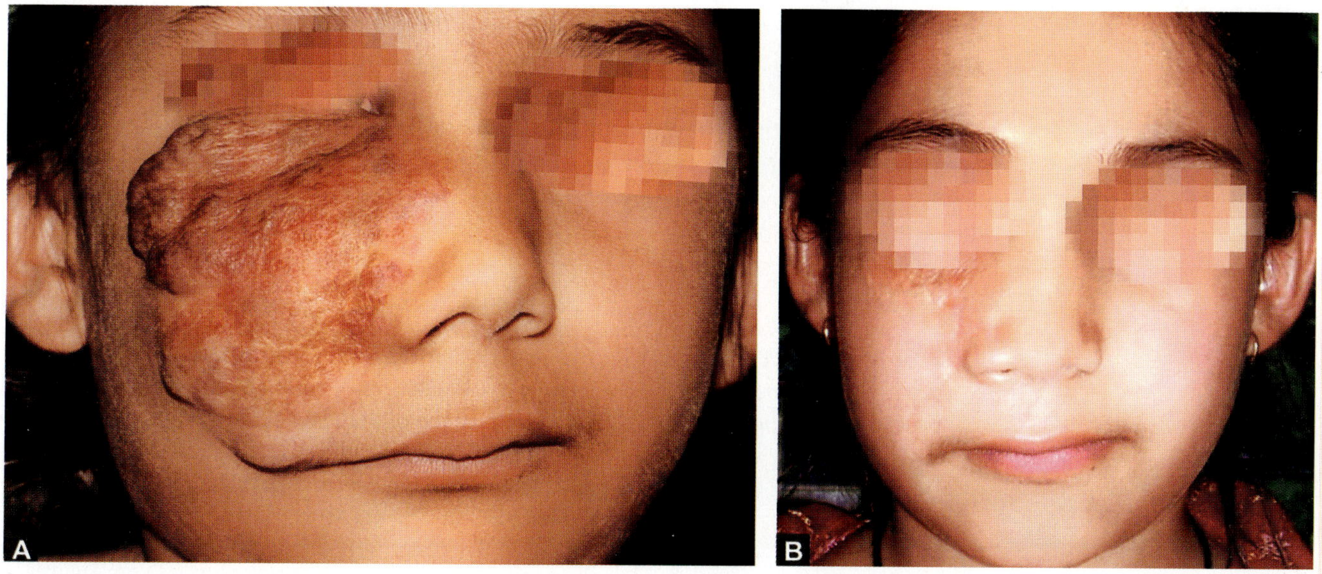

FIGURES 3.4A and B
A CHI at the age of 5 yrs., following an injection of a sclerosent at 1 yr, age: (A) The deformity as it presented; (B) The result after 3 serial excisions

Surface Applications

Surface applications have recently entered the therapeutic fields.

Imiquimod ointment entered the therapeutic armamentarium for treating CHIs a few years ago. It is the surface application of Imiquimod 5 percent cream, an immune response mediator, which has been shown to be effective in superficial CHIs (Ho NT et al 2007, Jorg BF et al, 2008).

This treatment has been used safely and successfully in children as young as 8 months. The typical reported reaction is edema, erythema, scaling, and crusting, which may be indicative of clinical response. Since the mechanism of action appears to be similar to the mechanism of natural involution, it appears to be promising.

Becaplermin 0.01 percent (Platelet derived growth factor BB), (PDGF-BB) has recently been reported as curative.

However, it is good to remember that spontaneous involution has stood the test of time.

SUMMARY

Of all the vascular lesions that are being dealt with in this publication, the capillary hemangioma of infancy has two unique characteristics. Of the four groups being considered, it is the only one, characterized by endothelial proliferation justifying the suffix '-oma' in its nomenclature. It is also the only one characterized by phase of proliferation followed by a phase of involution, both phases being completed in childhood.

It is the commonest intraorbital tumor of infancy and responds to steroid therapy in the proliferative phase.

Diagnosis is essentially clinical. If in doubt, Sonography and MRI are the most useful in confirming the diagnosis and avoiding exposure to radiation. Specific indications for surgical and other therapeutic interventions are required under selected circumstances.

Though no authentic nationwide study has been carried out in the Indian population, it is almost certain that the incidence is much lower than in the western world. It is possible that all the observations made in this chapter may not be fully relevant to all ethnic groups.

BIBLIOGRAPHY

1. Bartoshesky LE, Bull M, Feingold M. Corticosteroid treatment of cutaneous hemangiomas: how effective? A report on 24 children. Clin. Pediatr 1978;17:625.
2. Bruckner AL, Frieden IJ. Hemangiomas of infancy. J Am Acad Dermatol 2003;48(4):477-93.
3. Ho NT, Lansang P, Pope E. Topical imiquimod in the treatment of infantile hemangiomas: a retrospective study. J Am Acad Dermatol 2007;56(1):63-8.
4. Jorge BF, Del Pozo J, Castineiras I, et al. Treatment of ulcerated hemangiomas with a noncoherent pulsed light source: brief initial clinical report. J Cosmet Laser Ther 2008;10(1):48.
5. Lister WA. The natural history of strawberry naevi. Lancet, (quoted by John B Mulliken) 1938;1:1429.

6. Mc Carthy's Plastic Surgery pg. neous. Thompson HG and Burrows PE: Vascular Malformations. Mastery of Pl and Recons. Surg. (Pg. 352) Little Brown and Company, Boston/New York/Toronto/London
7. Mulliken JB. Cutaneous vascular anomalies Plastic Surgery. Joseph G Mc Carthy (Ed) 1990;3191.
8. Mulliken JB, Glowacki J. Hemangiomas and vascular malformations in infants and children: a classification based on endothelial characteristics. Plast. Reconstr. Surg 1982;69:412.
9. Patterson AB. Spontaneous cure of a naevus maternus-large vascular tumor occupying side of neck. South Med Rec 1894;24:477 (from coverse).
10. Pusey WA. The use of carbon dioxide snow in the treatment of nevi and other lesions of the skin. JAMA 1907;49:1354.
11. Ritter MR, Butschek RA, Friedlander M, Friedlander SF. Pathogenesis of infantile hemangioma: new molecular and cellular insights. Expert Rev Mol Med 2007;9(32):1-19.
12. Thompson HG, Burrows PE. Mastery of plastic and Reconstructive Surgery. Vascular malformations 1994:352.
13. Zak TA, Morin DJ. Early local steroid therapy of infantile eyelid hemangiomas. J Pediatr Ophthalmol Strabismus 1981;18:25.

4

SMALL CHANNEL LOW FLOW VASCULAR MALFORMATIONS

CAPILLARY, LYMPHATIC, VENULE COMBINATIONS (CLVCS)

KS Goleria

THE MIX-UP OF CHANNELS

This group involves the vascular malformations of small channel low flow systems — capillaries, lymphatics, and venules — singly or in combinations. These channels are histologically indistinguishable but for their contents. Malformations of Lymphatics (LMs) and Capillaries (CMs) may occur in pure form but the admixture, Capillary Lymphatic Malformations (CLMs) are more common. Venule malformations usually express themselves in combination with CLMs and when radiologically or clinically distinguishable are labeled as Capillary Lympho Venous Malformations (CLVMs) (Fig. 4.4). Logically, capillaries lead to venules. It will be fair to say that all low flow lesions have to be an admixture of these three channels and the labeling mentioned above reflects significant recognizable presence of the individual elements.

Lymphatic malformations can possibly have an independent existence and are usually the preponderant component of the mixed lesions. They are the earliest to have received recognition, when in the 19th century, Wagner identified lymphangiomas as a distinct identity. However, from the biological behavior point of view, all these three entities have some shared features and some specific characteristics. Both of these significantly affect their management.

BIOLOGICAL BEHAVIOR

The small channels low flow lesions, particularly the lymphatic malformations are characterized by incessant growth and scant respect for tissue planes. They continue to grow aggressively, at least till puberty and frequently longer though less aggressively. Lymphatics are the most aggressive. According to the current classifications and nomenclature they are labeled as 'lymphatic malformations'. However, because of the aggressiveness of their growth pattern and the frequency of their recurrence lymphangioma, the name given to them by Wagner, is frequently and interchangeably used. They grow against all odds and violate most tissue planes. Their surroundings are affected by their gentle, but persistent and compressive pressure, which can obstruct low pressure physiological channels in the head and neck and even affect the airway.

Over a period of time, particularly when the lymphatic component predominates, they distort, weaken and demineralize the skeleton.

On the other hand, the capillary malformations of the skin surface do not extend beyond their original limits, but induce skin hypertrophy and hyperkeratinization. They are associated with increased skeletal growth and bone formation.

Formations of pure venules are uncommon. But if we have capillaries, the venules have to be there and in most lymphangiomas involving the mucous membranes bluish vascular excrescences are easily seen (Fig. 4.1). The venules, no doubt have a role to play in the biological behavior of capillary malformations.

In all these combinations, two channels predominantly affect both the clinical course and the approach to management, viz. the capillary malformations and the lymphatic malformations. This chapter is therefore divided into these two parts:

CAPILLARY MALFORMATIONS (CMs)

The Specifics of Biological Behavior and Management

Capillary Malformations (CMs) must be distinguished from Capillary Hemangiomas of Infancy (CHI). Even though, both arise from capillaries, they can be clearly differentiated from each other.

The CHIs as emphasized in the chapter dedicated to them, are not uncommonly multiple and are **distinguished by the presence of endothelial hyperplasia**. Usually, the lesion first appears a few weeks after birth, followed by a phase of rapid proliferation. By the age of 8 or 9 months, the onset of involution is noticeable. Proliferation comes to an end at about 2 years of age. The involution is complete by 5 years but may sometimes be delayed till 8 years of age.

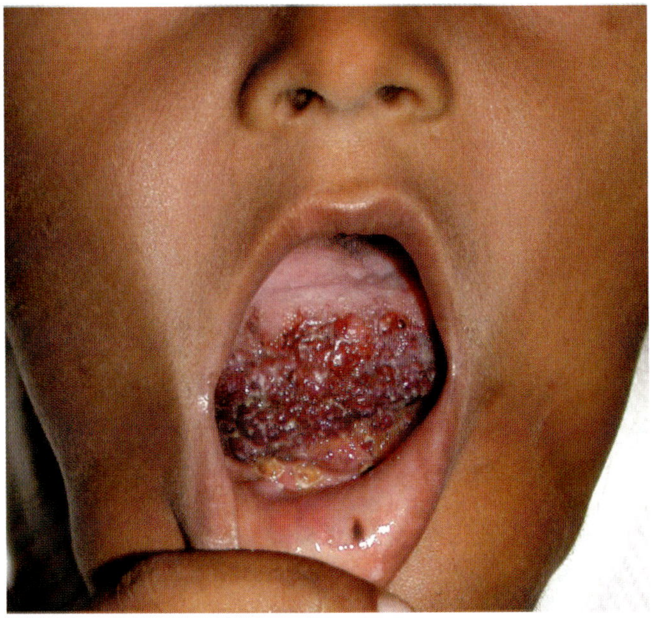

FIGURE 4.1
Extensive lymphangioma incorporating all the three small channels, lymphatics, capillaries and the venules

CMs too, are multiple entities, usually present at birth, and located in the dermis. They continue to grow steadily with age, covering a larger area—but not involving fresh areas. The affected area gradually hypertrophies and becomes nodular. The lesions do not involute. A large number have been described, most of them considerably disfiguring. Some involve genetic and neurogenic factors.

Of common concern is the 'Port-wine Stain'—essentially a surface capillary malformation and its sister lesion the 'Sturge-Weber syndrome', confined to the area of distribution of the trigeminal nerve. These are surface capillary malformations, usually present at birth. They, unlike the CHIs, are a conglomeration of ecstatic channels lined by flat non-proliferative endothelium. Thickening of the post capillary venule wall is common and bridged fenestrations can be seen in this region by electron microscopy. These fenestrations are commonly found in the venous capillaries surrounding the sweat glands and are believed to constitute areas of accelerated exchange between the circulation and the surrounding tissue.

They relentlessly continue to grow, not because of the growth of channel size, nor because of endothelial proliferation but because of channel proliferation, skeletal hypertrophy and hyperkeratinization of the skin. The growth of the lesion in the area it occupies is relentless. Lack of sympathetic innervation regulating the blood flow in the vessels is believed to produce progressive ecstasia.

CMs are commonly associated with developmental defects.

A very large percentage of these lesions are restricted to the face, and are usually referred to as 'Sturge-Weber syndrome'.

The Sturge-Weber Syndrome

Enjolras, Riche and Merland (1985) proposed that this complex represents an error of morphogenesis within a specific region of the neural crest giving rise to abnormal vasculature in the upper facial dermis, choroid and pia-arachnoid. According to these authors, 45 percent of these lesions are restricted to one of the three trigeminal areas and 55 percent overlap sensory dermatomes, cross the midline or occur bilaterally.

Involvement of V1 and V2 regions carries a high-risk of glaucoma and these infants need periodic prophylactic checks (at least every 6 months and at least till the age of 2 years), to facilitate early detection. When the distribution is confined to V3 area alone or to other parts of the body, this risk is not significant.

These lesions are associated with leptomeningeal malformations which can be capillary, venous or arteriovenous and being space occupying, can cause neurological signs and symptoms. The choroidal lesions can cause glaucoma, retinal detachment and loss of vision. Mineral deposition below the leptomeningeal malformations and capillary and venous malformations are known to be associated with this condition.

The adjoining mucous membrane is often concomitantly involved. Lesions in other parts of the body are referred to as Port-wine stains. These may be independently or simultaneously present. These scattered lesions are not associated with the complications associated with the lesions of the V1 and V2 regions.

A hypertrophy of both the skeleton and soft tissue (including connective tissue and skin) is often associated with all these malformations — almost invariably with the passage of time. Onset of keratinization is usual at about 6 years of age but can even earlier. Increasing hypertrophy and hyperkeratinization can make these lesions

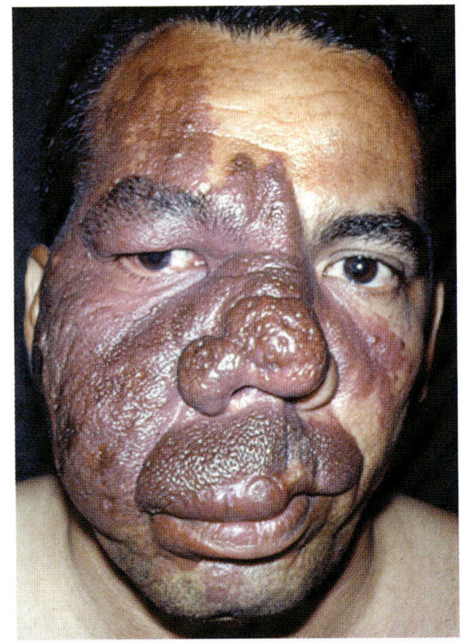

FIGURE 4.2
An untreated capillary malformation shows gross hypertrophy, marked keratinization and hyperpigmentation

even more ghastly (Fig. 4.2). At this late stage, surgical or laser ablation and a fresh skin cover are the only available and yet essentially poor options, particularly in the colored people, because of problems associated with color match.

Deep seated capillary malformations are often closely associated with microcystic small channel lymphatic malformations (CLMs) and their local effects are usually dictated by the predominant channel and are discussed later with microcystic lymphatic malformations.

Syndromes Involving Capillary Malformations on the Face

Hyperkeratotic cutaneous capillary venous malformation, associated with vascular malformations of the brain and affecting tissue around the eye is an autosomal dominant abnormality due to a mutation in the KRIT 1 gene and macrocephaly capillary malformation syndrome.

Typical capillary malformation must be differentiated from common macular stains of infancy usually seen in the nuchal region, the eyelids, the glabella and the lips. These usually fade away by the age of 1 year.

Management of Capillary Malformations

Cosmetics

In early lesions, a well planned and carefully executed use of cosmetics could be a good camouflage, socially acceptable, particularly in the fair population. However, it requires a repetitive painstaking effort, which may not suit all moods, all occasions and all complexions. Sometimes, the essentially repetitive effort wears out the victim.

However, as the lesions are present since birth, children and the teenagers are the worst victims of unfriendly social interaction. This method is totally unsuited to their lifestyle.

Lasers

Lasers are the highly refined successors of the old technique of scarification-used in the management of port-wine stains more than a hundred years ago, and given up years ago. Laser photocoagulation provide useful cosmetic improvement. Being capable of selective wavelength related destruction, they have come in as an important tool in the management of surface capillary malformations. Ideally, laser therapy should be done early, before hyperkeratinization sets in at about the age of six years. Multiple sessions are usually needed. Laser therapy after the onset of keratinization gives poor results.

The patient's complexion and sometimes the occupation considerably affects the quality of the benefit.

The therapeutic results on the fair skin have been significantly better than on colored skin. With the advancement of laser technology, the area of its applications is no doubt increasing as is the quality of the result. Laser therapy can be often fruitfully combined with surgery. The scope of lasers in the small channel low flow systems has been dealt with in Chapter 6.

Surgery

For surface lesions, replacement with neighboring skin whenever possible and whenever it can be esthetically done, gives the best color match and an esthetic result. A median forehead flap is ideal to resurface parts of the nose. Universally, a post auricular, full thickness skin graft is an excellent match for the eyelids.

The patient shown in Figure 4.3A, a fair complexioned girl, was seen about 20 years ago, in the pre-laser era, for a V2 Sturge-Weber syndrome. One attempt at cryotherapy, produced a result seen two years later (Fig. 4.3B) A serial excision and a skin replacement was planned. (Fig. 4.3C) shows the result 6 months following 1st serial excision and a median forehead flap. Figures 4.3D and E show the result 2 years after a couple of finishing procedures. The 'dog ear' was then corrected. She lost the dog ear and we lost the follow-up.

In female patients, considerable amount of skin of the lower face and neck can be mobilized for resurfacing the adjacent areas, either as a part of serial excision or after using the tissue expanders to give a good color match in most complexions. The problem of resurfacing is more complex in the male patients because of the hair distribution on the face.

Early interventions are advocated to prevent situations seen in Figure 4.2. Such patients do not only have a bad deformity but suffer from troublesome bleeding.

We thus see that lasers and surgery both have an important role to play in the management of capillary malformations. Lasers appear to be more useful in the younger age group before hyperkeratinization sets in. Surgery has a greater role to play in presence of hyperkeratinization and management of lesions affecting the eyelids and nose.

Surgery can also prove more useful in the female patients, where the skin of the face and neck is hairless, faicilitating serial excisions and skin replacement by a closely matching skin. Both modalities can be combined. A simultaneous persual of Chapter 6 which details the use of lasers will help in organizing a management plan.

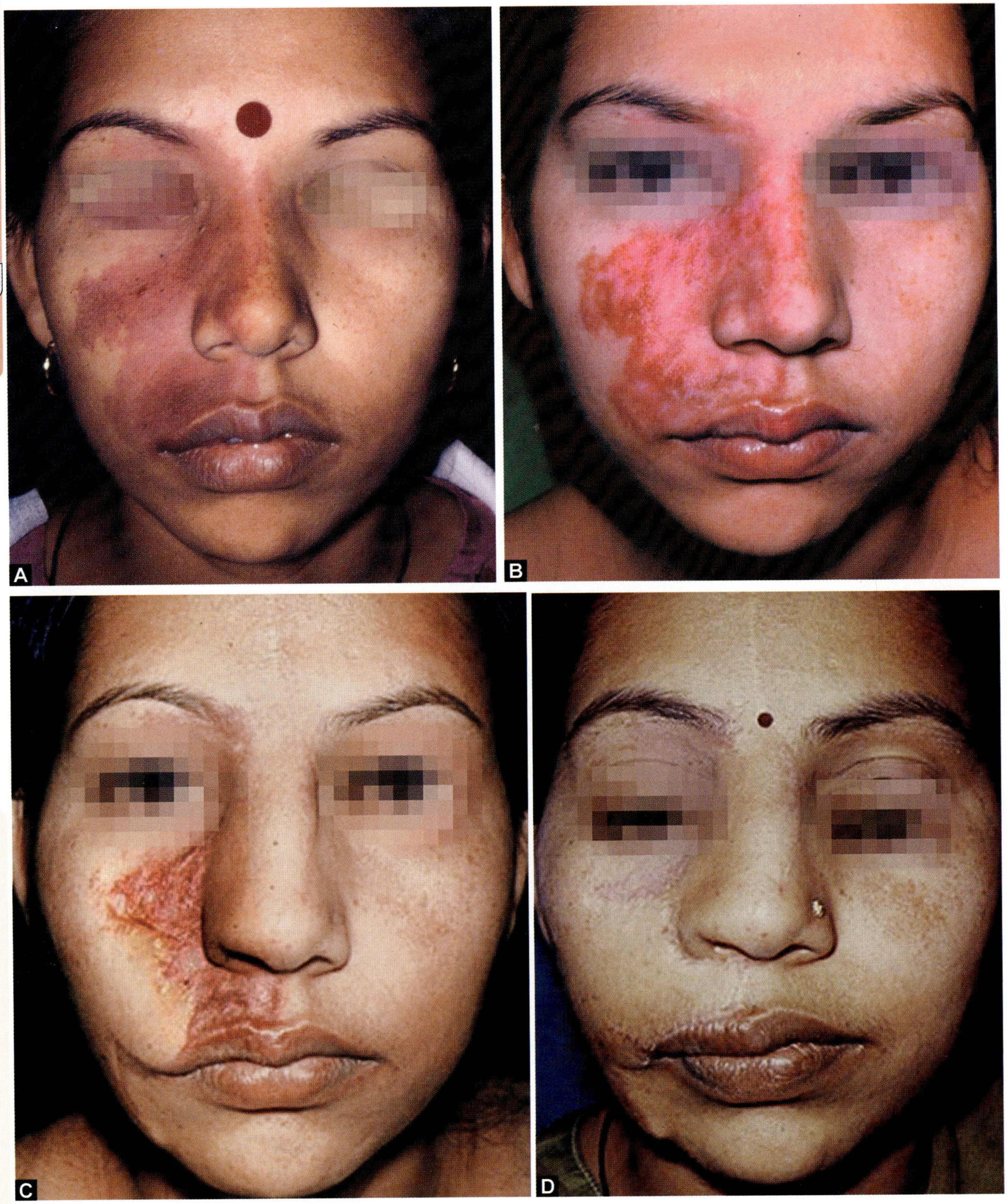
A
B
C
D

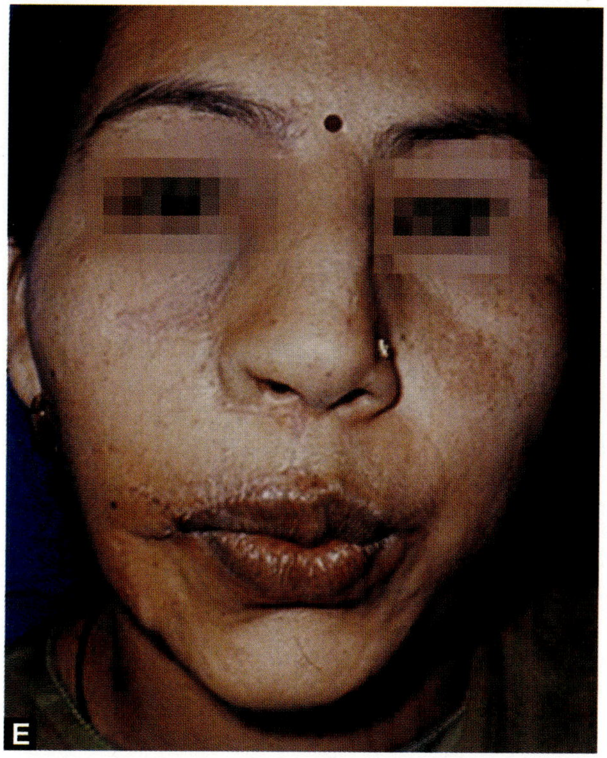

FIGURES 4.3A to E
Capillary malformation (CM) V2. Sturge-Weber Syndrome: (A) Preoperative status. Treated with cryotherapy; (B) 2 years. following cryotherapy; (C) 6 months following 1st serial excision and a median forehead flap; (D) 2 years following the finishing procedures; (E) the dynamics of the face unaffected

LYMPHATIC MALFORMATIONS (LMs)

Subclassification, Nomenclature and Biological Behavior

Until now when dealing with CLVCs we have essentially dealt with the small channel systems.

However, based on their physical characteristics and their biological behavior, the lymphatic malformations are divided into three groups, the macrocystic, the microcystic and the combined group.

In the older classification, large cystic lesions occurring mainly in the head, neck and axilla were labeled cystic hygromas. The large channel lesions were mentioned in literature. They were extremely rare. Their biological behavior was similar to that of cystic hygromas. In the modern nomenclature both have been grouped as the macrocystic lymphatic malformations.

The Macrocystic and the Microcystic Lymphatic Malformations

Macrocystic LMs

The biological behavior of the large channel macrocystic LMs is distinctly different from the small channel micrrocystic LMs. If totally removed recurrence is uncommon.

A good response is also reported to the use of a number of sclerotic agents, e.g. Inj. Bleomycin, Inj. of Tisseel Fibrin Glue, Doxycycline, Bleomycin, OK-432 (Picibanil), etc.

Microcystic LMs

The small channel lesions do not show a consistent or lasting response to the use of these agents. Even after a surgical ablation aggressive recurrence is usual and is often referred in literature as relentless. However, long follow-ups suggest, that if the lesion is kept under control by periodic ablation, (to ensure prevention of other disabling consequences), the tendency to recur begins declining after puberty and appears to become less and less as the age advances. Benefits of interventions after puberty appear to be lasting.

Both the Macrocystic and the Microcystic Malformations can coexist

The later can be associated with the other small channels, the capillaries and the lymphatics.

The 3-year-old illustrated in Figures 4.5A to C is of this combination and the case study that follows deals with its management.

The most common of the lot, the microcystic group comprises of small channeled lymphatics and continues to be labeled as lymphangioma. However, since there is no evidence of increased endothelial turnover, the use of the term 'Lymphangioma' is being replaced by 'Lymphatic Malformation'.

Microcystic Lymphatic Malformations

Amongst all the small channel systems, microcystic lymphatic malformations are by far the most common. The term 'LM' or 'Lymphatic Malformation' when used without a prefix is considered a synonym of this malformation'.

Their *biological behavior* has been described in the beginning of this chapter. They are characterized by an incessant growth (until puberty and sometimes longer) and scant respect for tissue planes. They exert gentle, but persistent compressive pressure, which can obstruct low pressure physiological channels in the head and neck and even affect the airway. Over a period of time, they distort, weaken and demineralize the skeleton. Aggressive recurrences are common in the younger age groups.

These lesions may be supercial or deep. Both groups can coexist. They are usually present at birth but remain undiagnosed, particularly because they are colorless. Superficial lesions are missed if they are small or deep, particularly if the infant is plump.

When mixed with other small channels, they dominate the scene, leave an imprint of their characteristics on the lesion and create identities based on the combinations such as CLMs (Capillary Lymphatic Malformations) or more uncommonly the CLVMs (Capilary Lymphatic Venous Malformations).

The Management

Influencing Factors

The lesions are congenital. The speed of growth waxes in the early childhood and wanes usually after adolescence . The pattern of growth and its management is affected by the constraints of space. The constituent channels are in varying proportions and the optimal therapeutic modality for each of them may be different. Previous therapeutic attempts too, may leave their problems.

I have therefore chosen to cover this topic in the form of 3 case studies.

Case study 1 deals with a lesion involving all the small channels.

CASE STUDY 1

Capillary-Lymphatic-Venous-Malformation (CLVM)

Figure 4.4 is a good example of a CLVM. Using the old terminology, it could also be labelled as a Klippel-Trenaunay syndrome of the face.

The lesion was present at birth and treated locally. He gave a history that at the age of 2 days, a 'Protuberant pedunculated cystic swelling, protruding from the right angle of the mouth' was excised. The child was administered Inj. Bleomycin intralesional at 3 months and 6 months of age. Figures 4.4A to C are pictures from the family album showing the still growing deformity.

He was seen by us at the age of 7 months. Local examination revealed an abnormal right angle of the mouth with a fibromucoid mass just behind the angle and a diffuse lymphangiomatous lesion of the right cheek, lower face and neck. The patient was referred to a senior colleague pediatric surgeon. He was referred back after 2 years. His status after 8 injections of Bleomycin is seen in Figures 4.4D to G. The mother's assessment of the Bleomycin therapy was, 'initially 50 percent better, no further response' thereafter. CT and MRI studies revealed lymphangiomatous tissue predominating in the subcutaneous tissue and tongue, particularly its base (Figs 4.4H to J) and extensive vascular involvement from subtemporal region to floor of mouth (Figs 4.4K and L). The few phleboliths seen in these characterize the venous elements.

Case Study 1: A case of 'Capillary, Lymphatic, Venous Malaformation - CLVM' (Figures 4.4A to T)

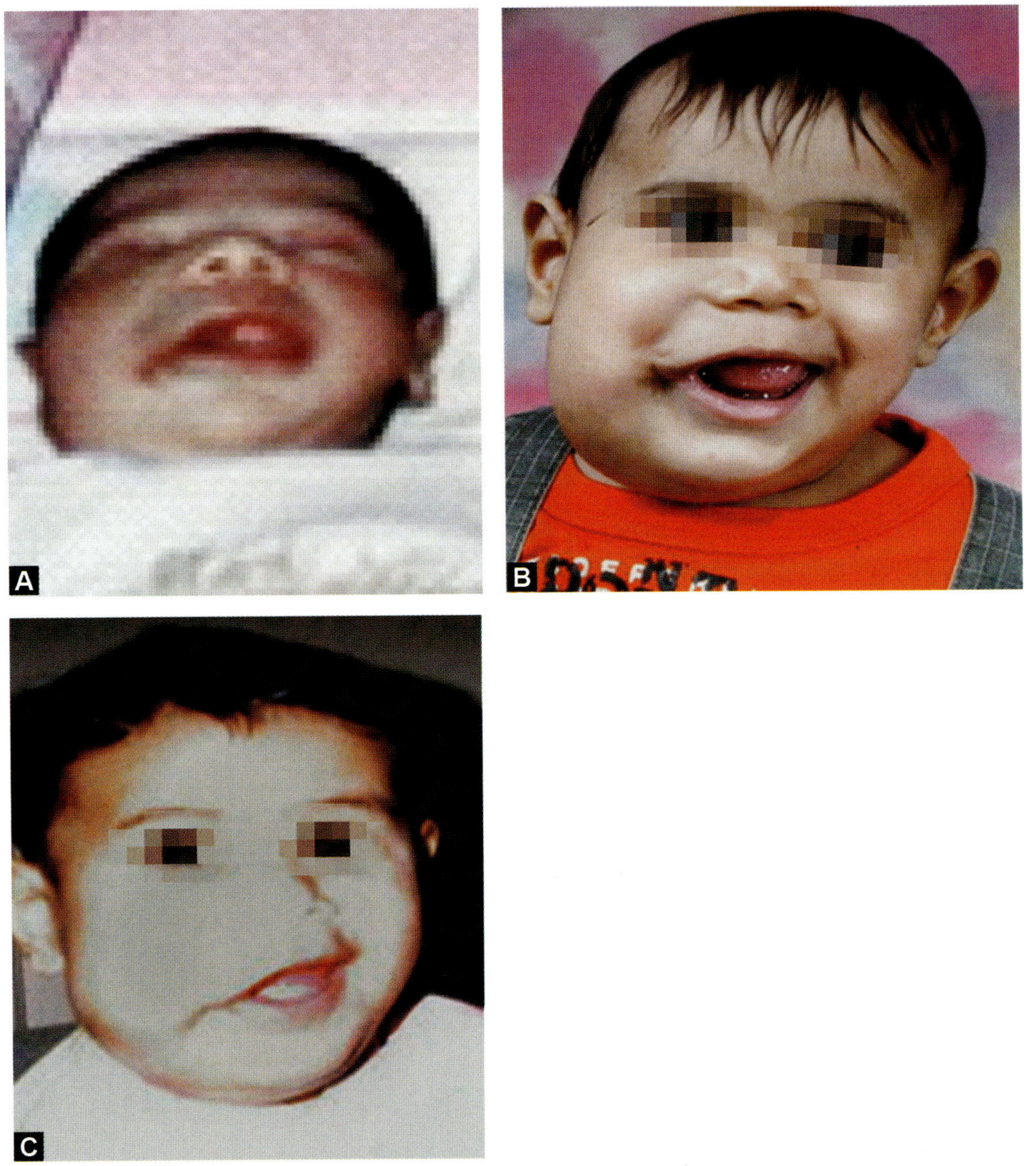

FIGURES 4.4A to C

(From the family album) at 1 month, 1 year and 2 years

Case Study 1: A case of 'Capillary, Lymphatic, Venous Malaformation - CLVM' (Contd...)

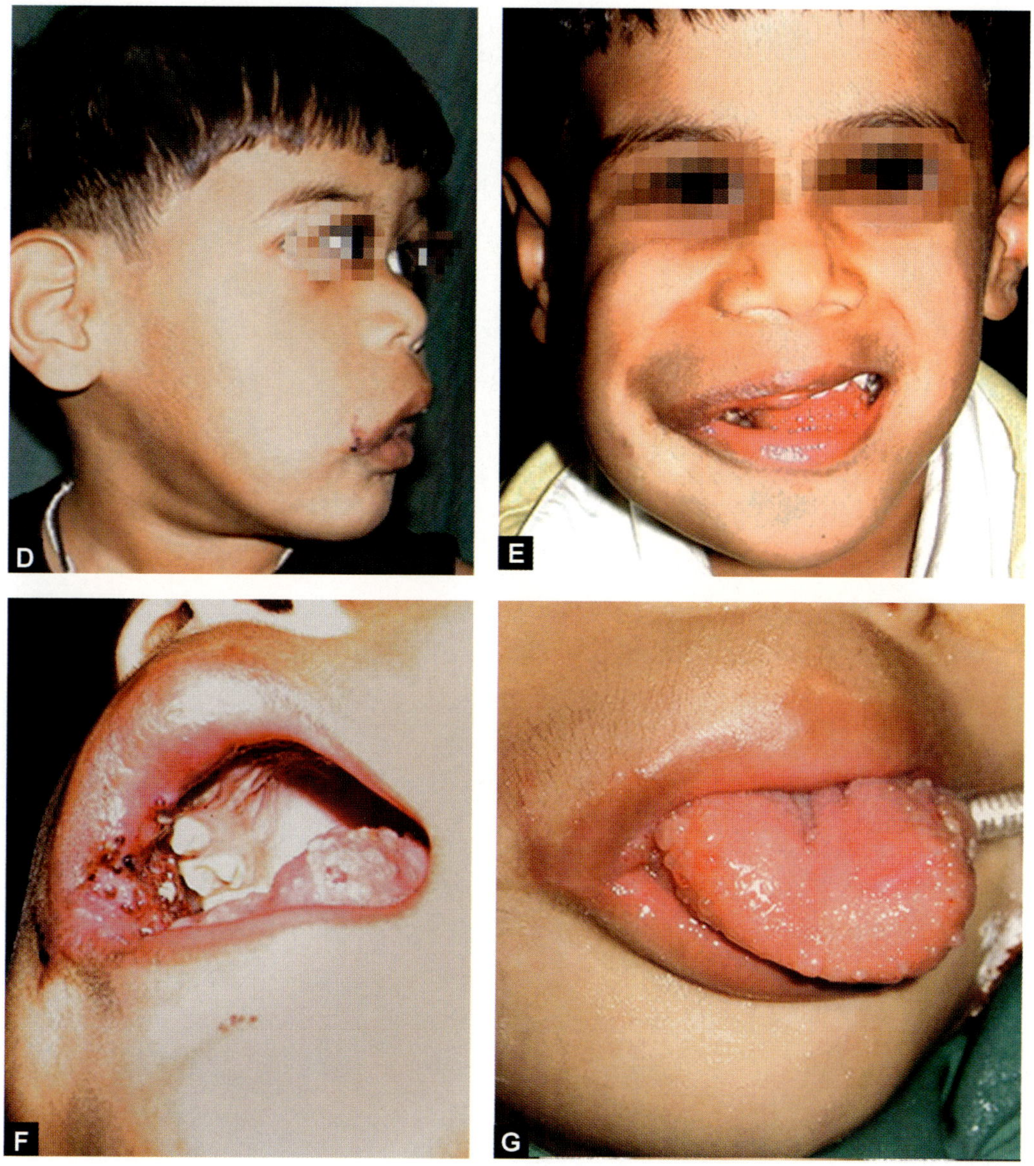

FIGURES 4.4D to G

Status at the age of 3 years. Swelling and deformity at right side of face, anterior open bite and the macroglossia

Case Study 1: A case of 'Capillary, Lymphatic, Venous Malaformation - CLVM' (Contd...)

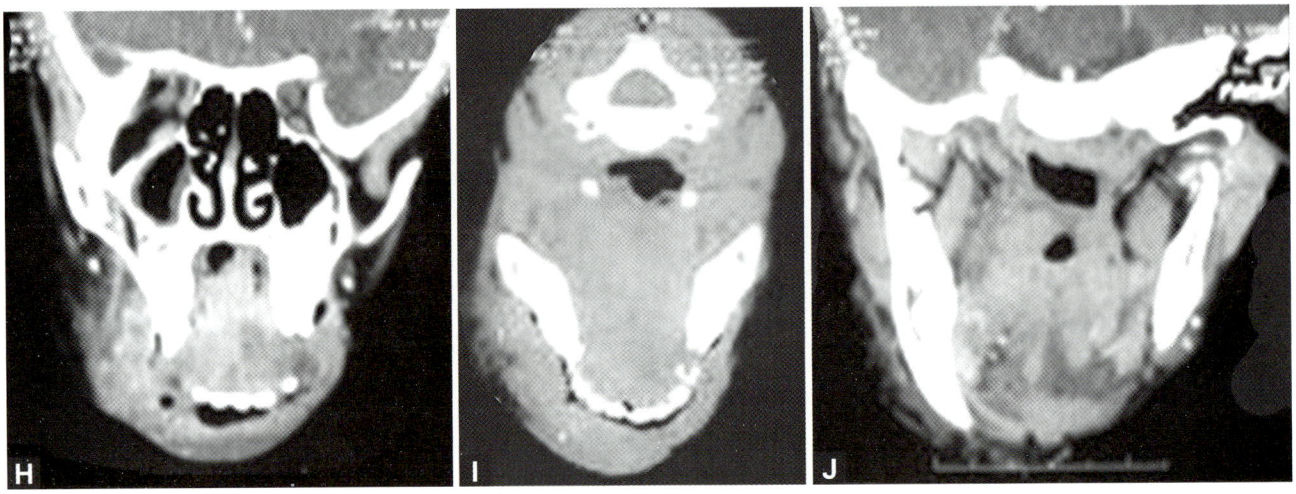

FIGURES 4.4H to J
Axial CT scans

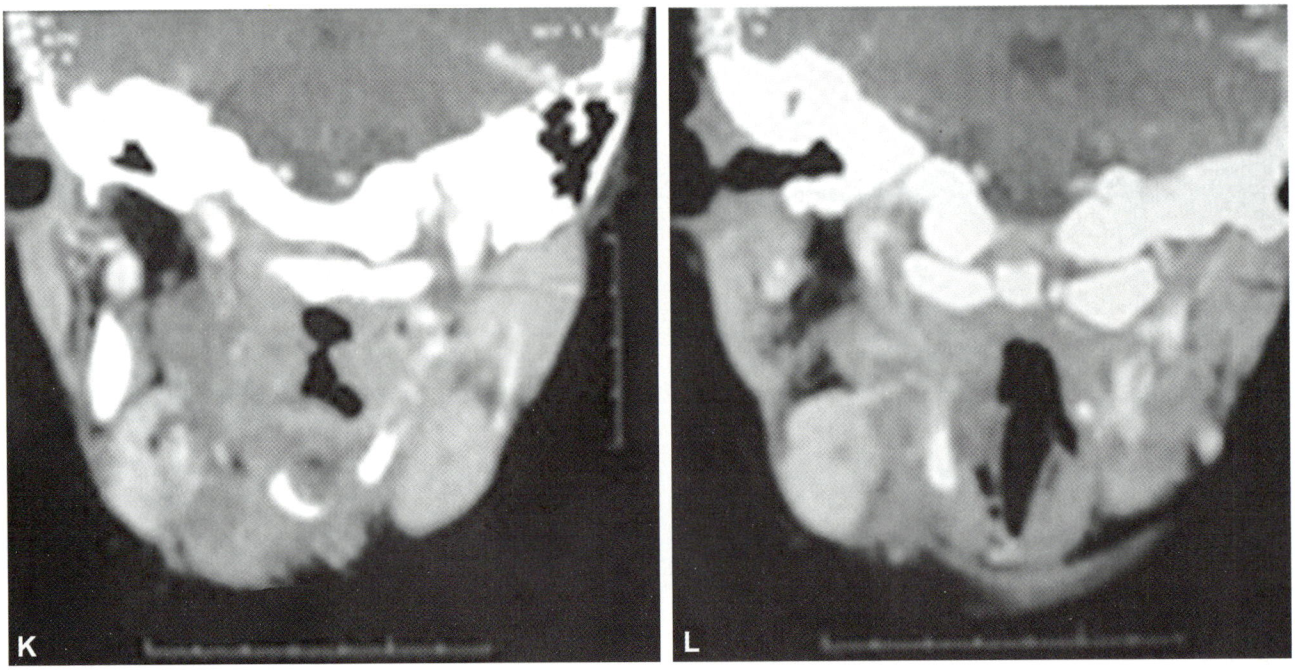

FIGURES 4.4K and L
Coronal scans. Deeply located venous component characterized by the phleboliths

Case Study 1: A case of 'Capillary, Lymphatic, Venous Malaformation - CLVM' (Contd...)

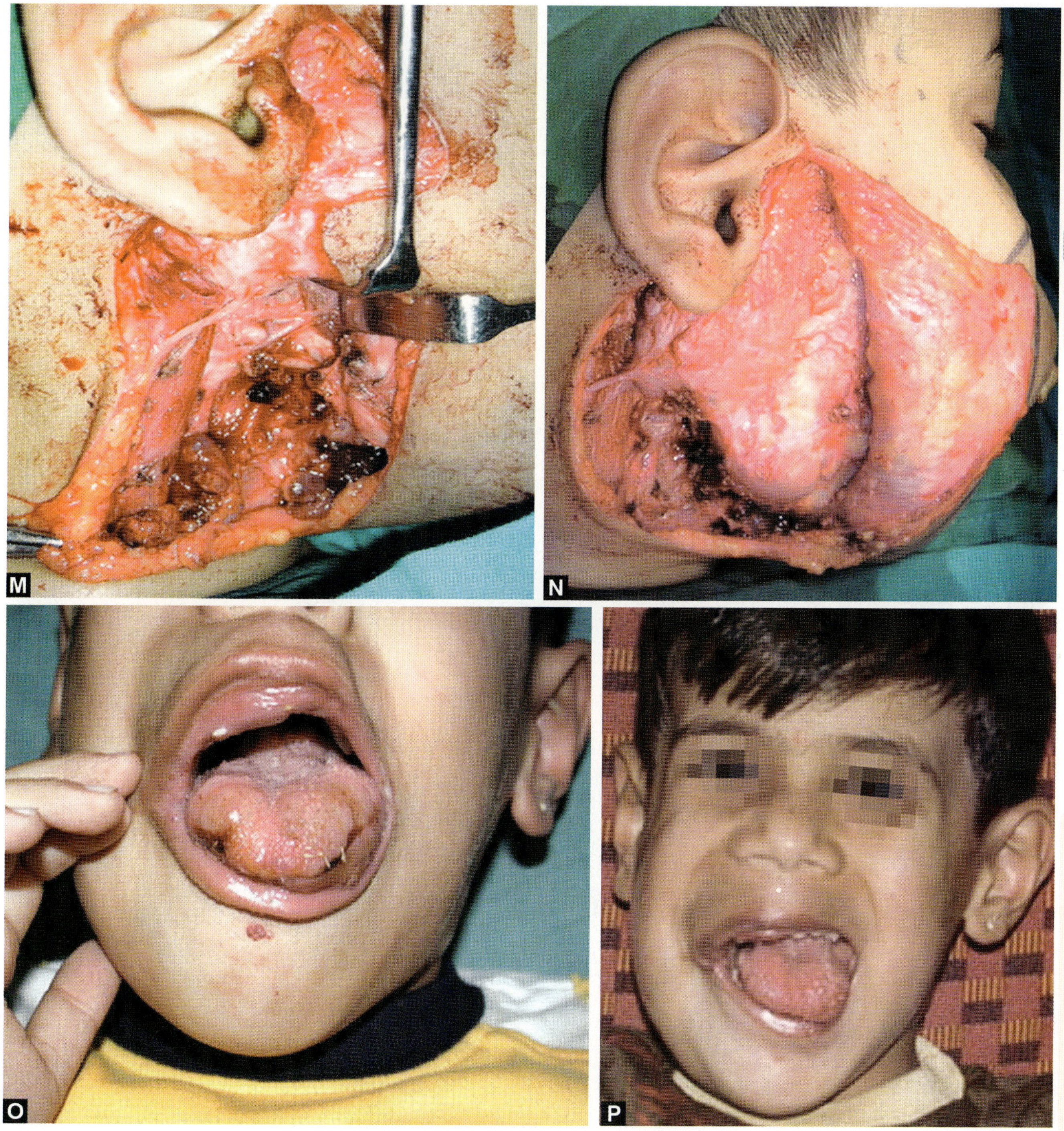

FIGURES 4.4M to P

(M and N) Superficial and deep (subtemporal) exposure provided by a parotid incision;
(O) Soon after RF of the surface lesions;
(P) 10 months later

Case Study 1: A case of 'Capillary, Lymphatic, Venous Malaformation - CLVM' (Contd...)

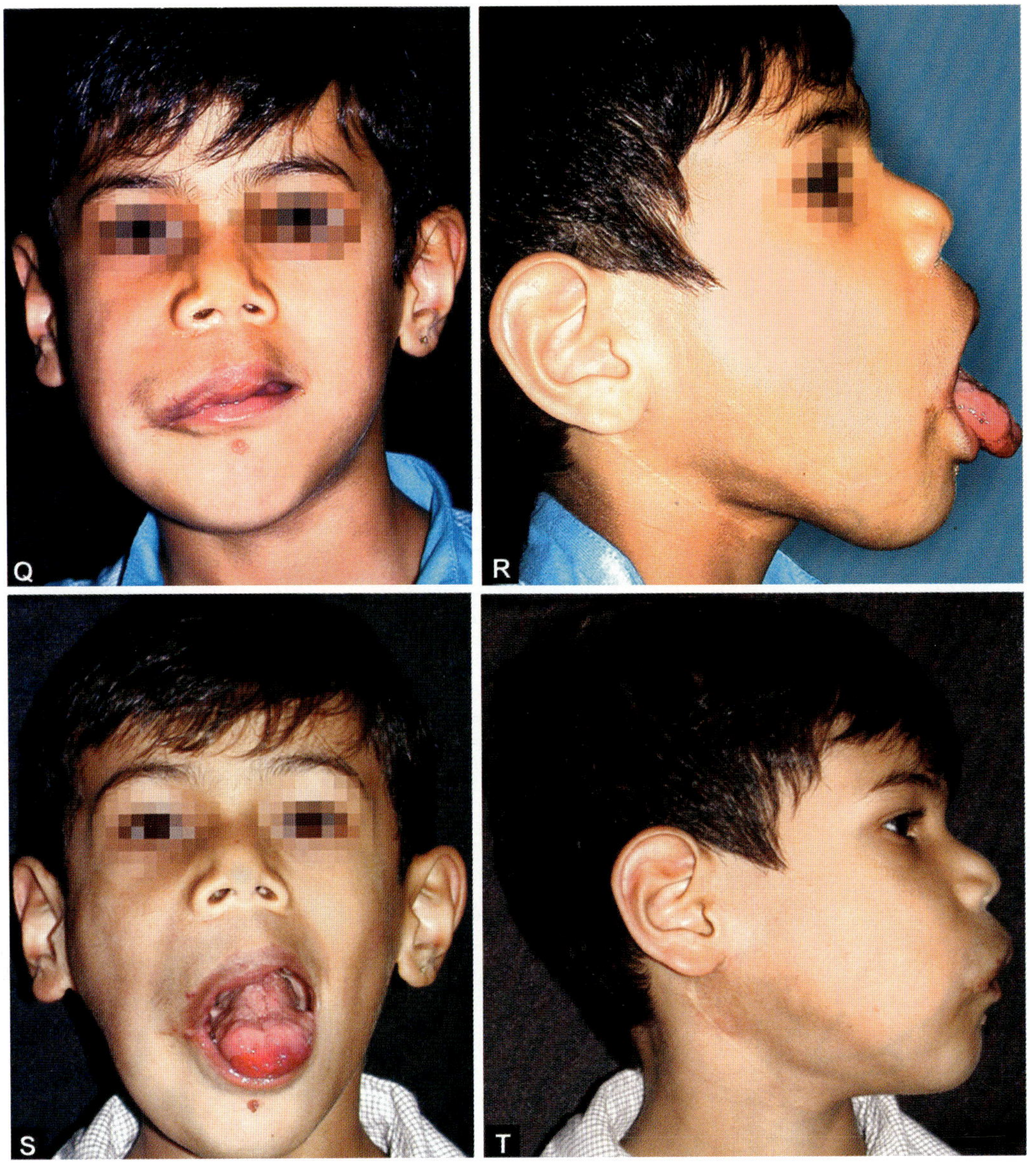

FIGURES 4.4Q to T
(Q and R) 1½ years later
(S and T) 3 years later.

FIGURES 4.4A to T
A case of 'Capillary, Lymphatic, Venous Malaformation - (CLVM)

The child was taken up for surgery (Figs 4.4M and N). The lymphatic areas and the venous areas were in parts intermingled and interspersed with areas of fibrosis, probably caused by Bleomycin injections. The venous malformation was excised. The bipolar cautery was used to ablate the exposed lymphatic malformations and the RF superpulse was used for the submucosal and the subcutaneous lesions. Figure 4.4O shows the immediate postoperative result and Figure P the result 10 months later.

Figures 4.4Q and R show the status one and a half year later. At about this time, he began developing recurrent tonsillitis associated with inflammatory areas in the adjacent tongue resulting in a predominately right sided macroglossia. A tonsillectomy and adenoidectomy were carried out. Simultaneously, the surface lymphangiomatous areas along the left borders of the tongue were excised and considerable portion of adjacent deeper lymphangiomatous elements were ablated with complete relief (Figs 4.4S and T).

CASE STUDY 2

Bilateral Macrocystic and Central Microcystic Lymphatic Malformation—

Illustrating the coexistence of the macrocystic and microcystic lymphatic malformations with different biological behavior.

Figures 4.5A to C shows a 3-year-old child, with bilateral Macrocystic lymphangiomatous lesions (Cystic Hygromas) and an extensive Microcystic small channel lymphatic capillary malformation (LCM) of the midline structures of the lower half of the face, associated with Macroglossia and mandibular enlargement. CT studies Figures 4.5D to G show a heterogeneous, enhancing, irregular, hypodense mass lesions in the bilateral parotid regions. The gland tissue was hardly distinguishable. They also show the small channel lesion of the midface, with a fairly symmetrical compression of the nasopharyngeal and laryngeal airspace. Figures 4.5H and I show a significant expansion of the mandible with jaw jutting forwards over the sternum, and no bone destruction.

This bone expansion is characteristic of all small channel low flow malformations, lying in a space bordered by bone. These skeletal changes appear to be an expression of the response of the skeletal tissue to the gentle expansive pressure of the expanding soft tissues.

The macrocystic lesions exhibit a lasting response to surgery and the surgery can be carried out early in infancy. Figure 4.5J shows the dissection on the left side. The right side was operated a few months later together with debulking of the lymphatic malformation of the tongue. The postoperative result is seen in Figure 4.5K. Figure 4.5 L taken 3 years later shows the lasting benefit following ablation of the Macrocystic lesions but the characteristic regrowth of the microcystic lesion.

Case Study 2: Bilateral Macrocystic and Central Microcystic Lymphatic Malformation (Figures 4.5A to Z)

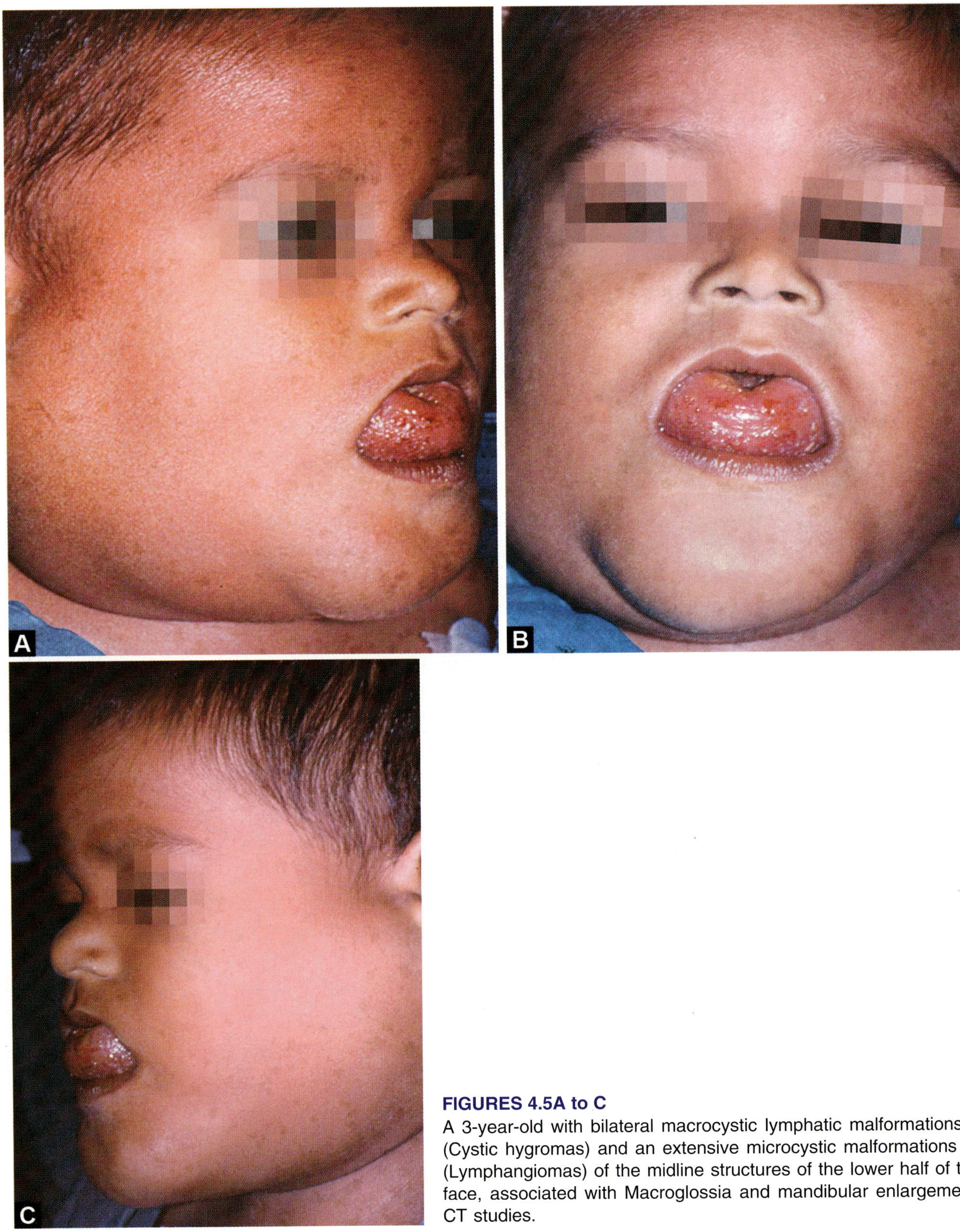

FIGURES 4.5A to C

A 3-year-old with bilateral macrocystic lymphatic malformations (Cystic hygromas) and an extensive microcystic malformations (Lymphangiomas) of the midline structures of the lower half of the face, associated with Macroglossia and mandibular enlargement. CT studies.

Case Study 2: Bilateral Macrocystic and Central Microcystic Lymphatic Malformation (Contd...)

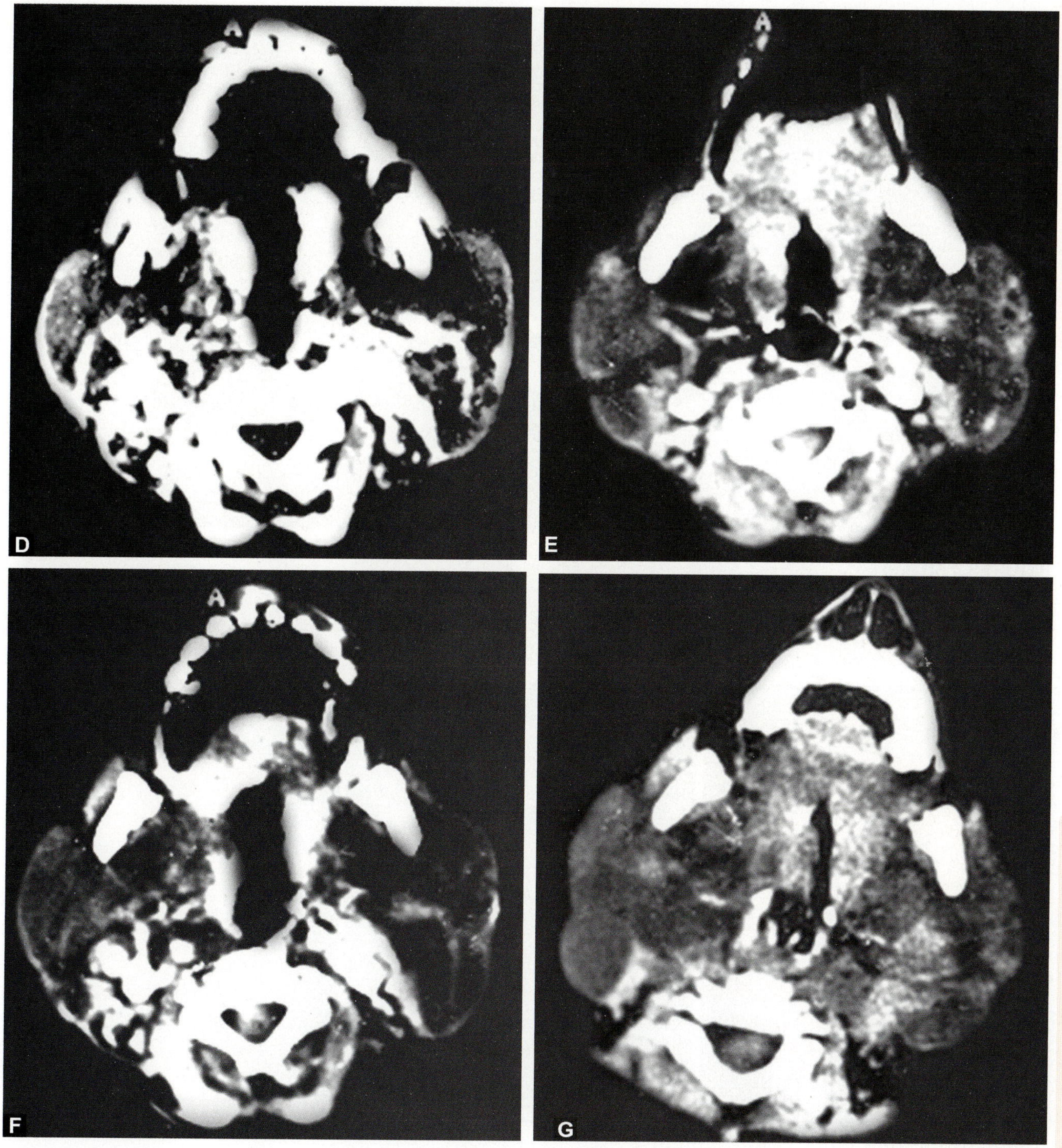

FIGURES 4.5D to G

Show a heterogeneous, enhancing, irregular, hypodense mass lesions in both the parotid regions and a fairly symmetrical compression of the nasopharyngeal and laryngeal airspace.

Case 2: Bilateral Macrocystic and Central Microcystic Lymphatic Malformation (Contd...)

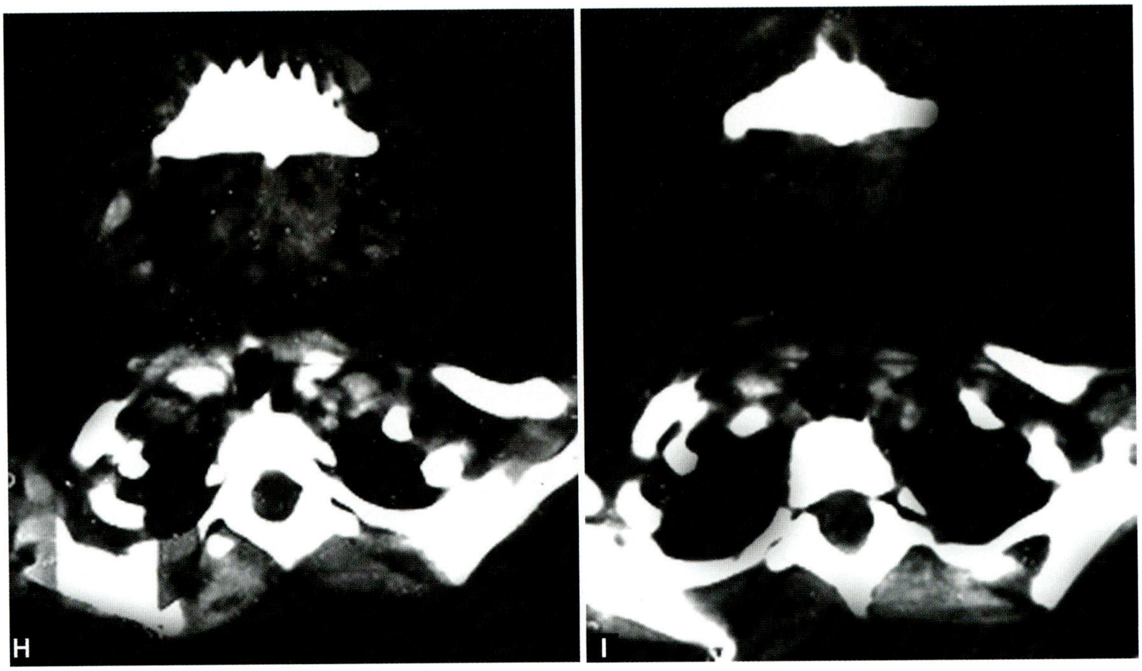

FIGURES 4.5H and I
A significant expansion of the mandible with jaw jutting forwards over the sternum, no bone destruction.

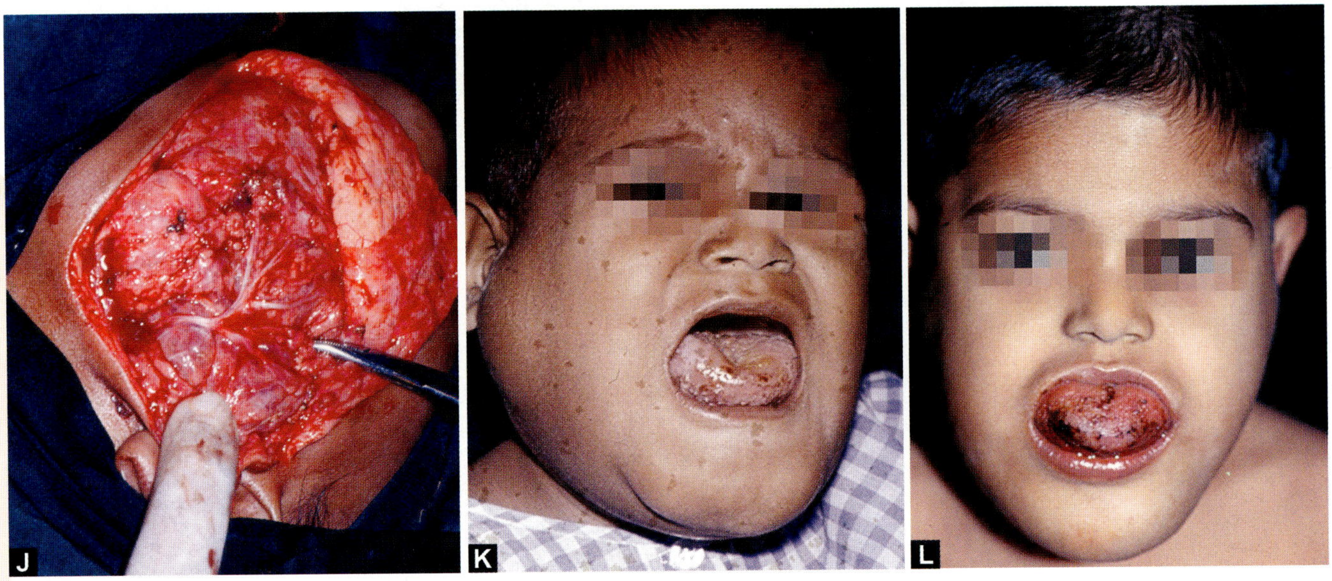

FIGURES 4.5J to L
(J) The operation field after clearing the right macrocystic lesion; (K) Appearance after both the macrocystic lesions were ablated and after a significant debulking of the midline microcystic lesion; (L) Three years later we see the regrowth of the microcystic lesion (Lymphangioma) and the lasting benefit of the surgical ablation of the bilateral macrocystic lesions.

These macrocystic lesions have been reported to respond to the intralesional use of Doxycycline, Bleomycin, Picibanil (OK-432) and Tisseel Fibrin Glue. Each has its own limitation and my personal preference is still for surgery. Within six months of the diagnosis the child had the removal of both the macrocystic lesions and a debulking of the microcystic lesion of the tongue.

Three years later (Figs 4.5M to O), we see the lasting relief from the macrocystic lesions and a good definition of the lateral sides of the face. However, there is massive hypertrophy of the midline structures (Figs 4.5L to O). Using both the transoral approach and the external midline of the neck approach. A considerable debulking of the LM was carried out. However, the growth has continued and the result 2 years later is seen in (Figs 4.5P and Q). Figures P and Q show the patient a year after six sessions of RF superpulse (surface therapy) spread over one year. Note the significant reduction of the mass of the malformation. The lymphatic malformation of the tongue has also benefited considerably (Figs 4.5R and S).

He was now put on periodic surface RF therapy over a period of three years. The effective control of the lesion is illustrated 3 years later (Figs 4.5T to U).

Whereas the gums were not affected, the adjacent mucosa was heavily infiltrated (Fig. 4.5U) masking the distorted and damaged dentition as seen in the OPG (Figs 4.5V and W). The Figs 4.5V and W show the residual dentition with severe damage and infection underlying the visible pathology.

The lateral ceph also shows the projection of mandible (Figs 4.5V and W).

The small channel lesion has caused thinning of the mandible and its expansion, making the bone jut forward even at the age of 3 years (Figs 4.5 H and I). With growth, the chin looks very prominent mainly because of its expansion both in the antero-posterior (Fig. 4.5W) and the transverse dimensions. The same patient is also shown in Figure 4.1, where one sees a significant presence of the Capillary Malformation (CMs) which could account for the thickening and irregularity of the bone along the outer surface of the chin. The LM has involved the mucosa adjacent to the gum and its hypertrophy has buried the poor quality decayed teeth which are almost invisible on a clinical examination. The correction of the established skeletal deformity by a set back of the chin accompanied by ablation of the residual malformation in the tongue has improved the balance of face as seen in Figures 4.5X to Z showing the final result.

LMs—Treatment Modalities—RF an Effective Addition

RF has been cited as a treatment modality in both the case studies cited above. A few words on this effective modality are relevant at this stage.

The microcystic lesions, have traditionally been treated with sclerosants or surgery. Specially when extensive, they do not respond well to sclerosants and even to surgery, unless almost a total ablation is achieved–a difficult task.

Superficial lesions, particularly on the face do present themselves for aesthetic reasons. These pervade the soft tissues with ill defined borders, have a boggy feel, cause a bulge and, sometimes have a faint bluish tinge. The anatomical borders are often not clearly defined. A steady growth is usually seen. Neither surgery nor sclerotics give really satisfactory results. Recurrence is common. Radical approach can produce deformities. Conservative approach invites recurrence.

Case Study 2: Bilateral Macrocystic and Central Microcystic Lymphatic Malformation (Contd...)

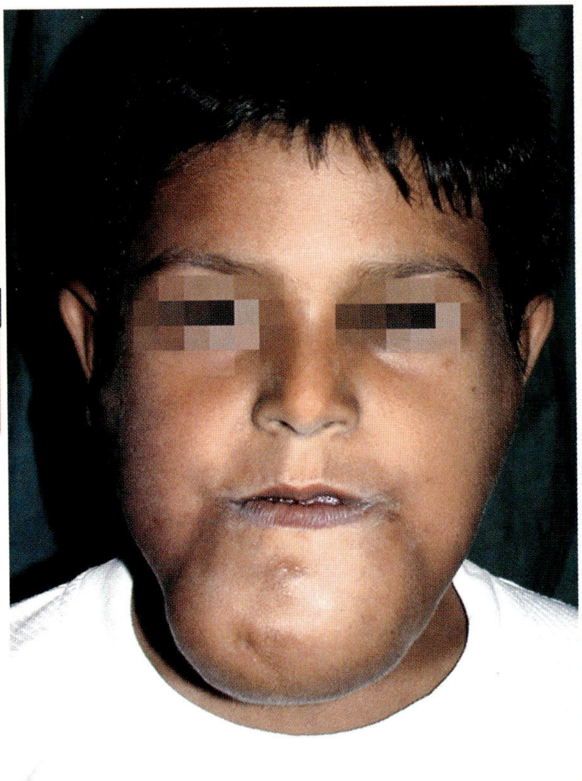

M

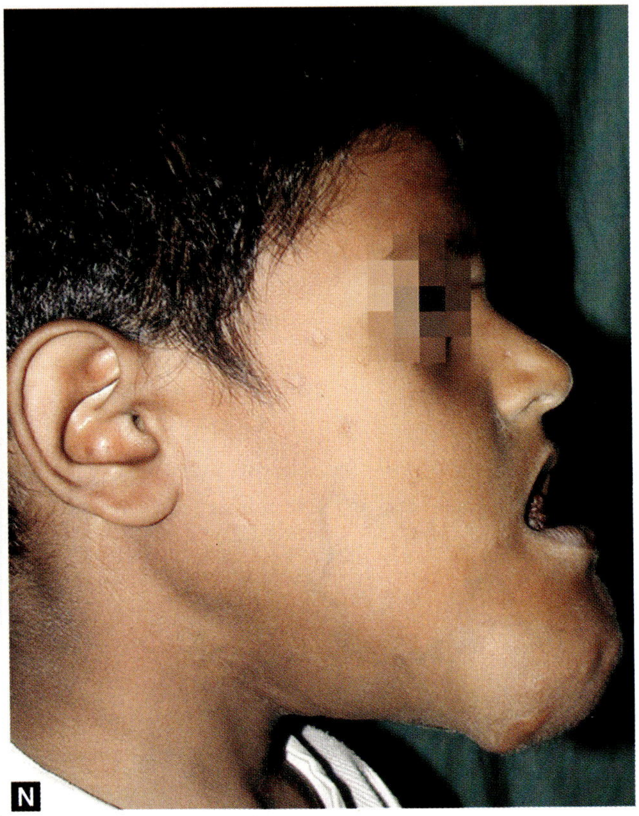

N

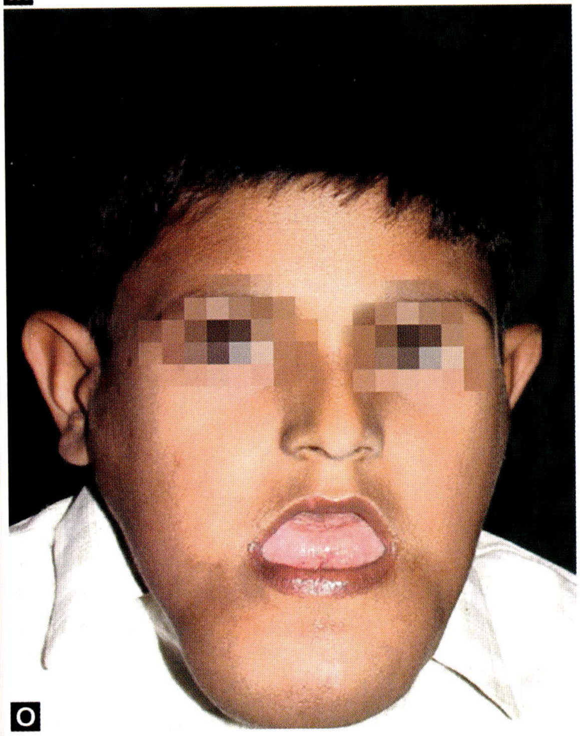

O

FIGURES 4.5M to O
6 years later—Massive growth of the microcystic lesion associated with significant mandibular expansion and hypertrophy

Case Study 2: Bilateral Macrocystic and Central Microcystic Lymphatic Malformation (Contd...)

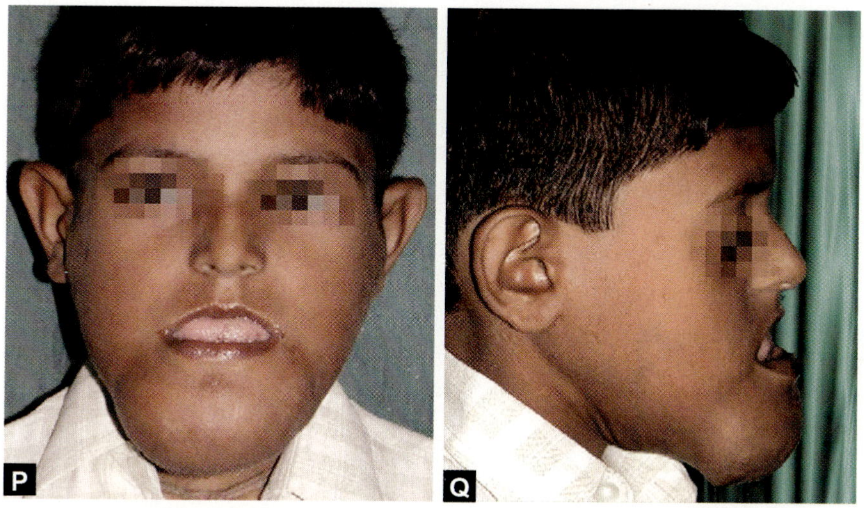

FIGURES 4.5P and Q
(P and Q) Patient after 6 sessions of RF superpulse spread over one year. Note the sigificant reduction of the mass of the malformation.

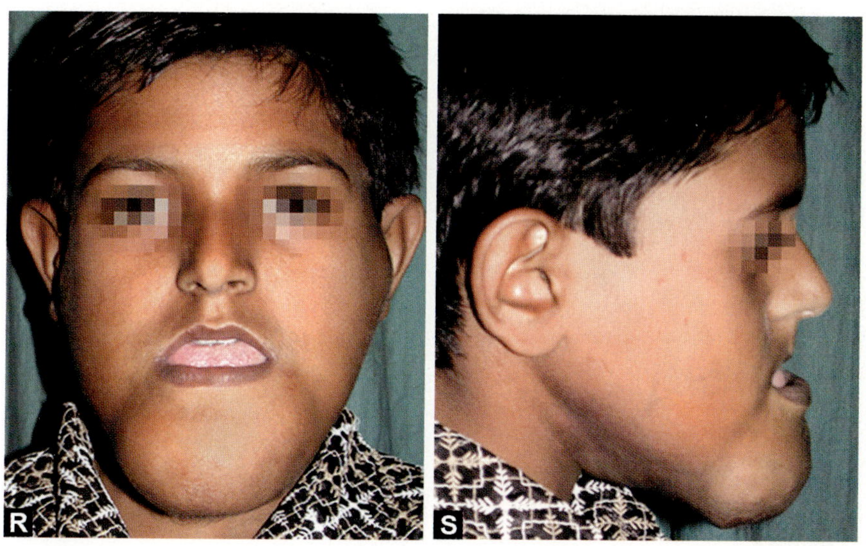

FIGURES 4.5R and S
(R and S) The correction of the established skeletal deformity by a set back of the chin accompanied by ablation of the residual malformation in the tongue. S shows the corrected profile

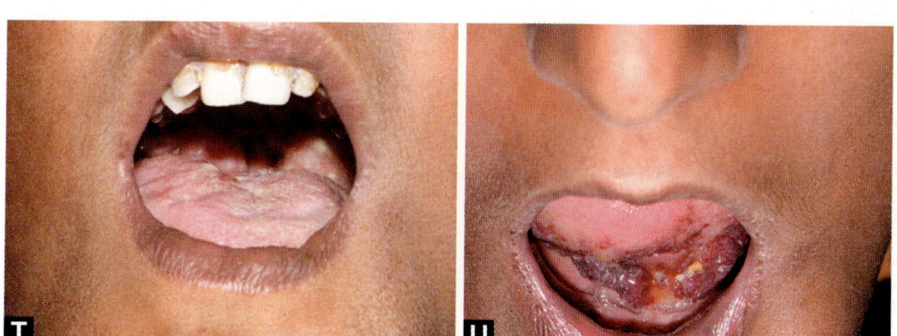

FIGURES 4.5T and U
Figs T and U Show the significant reduction in the size of the lymphatic malformation of the tongue and the mouth over a period of three years of periodic RF Therapy.

Case Study 2: Bilateral Macrocystic and Central Microcystic Lymphatic Malformation (Contd...)

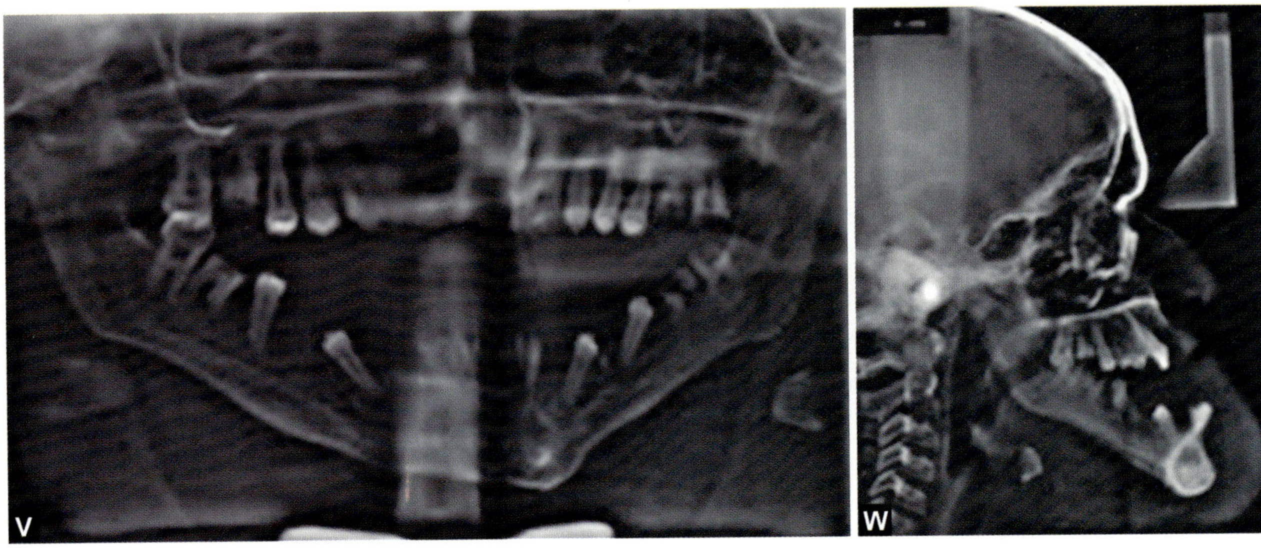

FIGURES 4.5V and W
(V) The OPG shows the dental distortion; (W) Lateral cephalogram show both, the distorted dentition and projection of the mandible.

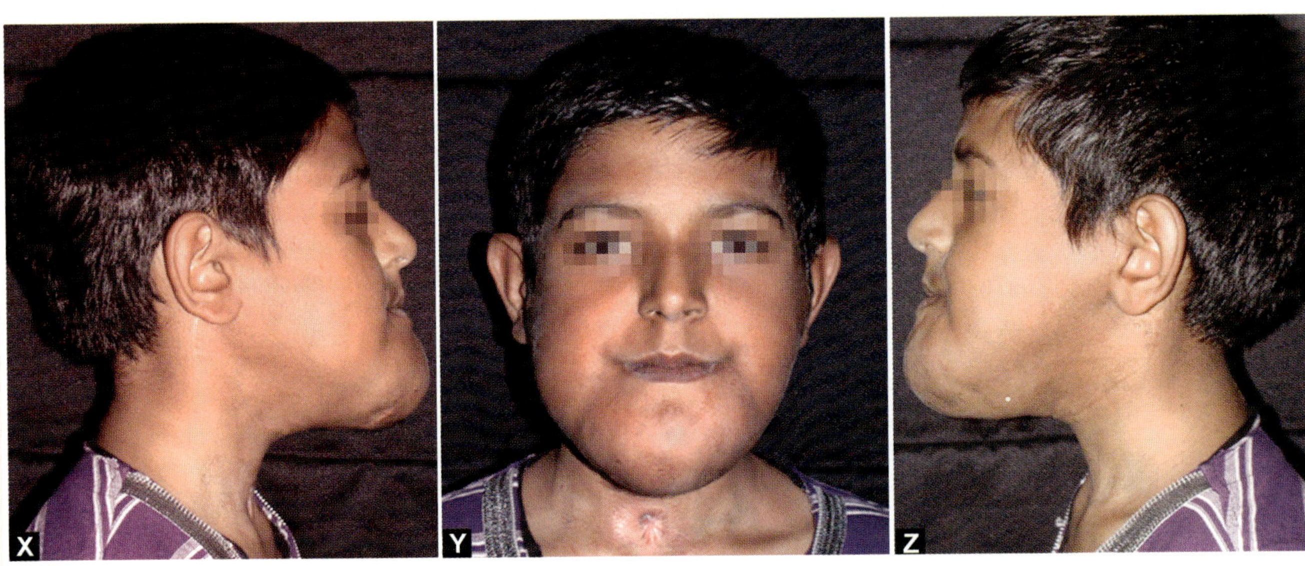

FIGURES 4.5X to Z
The final status after correction

FIGURES 4.5A to Z
Bilateral Macrocystic and Central Microcystic Lymphatic Malformation

The use of radiofrequency (RF) (Fig. 4.6) in the superpulse mode has revolutionized the management of the superficial Microcystic Lymphatic Malformations. The treatment can be given as an office procedure. The treatment if needed, to cover a larger lesion, a residual lesion or a recurrence can be repeated.

During the growth phase, if we can effectively ablate parts of the lesion, under fluoroscopic control, and modulate soft tissue growth, we will be able to prevent both functional disability and deformity.

Deeply Located Lymphatic Malformations

The deep lesions are usually first noticed for a a bulge. A steady relentless growth is a common feature. They expand the skeleton, weaken and deform it. Coexistence with capillary malformations (CMs), the venules and even the venous malformations is known. Small deep lesions if not aggressive, may easily remain, unnoticed, but if large can be very troublesome.

However, in general the deep microcystic lesions of head and neck pose tough problems in management, because of tissue crowding in a limited space. Here, we normally have vital anatomical structures which include the conduits of blood (particularly the low pressure veins) and the compressible passages for air, water and food. If we add to this, a bulky benign tumor growing relentlessly with an effective pressure, enough to expand and distort the bone, the combination required to cause maximum surgical problems is in place. The only saving grace for the operator is the compressibility of the LMs.

In addition, these lesions particularly when located in the suprahyoid region, pose a serious challenge to the anesthetist–difficult intubation and post-anesthetic management.

These lesions also pose problems in the effective use of obliterating agents (sclerotics) locally. There may be some relief, but rarely cure. The access is deep and the ramifications many. The lesion is not confined to specific planes and grows in various directions. The deformities are often compounded by tissue hyperplasia, particularly skeletal.

Using RF probes under imaging control, is a promising new tool to destroy the deep seated lesions.

In childhood, even after debulking, the rapid re-growth of the lesion becomes frustrating. It is only after puberty and after the growth slows down or ends, that final interventions can lead to reasonable results.

The management of these malformation is challenging.

The following case study illustrates almost everything that can go wrong and the challenges posed by their management.

CASE STUDY 3

Lymphatic Malformation with Iatrogenic Problems (Fig. 4.6)

Figures 4.6 A to F present the various aspects of her deformity. She was treated elsewhere since childhood with a diagnosis of 'Cystic Hygroma'. She had already undergone six surgical procedures elsewhere and had developed a number of iatrogenic deformities. A CT study, a year earlier and prior to the last surgery had reported the possibility of a 'benign oropharyngeal soft tissue tumor with no bone destruction'. No operative details were available. The attributed diagnosis was probably based on the growth of the lymphangioma and the bone destruction induced by earlier surgery, the combination simulating the behavior of a neoplasm.

Figures 4.6A to C show her appearance on the first presentation; Figures 4.6D to F show the deformity of the lower jaw, the preexisting macroglossia and facial palsy, apparently postsurgical. Figures 4.6G to J show the deformities of the facial skeleton. Note that the malunited left and the ununited right osteotomy-sites of the body of the mandible and the associated deformity and malocclusion.

The anterior part of tongue had been ablated. The patient had severe impairment of sleep, speech and swallowing.

Bilateral osteotomies of the body of the mandible had been carried out presumably to control prognathism. There was a nonunion on one side, a partial malunion on the other and an associated significant deformity and malocclusion.

The macroglossia continued to impair oropharyngeal function. The impairment of sleep and speech, could be attributed to this deformity. In addition, the patient had developed a left sided complete facial palsy.

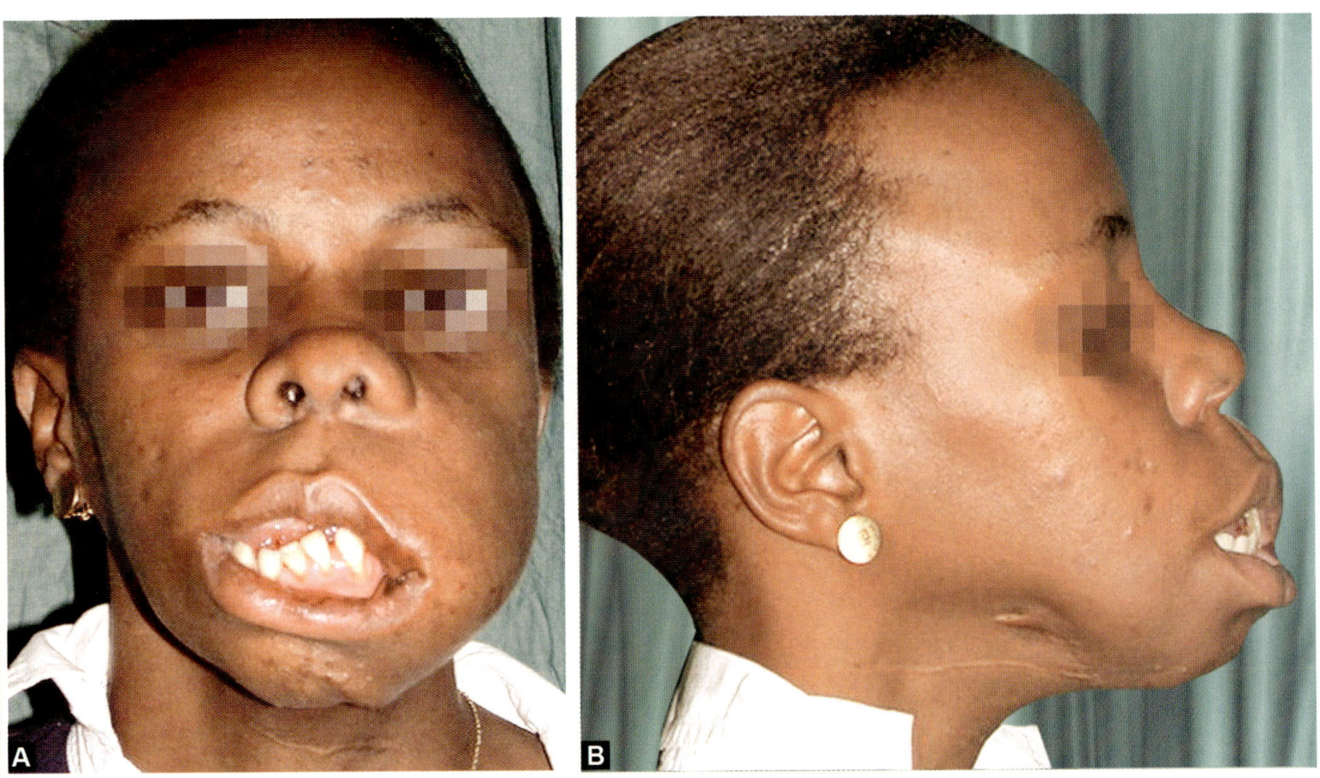

FIGURES 4.6A and B
Facial asymmetry and occlusal plane deformity

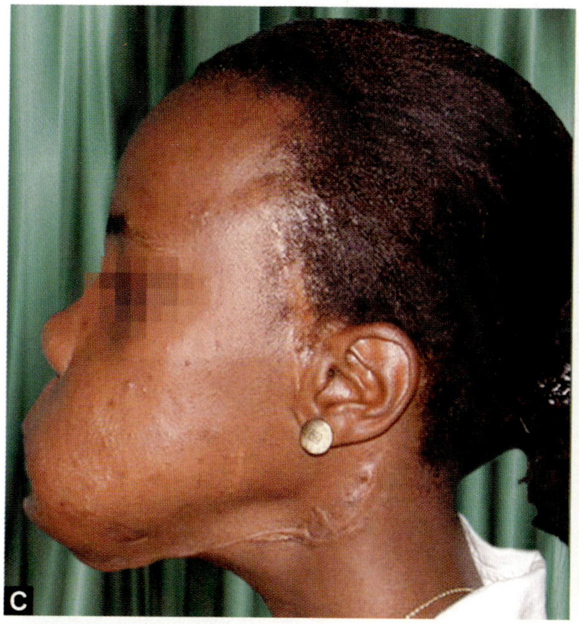
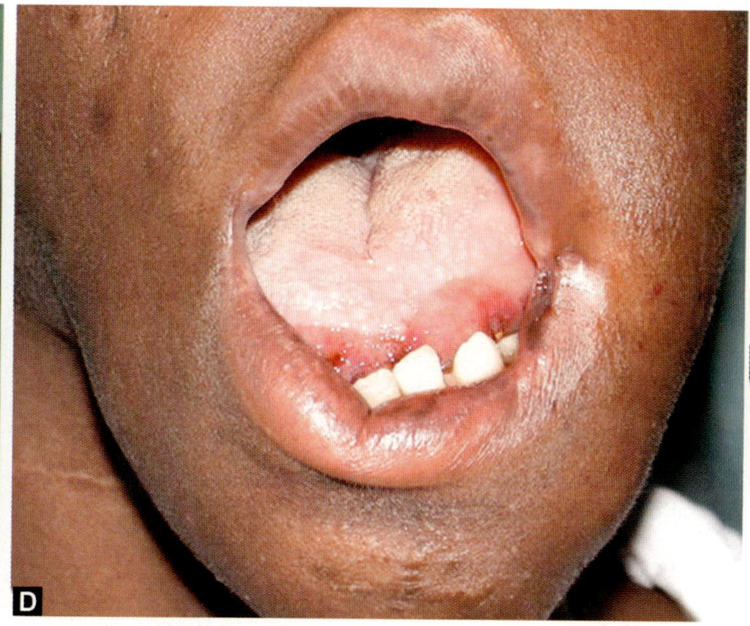

FIGURES 4.6C and D
(C) The overgrowth of left jaw; (D) The macroglossia

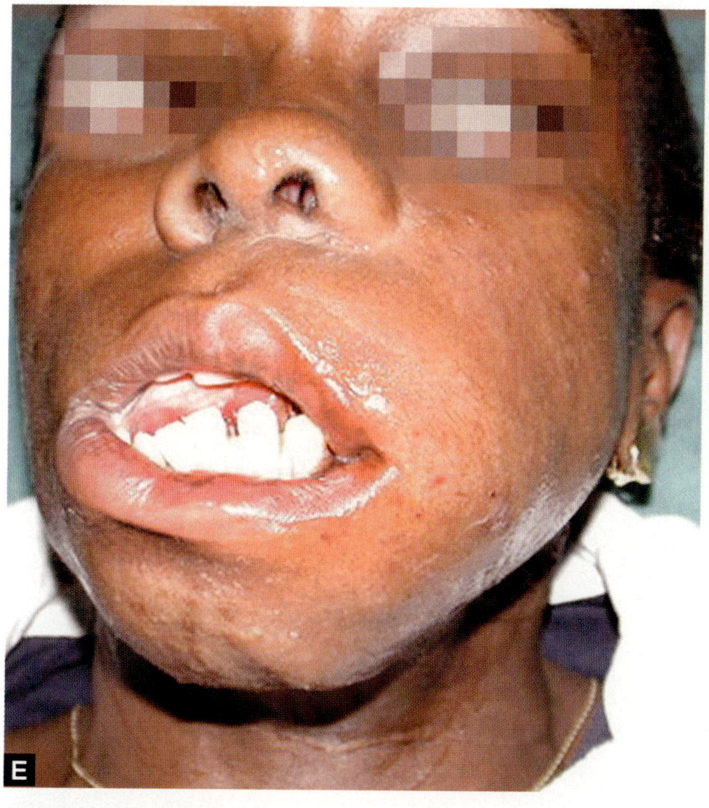
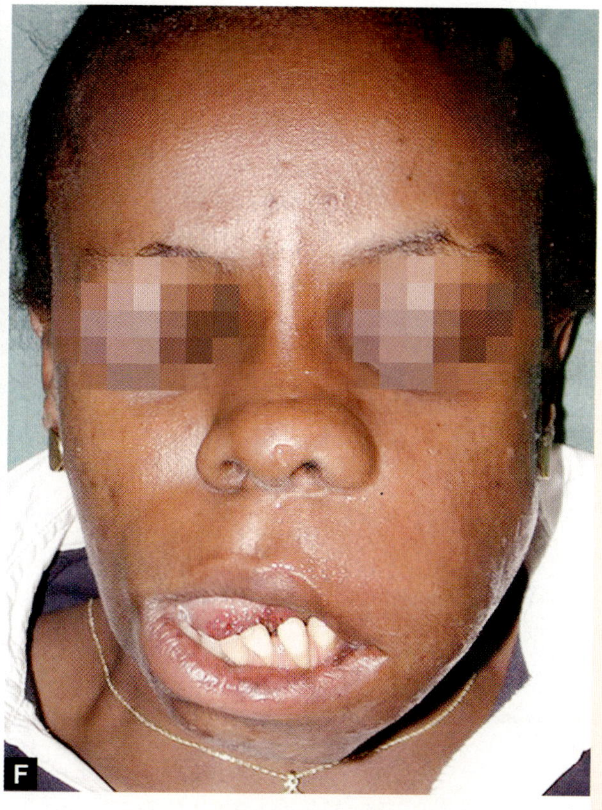

FIGURES 4.6E and F
The left sided facial palsy and the jaw deformity

FIGURES A to F
The appearance when 1st seen

Case Study 3: Lymphatic Malformation with Iatrogenic Problems (Contd...)

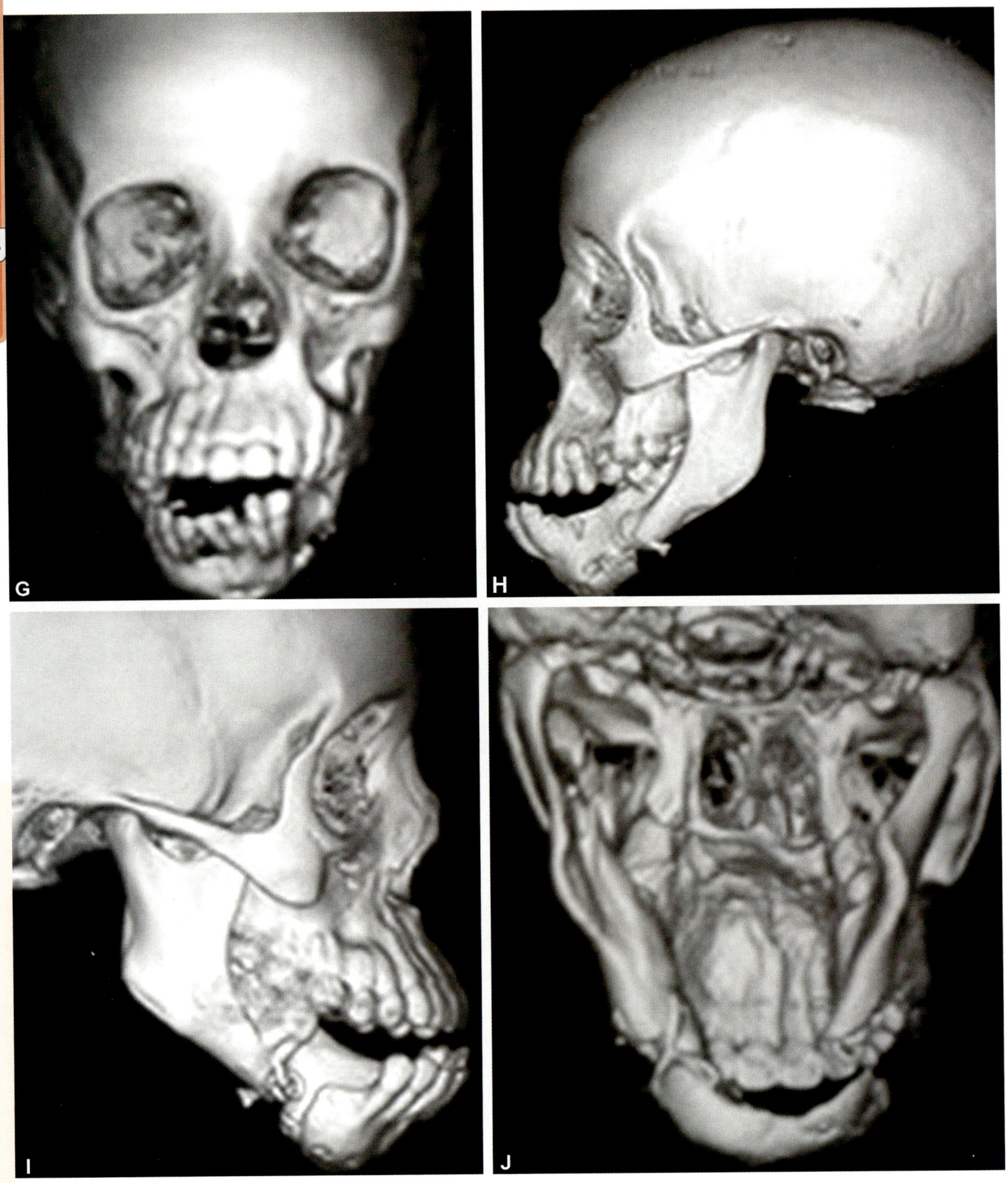

FIGURES 4.6G to J
The skeletal deformities. The scans illustrate the deformities of the facial skeleton, show overgrowth on the left side, mandibular osteotomies, nonunion on the right, malunion on the left, prognathism and the implants

Case Study 3: Lymphatic Malformation with Iatrogenic Problems (Contd...)

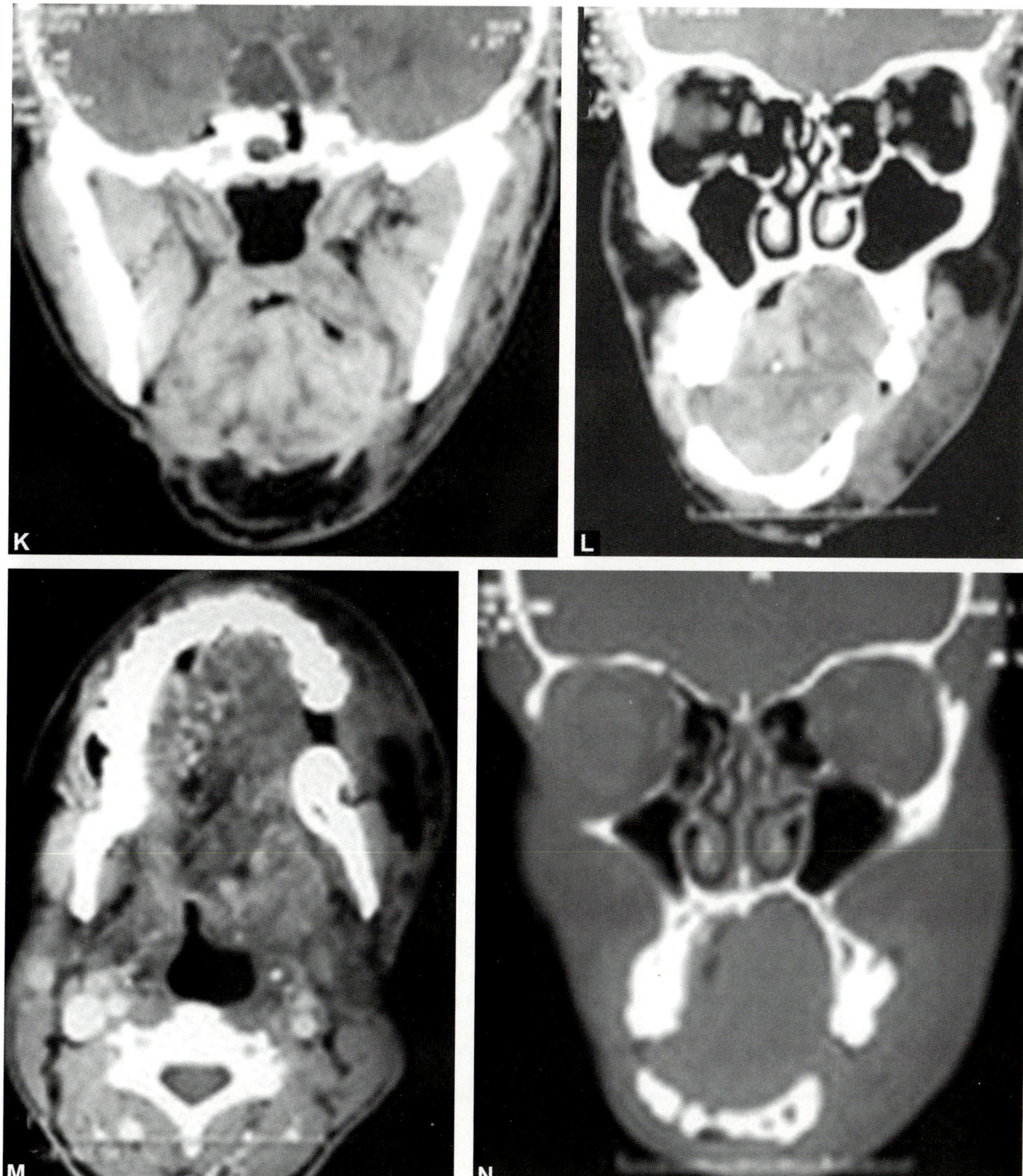

FIGURES 4.6K to N
show a soft tissue mass involving tongue, tonsillar fossae, nasopharynx, parapharyngeal spaces, and the left cheek.

Assessment

The first step in the management of such a problem has to be a careful assessment. Apart from the clinical assessment, a CT study (Figs 4.6K to N) showed a soft tissue mass involving the tongue, extending into tonsillar fossae, anterior aspect of nasopharynx and parapharyngeal spaces, with an extension to the left cheek. The appearances were consistent with the diagnosis of a microcystic lymphatic malformation. The skeletal findings are consistent with a postsurgical iatrogenic deformity with an underlying expansile benign lesion.

Preoperative Preparation

Planning the skeletal correction was the next step. It involved mock surgery on the dental models and the preparation of an appropriate splint for inter-maxillary fixation. Figure 5.6 O, on the left model depicts the existing jaw alignment. On the right is seen the desired jaw alignment, with the proposed splint mounted on the model.

Coping with Soft Tissue Impediments

This was followed by measures to cope with the soft tissue impediment to airway, speech, intubation and skeletal correction. To this end the use of RF superpulse did help. Figures 4.6P and Q are almost identical CT sections taken before and after 5 sessions of RF super pulse, each 4 days apart showing distinct benefit with the help of a CT study. An effort was now made to cope with the soft tissue impediment to airway, speech, intubation and skeletal correction. To this end, the use of RF superpulse did help modestly.

A Difficult Intubation

Then there was the tough problem of intubation. Even with highly experienced anesthesia team, attempts at transendoscopic intubation failed. However, a transnasal intubation could be achieved with difficulty.

The Operation

The Surgical objectives were two-fold—to overcome the obstruction to the Respiratory and the Alimentary passages and to correct the facial deformity. The facial deformity too had two components, an iatrogenic skeletal deformity and the lymphangiomatous infiltration of the left side of the face.

The surgical approach available was intraoral (particularly splitting the tongue in the midline) and externally through the old scars. The intraoral approach is particularly useful when the gum margin incision is relevant, This incision provides a direct access to the skeleton and minimizes collateral damage to the soft tissue.

The Reduction of Lymphangiomatous Mass

The midline of the tongue is its most avascular area and is the favored site for an incision to explore the tongue. It also helps the protection of the nerve supply and the main blood supply of the tongue. Using this incision, we were able to access a large part of the central mass and using RF and RF superpulse to ablate and significantly reduce the soft tissue lymhangiomatous mass, obstructing the respiratory and the alimentary passages. All the residual lesions were similarly treated.

Case Study 3: Lymphatic Malformation with Iatrogenic Problems (Contd...)

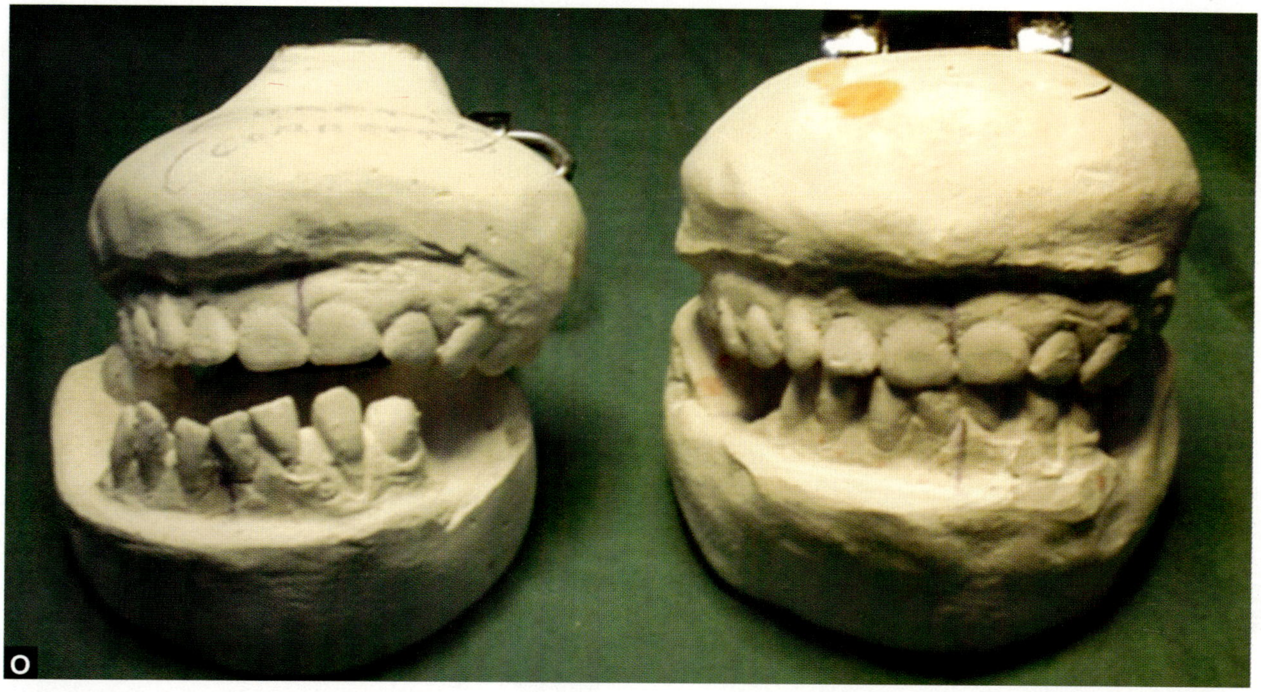

FIGURES 4.6O
Mock surgery on the dental models to plan the future occlusion and preparation of postoperative occlusal splint (*in place in the corrected model*)

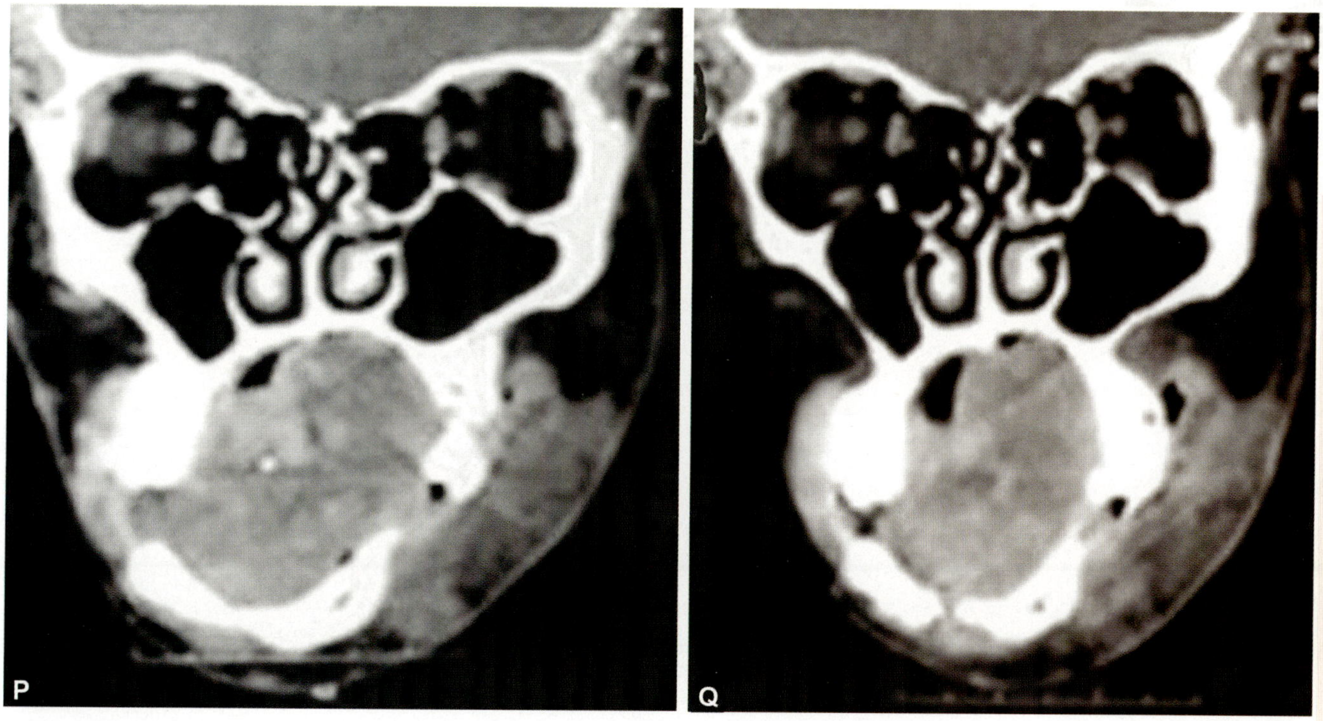

FIGURES 4.6P and Q
Almost identical CT sections taken before and after five sessions of RF superpulse, with a gap of four days between each session

Case Study 3: Lymphatic Malformation with Iatrogenic Problems (Contd...)

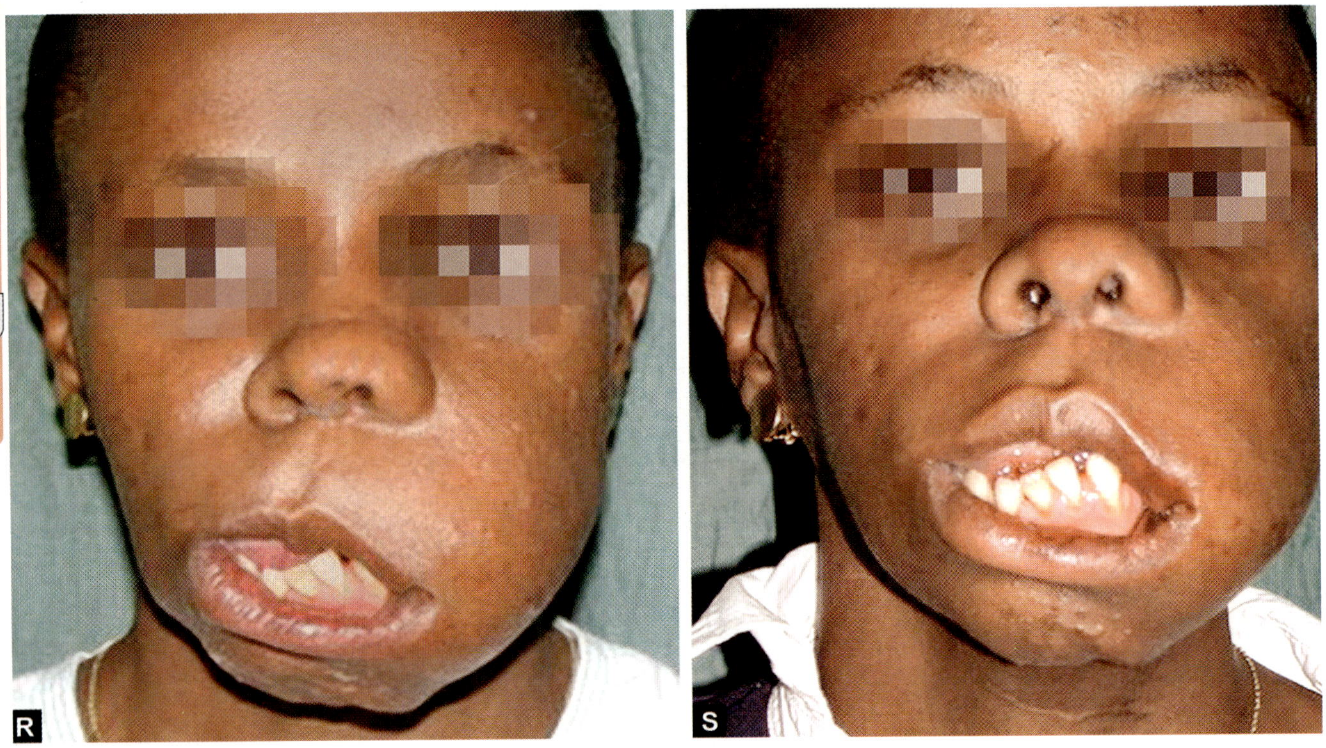

FIGURES 4.6R and S
Pre and post RF of the face

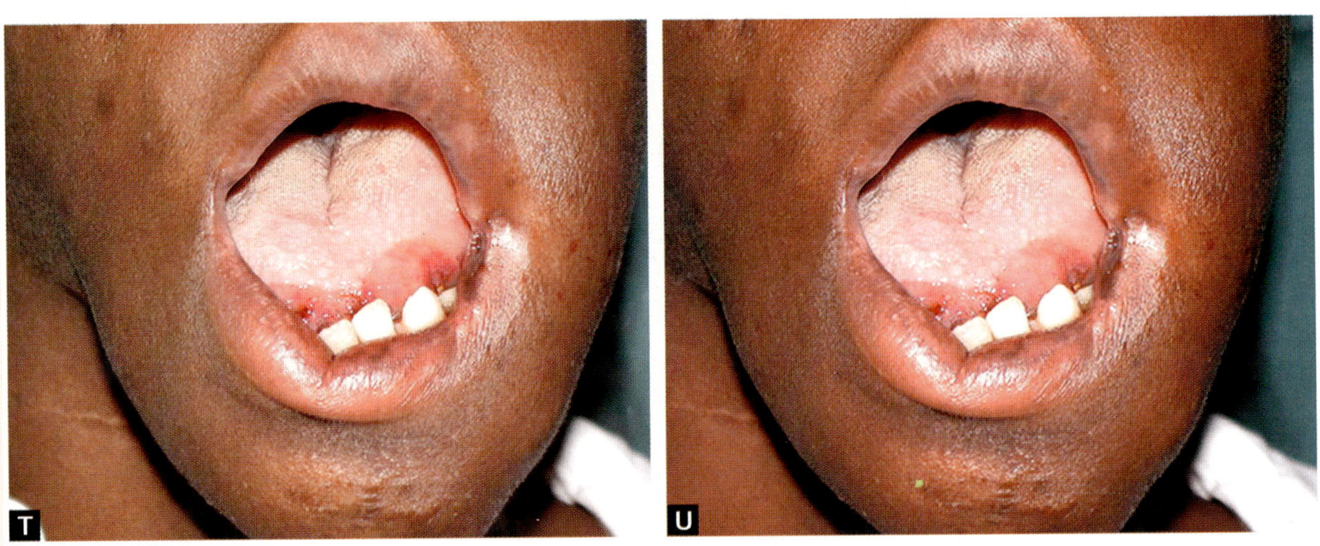

FIGURES 4.6T and U
Pre and post RF to the tongue

Case Study 3: Lymphatic Malformation with latrogenic Problems (Contd...)

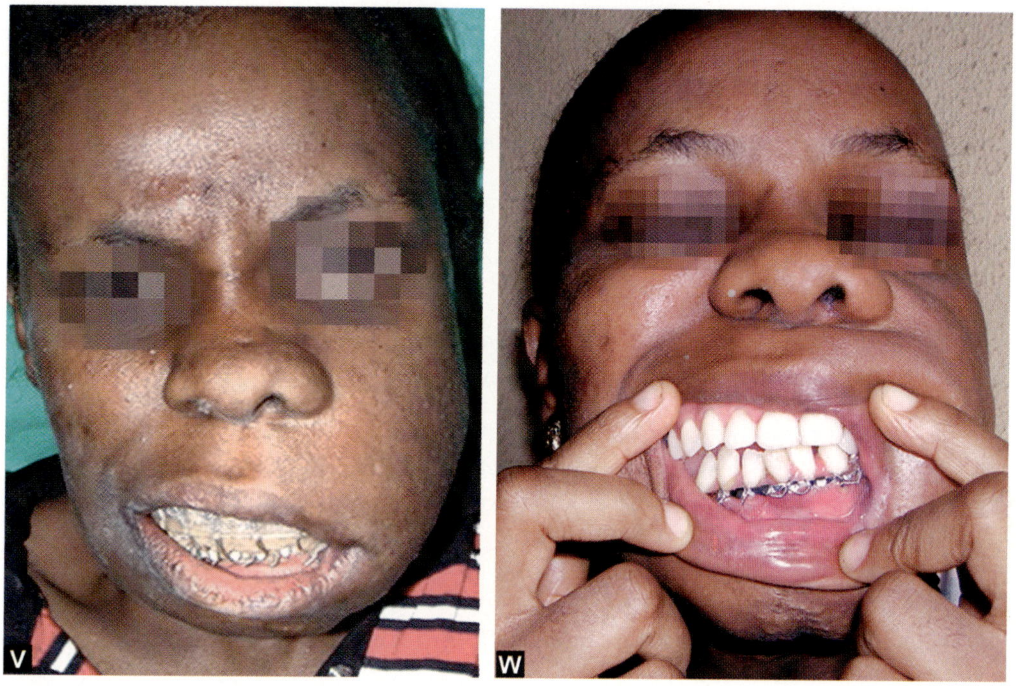

FIGURES 4.6V and W
(V): Immediate postoperative status; (W): Shows the occlusion 6 months later

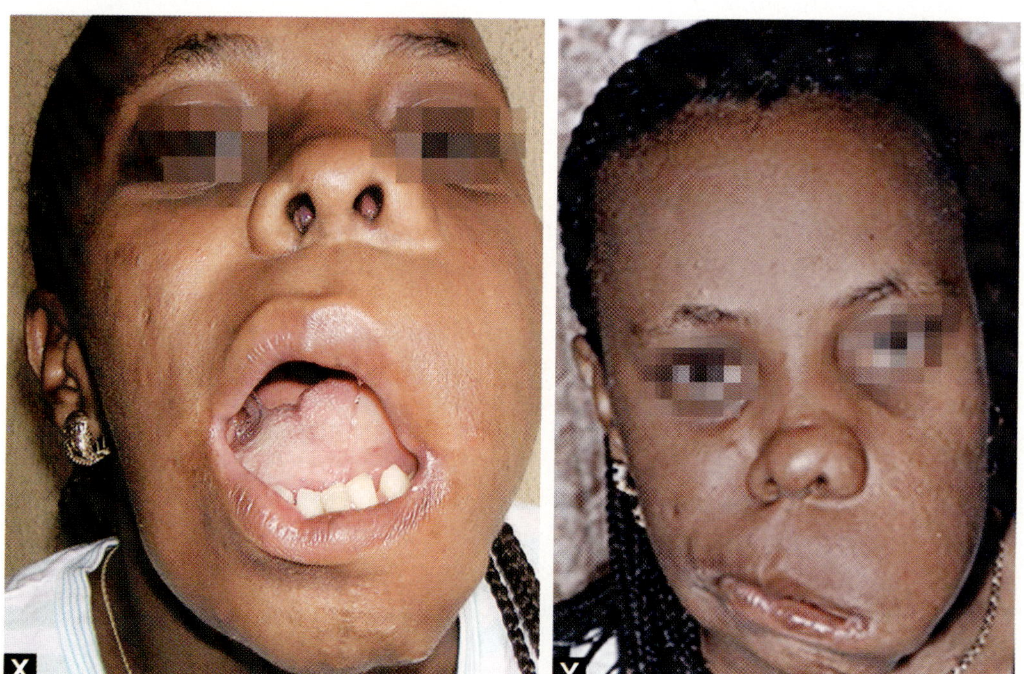

FIGURES 4.6X and Y
(X): Shows the tongue 6 months later; (Y): Shows the face in repose 1 year later

FIGURES 4.6A to Y
Lymphatic Malformation with latrogenic Problems

The Skeletal Correction

Both the osteotomy sites were accessed through the existing external scars. The right fracture site was exposed and debrided, the ineffective fixation removed and the skeleton suitably mobilized. The left malunited fracture of the mandible was osteotomized, and a 4 mm wide strip of bone excised, the segments aligned, plated and immobilized in the predetermined position with a titanium plate. Iliac bone graft was packed in the defect.

It was noted, that the mandible was thin and osteoporotic, a characteristic associated with microcystic lymphatic malformations.

Postoperative Care

Though the surgical intervention was smooth, intensive care was required for almost a week to stabilize the airway threatened by edema and to **retrain and restore deglutition.** The latter was a tough task because of the massive lymphangiomatous infiltration in the base of the tongue and in the parapharyngeal tissues had been ablated, resulting in a massive edema in a restricted space, severely impairing function. However, thereafter, the recovery was smooth. Figure 4.6V shows the improvement in occlusion and the change in appearance soon after surgery.

Follow-up Surgery Still Needed

She still needs an intervention to correct the long standing facial palsy in order to balance her face.

SUMMARY

The small channel low flow vascular malformations are usually present at birth and steadily proliferate. Even after ablation, the residual lesions proliferate rather rapidly. This process appears to slow down with age and disappear after puberty.

Some capillary malformations (CMs) on the skin surface are located in the upper two-thirds of the face, involve genetic and neurogenic factors, require careful monitoring of the eye for glaucoma, at least through the first two years of life. They are best treated by lasers in childhood before local keratization sets in.

If not treated early, their proliferation is associated with an ugly hypertrophy and deformity. Their presence is also associated with hypertrophy of the adjacent skeleton. Both these changes are attributed to the 'increased blood supply'. When local hypertrophy and hyperplasia are well established, skin replacement becomes the only viable option.

The macrocystic LMs respond well to surgical ablation even at a very young age.

The small channel LMs need periodic ablation to control growth, impairment of function and deformation of the skeleton. The best tool for this purpose is RF superpulse for surface lesion and RF cautery for surgically or endoscopically exposed lesions.

The microcystic lesions are usually present since birth. But their presence is easily missed in a chubby infant or in a deeply located lesion. However, it is important to keep the patient under observation and to ensure timely and effective interventions, balancing the therapeutic measures with psychological support and attention to the educational and psychological needs of the patient.

The management of these microcystic LMs can be complex, depending on the location, the combinations (with CMs and VMs), the secondary effects on normal structures (displacement, compression or infiltration) and skeletal deformities resulting from expansion or hypertrophy.

When on the surface, they proliferate and cause a diffuse, slowly enhancing swelling, which responds well to RF superpulse therapy. When located deep, they proliferate, sometimes profusely. They often go around and displace vital structures and thereby render their accessibility too difficult. They also expand, thin out and distort the skeleton. They need early and sometimes periodic therapeutic interventions to ablate and modulate their growth. The final interventions required are around puberty or soon thereafter.

The use of RF superpulse for the surface lesions, controls and cures without any distortion or visible scarring.

RF (cautery) is an effective tool for ablating the deep lesions. It is useful in controlling and modulating the growth during the proliferative phase. CT guided RF using special probes, promises to be an effective technique of ablation of deep lesions with precision and without extensive surgical exposure. This scope appears to be limited, only by their accessibility and their proximity to vital structures and hence significantly limited in head and neck region.

BIBLIOGRAPHY

1. Boyd JB, Mulliken JB, Kaban LB, Upton J, III, Murray JE. Skeletal changes associated with vascular malformations. Plast. Reconstr. Surg 1984;74:789.
2. Clodius L. Surgery for the facial port-wine stain: technique and results. Ann. Plast. Surg 1986;16:457.
3. Conway H, McKinney P, Climo M. Permanent camouflage of vascular nevi of the face by intradermal injection of insoluble pigments (tattooing): experience through twenty years with 1022 cases. Plast. Reconstr. Surg 1967;40:457.
4. Conway H. Evolution of treatment of capillary heman-giomas of the face with further observation on the value of camouflage by permanent pigment injection (tattooing). Surgery 1948;23:389.
5. Enjolars O, Richle MC, Moland JJ. Facial port urine stain and sturge-Kleber syndrome. Pediatrics 1985;76:48.
6. Jarzab G. Clinical experience in the cryosurgery of haemangioma. J Maxillofac. Surg 1975;3:146.
7. Mihm, Martin Jr, North Paula E. Histopathological Diagnosis of Infantile Hemangiomas and Vascular Malformations. Facial Plastic Surgery Clinics of North America. Vascular Birthmarks of the Head and Neck. November 2001. WB Saunders Company.
8. Mihm, Martin Jr, North, Paula E. The Surgical Pathology Approach to Pediatric Vascular Tumors and Anomalies. Hemangiomas and Vascular Malformations of the Head and Neck. Wiley-Liss 1998.
9. Ohtsuka H, Shioya N, Tanaka S. Cryosurgery for hemangiomas of the body surface and oral cavity. Ann. Plast. Surg 1980;4:462.
10. Reder F. Hemangioma and lymphangioma, their response to the injection of boiling water. Med. Rec. NY 1920;98:519.
11. Servelle M. Klippel and Trenaunay's syndrome. 768 operated cases. Ann. Surg 1985;102:365.
12. Shafirstein Gal, Baumler, Wolfgang, Lapidoth, Moshe, Ferguson, Scott BS, North, Paula E, Waner, Milton. A New Mathematical Approach to the Diffusion Approximation Theory for Selective Photothermolysis Modeling and Its Implication in Laser Treatment of Portwine Stains. Lasers in Surgery and Medicine. Wiley-Liss, Inc 2004.
13. Smoller BR, Rosen S. Portwine stains: A disease of altered neural modulation of blood vessels? Arch. Dermatol 1986;122:177.
14. Squire B. An improvement in the treatment of portwine mark by linear scarification. Br. Med. J 1879;2:732.
15. Thomson HG, Wright AM. Surgical tattooing of the port wine stain. Operative technique, results, and critique. Plast. Reconstr. Surg 1971;48:113.
16. Wegner G. Ueber Lymphangiome. Arch. klin. Chir, Berl 1876-77;20:641.

HEMANGIOMAS AND VASCULAR MALFORMATIONS OF THE ORBIT

5

Nirmala Subramanian

INTRODUCTION

Vascular lesions of the orbit and periorbital region are quite rare. They frequently pose a challenge, both to the diagnosis and management, mainly because of anatomical constraints. The advances in imaging techniques and histochemistry have helped to clear the confusion which existed in the nosology of these lesions. Mulliken and Glowacki, 1982 and GJ Harris, 1999[1,2] introduced the biological classification which was based on clinical presentation, natural history and histopathology. This brought order to the classification of these lesions. They classified vascular lesions into Hemangiomas and Vascular malformations. Further assignment was based on clinical findings, imaging and histopathological criteria.

Hemangiomas are true neoplasm of unknown etiology, having vascular channels lined with proliferative cells. They are connected to normal vascular system. Vascular malformations are also congenital lesions which enlarge via ectasia of the channels and hypertrophy, but there is no proliferation of endothelial cells. Rootman came out with a classification based on the hemodynamics of the lesion[3] (Rootman J, 2003). Based on this, the Orbital Society in 1999 gave a classification of the vascular lesions of the orbit into vascular malformation and vascular tumors. Vascular malformations were further classified, according to the flow of blood, into no flow, venous flow and arterial flow (Table 5.1).

TABLE 5.1
Vascular lesions of the orbit and the periorbital region

New Growths	
Benign	Infantile Hemangioma Syndromic Hemangiomas
Malignant	
Congenital Vascular Malformations	
• No flow	
• Venous flow	
• Arterial flow	

Martin Mihm and Paula North introduced the first immunochemical marker for hemangiomas which confirmed that they are a unique group of disorder.

CAPILLARY HEMANGIOMAS OF INFANCY

Hemangiomas — the CHIs are one of the most common tumors of infancy. They are seen within 1 to 3 weeks of birth They are characterized by a proliferative phase followed by a phase of involution. They continue to grow till 12 to 24 months. Involution starts before a child is a year old. Both proliferation and involution coexist for a period of time; involution totally dominating by two years of age. Due to the mass effect, they can produce expansion of the orbit and displacement of the globe or infiltrate the skeleton. Their biological behavior is distinctly different from the vascular malformations which are also present at birth but are noticed later in the section dedicated to them.

The Capillary Hemangioma of Infancy is also called Infantile Hemangiomas in the Orbito palpebral area. It is the most common benign tumor seen in infancy. The orbital lesions being near the eyes, are noticed quite early. They grow rapidly as they are hemodynamically, a high flow system.

Depending on their anatomical location, the CHIs of the Orbito palpebral region are subdivided into: Superficial, Deep, Combined and Complex.

a. Superficial involve only the skin or conjunctiva.
b. Deep or orbital hemangiomas are located in the orbit.
c. Combined involve both the superficial and the orbital hemangiomas.
d. Complex involve other areas besides periorbital and orbital.

THE SUPERFICIAL CHI

The superficial CHI is spotted within three weeks of age as a red or a pale spot depending on the child's complexion. Invariably, the mother would say that the spot was a mosquito bite or a scratch which started growing. Initially it is flat but gets raised and is spongy to touch and may blanch. It may remain confined to the eyelid or involve the periocular areas. The color varies from red to violet. The margins are distinct but irregular. It continues to grow till the infant is 12 to 24 months old. Being near the eye, the infant is brought early (Figs 5.1A to C). In western literature, the incidence quoted is 10 percent. It is relatively uncommon in Asians. Incidence is higher in premature babies.

When the lesion is in the upper eyelid, some degree of mechanical Ptosis (Fig. 5.1A) is usually present. If the CHI covers the pupillary area (Fig. 5.6A) the child may develop amblyopia. It is important to get a complete ophthalmologic examination to rule out glaucoma and any other posterior chamber problem. When the CHI involves only the conjunctiva, the lid may get everted. There may be instances of bleeding or ulceration. No imaging is indicated for small lesions but for large lesions, it is advisable to rule out associated intracranial vascular anomalies.

THE DEEP CHI

Deep CHIs may be situated in the subcutaneous plane or deep to the orbital septum. They may have extensions into the retrobulbar space. They are generally extraconal

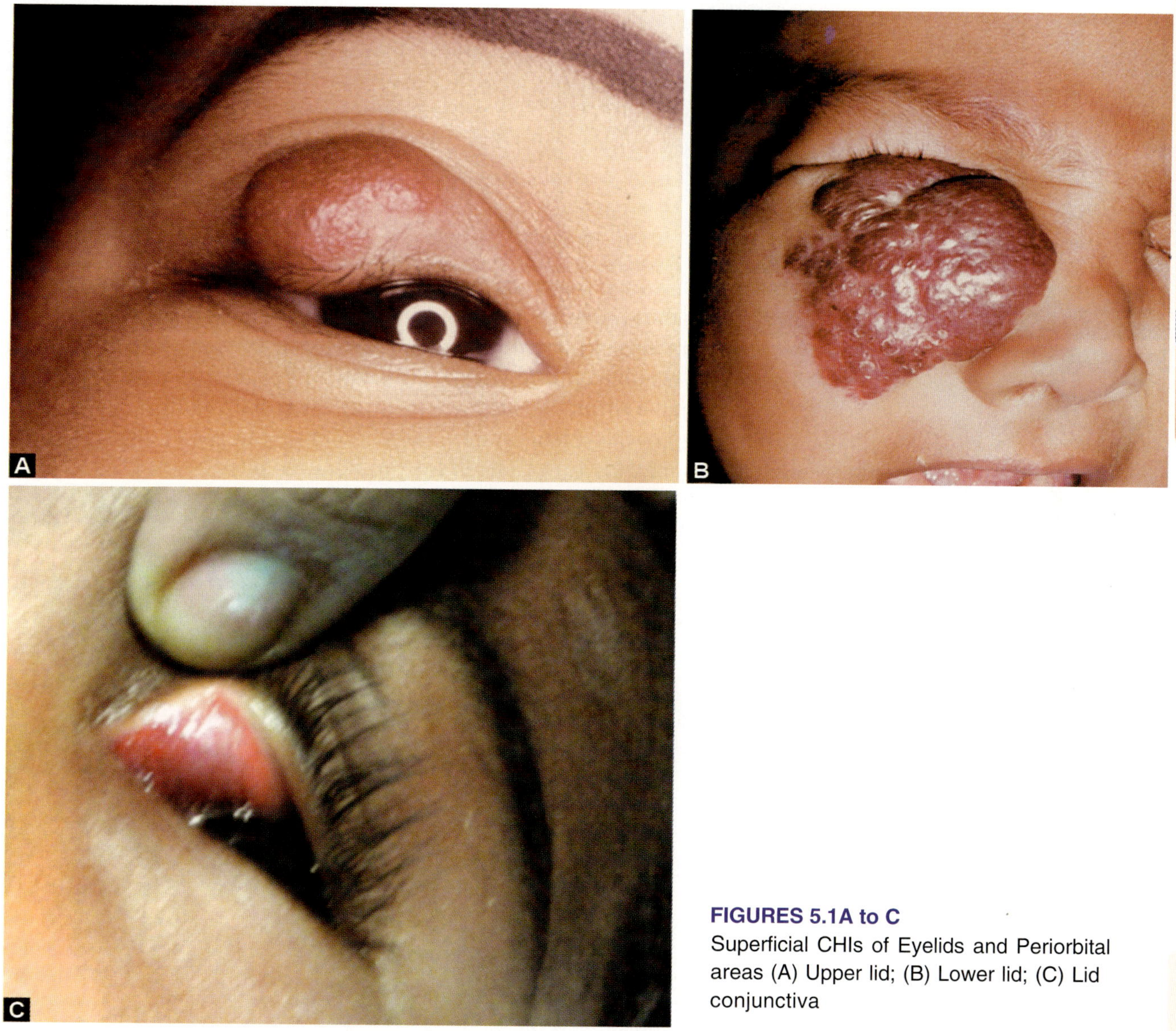

FIGURES 5.1A to C
Superficial CHIs of Eyelids and Periorbital areas (A) Upper lid; (B) Lower lid; (C) Lid conjunctiva

and may involve extraocular muscles. A child may be brought because of displacement or proptosis of the globe. The mother may notice an increase in the size of the lesion or an increase of proptosis when the child cries or strains.

These lesions do not involve the epidermis. The size and location may produce secondary problems, e.g. amblyopia, strabismus, astigmatism or compression of optic nerve. Involvement of the extraocular muscle is thought to contribute to strabismus. There may be dystopia if the bony orbit has been significantly enlarged by the orbital hemangioma. In the presence of proptosis, appropriate investigations for proptosis must be done to define the nature, location and extent of the lesions in the orbit.

Figure 5.2A shows an axial proptosis in a two months old child. A inferior transconjunctival orbitotomy was used to do a biopsy which ruled out other rapidly growing tumors of the orbit. A debulking of the fleshy vascular lesion was simultaneously carried out. Histopathology confirmed the diagnosis of a CHI. The picture at the age of ten months child (Fig. 5.2C) shows the reduction of proptosis and the presence of some conjunctival chemosis. It was difficult to access the vision.

COMBINED SUPERFICIAL AND DEEP CHI

The combined superficial and deep variety, involves periocular areas besides the orbital area. Presentation in the superomedial orbit as seen in Figure 5.3A is the commonest. Here we see a three month old infant with a superiormedial mass producing a ptosis. The swelling was first noticed a few days after birth. A well circumscribed solid hyperintense preseptal and medial periocular mass lesion with multiple flow void signals within, is a characteristic of capillary hemangioma of infancy. Marked enhancement is a characteristic of CHIs in the proliferative phase.

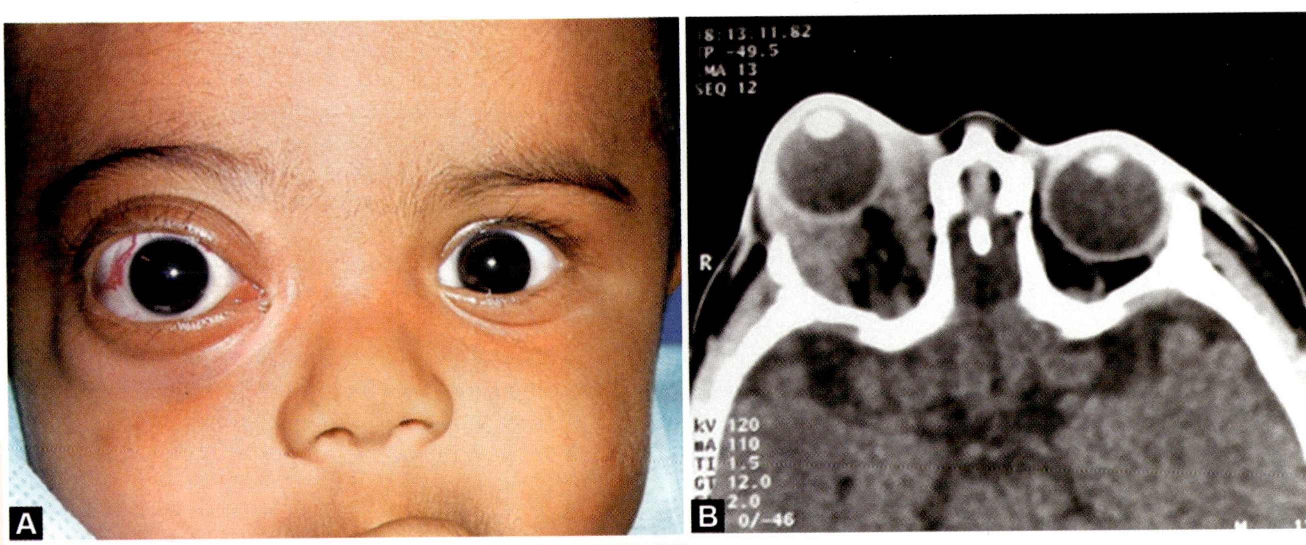

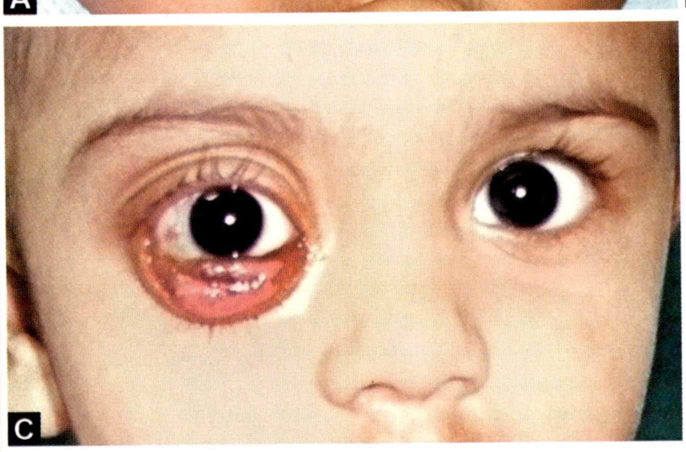

FIGURES 5.2A to C

A Deep Orbital CHI with axial proptosis: (A) Axial proptosis in an infant of two months who is taken up for biopsy and debulking; (B) CT Scan shows diffuse infiltrating mass filling and expanding the orbit; (C) The appearance at the age of ten months

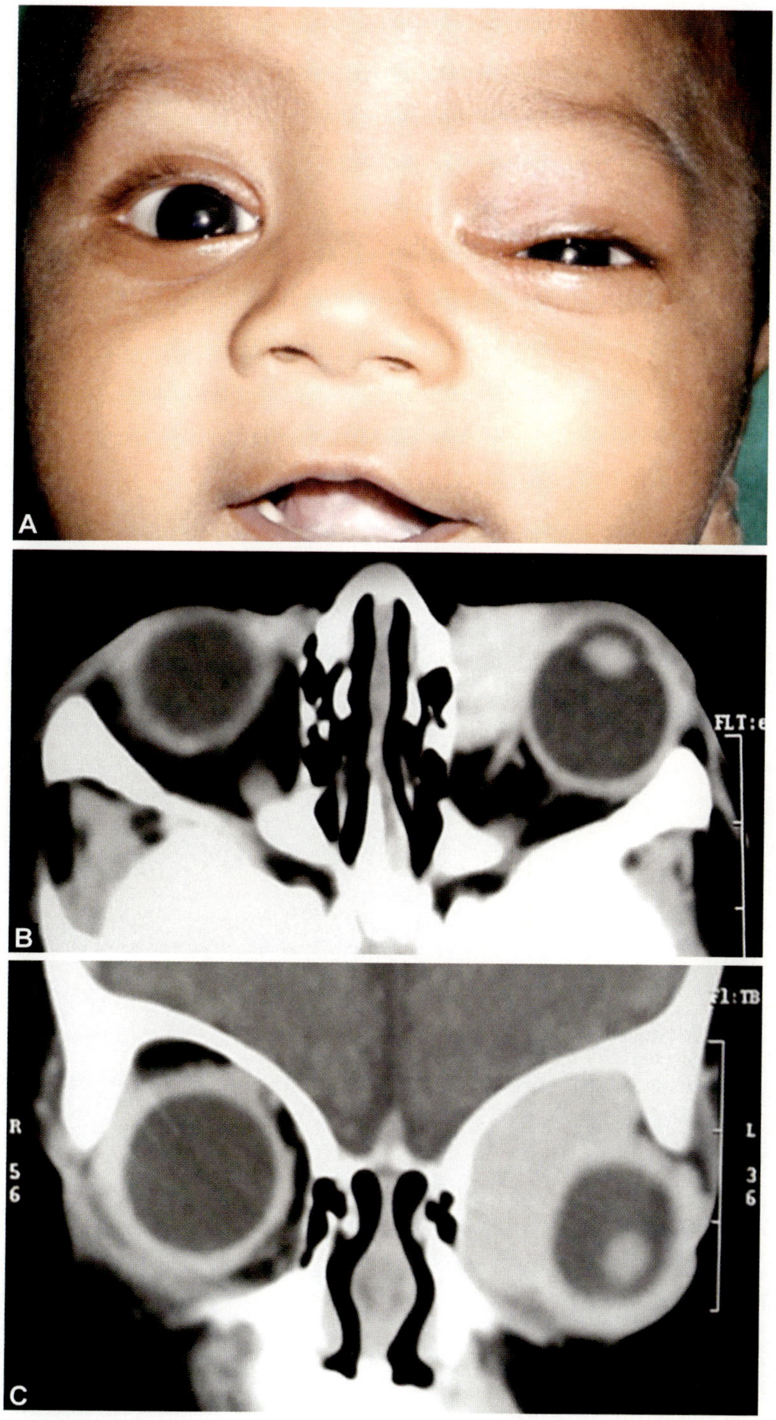

FIGURES 5.3A to C

Combined Superficial and Deep CHI: (A) Three months old infant with a superomedial mass and severe ptosis; (B and C) Axial and coronal post-contrast CT Scan of the orbit shows a well circumscribed brilliantly enhancing lesion in the left medial orbit displacing the globe laterally

COMPLEX CAPILLARY HEMANGIOMAS

Complex Capillary Hemangiomas involve the other parts of the face or may be multiple as seen in Figures 5.7A and 5.9A.

IMAGING CAPILLARY HEMANGIOMAS

Ultrasonography

The internal structure of a capillary hemangioma consists of small to medium-sized vascular channels. Sometimes larger vascular spaces may also be seen. A-scan USG shows irregular to high internal reflectivity due to vascular spaces and septae. In areas with more cellular composition or with large cavernous spaces there may be low reflectivity. The tumors are not well circumscribed and can be located in the lid or in the orbit. B-scan USG shows irregularly structured lesions with occasional cavernous spaces. Capillary hemangiomas are highflow lesions and vascularity can be demonstrated by A-scan and by Doppler.

CT Scan

In plain CT scan, heterogenous and hyperdense well defined or infiltrating mass is seen. They may be intraconal, extraconal or posterior to the septum. Orbital hemangiomas appear well defined .There may be indentation or expansion of the orbit due to mass effect. With contrast, there is marked enhancement. It may be homogenous or heterogenous depending on the phase of proliferation or involution.

MRI Imaging

MRI shows lobulations with septae and flow voids due to vessels within the lesion. The MRI characteristics are presented in Figures 5.4B to D.

Surgical Intervention

The Surgical approach to the orbital contents is referred to as orbitotomy. It is indicated in the management of the Deep CHIs very selectively:

a. If there is a threat to vision
b. An expansion of the orbit or other skeletal changes
c. Sometimes for the confirmation of the diagnosis.

The Surgical Approach

Surgical approach to the orbit depends on the location of the lesion. For lesions situated in the superomedial aspect of the orbit , an anterior superior orbitotomy is done. For inferomedial mass an anterior inferior orbitotomy is done. For lesions which are situated intraconally and are large in size, a Lateral Orbitotomy is advised.

Even if the CHI can not be completely removed, the tissue removed helps to establish the diagnosis of a CHI, and reduces the proptosis due to the debulking of the mass. Remaining lesion involutes with time as illustrated in Figure 5.5A which shows the course of the disease in an 11months old with proptosis and upward displacement of globe, noticed a few weeks after birth and gradually increasing.

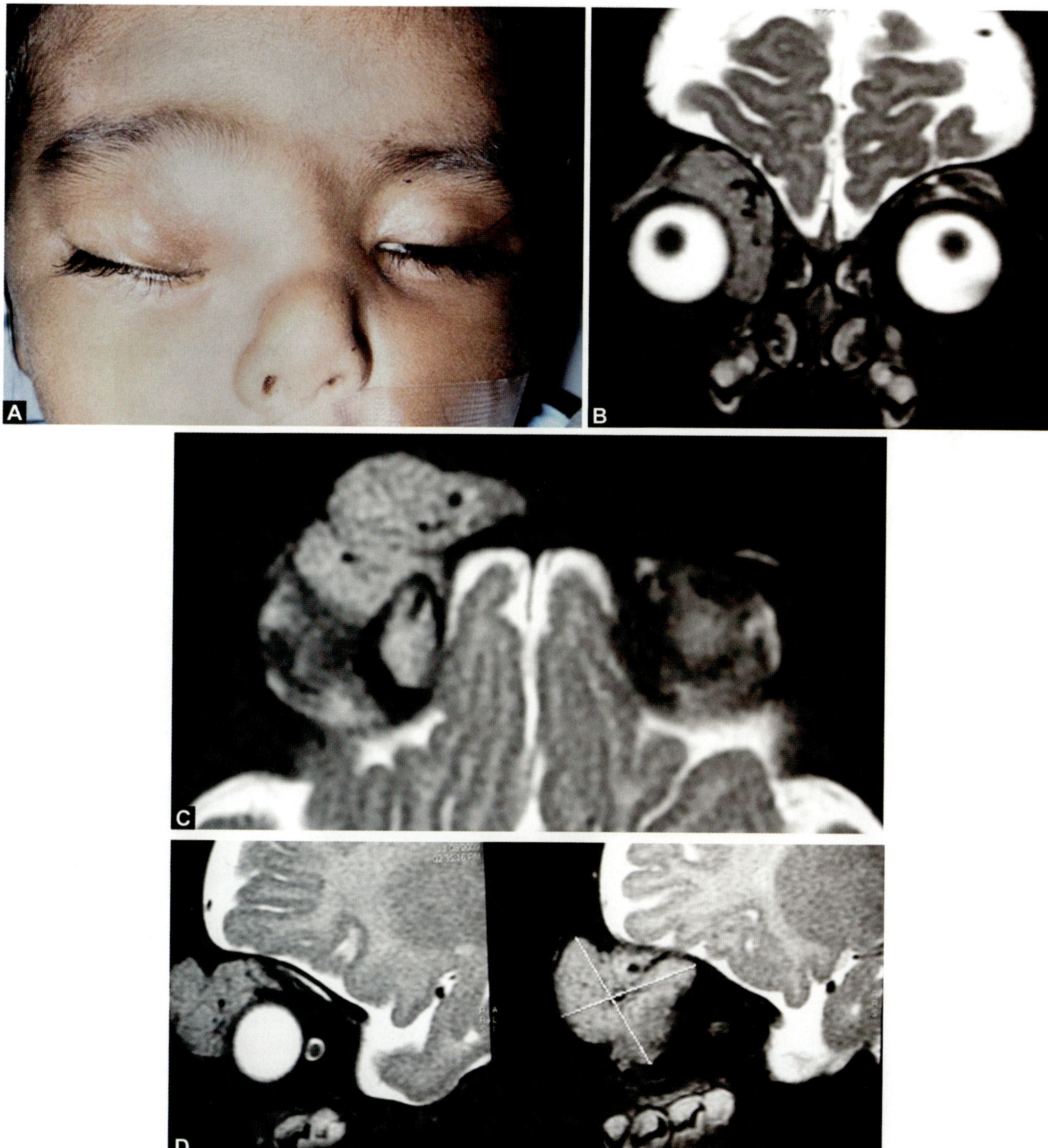

FIGURES 5.4A to D

Expansion of orbit due to mass effect as seen on an MRI: (A) Three-month-old infant with a mass in the superomedial area of orbit, producing ptosis; (B to D) MRI T2 fat suppressed images of the orbit: Axial, coronal and sagittal. A well circumscribed solid hyperintense preseptal and medial periocular mass lesion with multiple flow void signals within are characteristic of capillary hemangioma of Infancy

An intraconal and extraconal mass had displaced the eyeball with the optic nerve, encased in its anterior portion Figures 5.5B and C. The orbit was explored through a subciliary incision and the irregular fleshy mass excised piecemeal. Histopathology confirmed the diagnosis of a CHI. Significant clinical improvement was recorded seven months later in Figures 5.5D to F below. The scan in Figure 5.5G records the status three and a half years later showing that the lesion had cleared satisfactorily and there was no impairment of the function. Figures 5.5H to K represent the situation five years later shows a total clearance of the lesion, a total resolution of the initial skeletal deformity, and a total restoration of function.

The objective of the surgical intervention in a case of a CHI is decompressing the orbit by debulking, whenever considered necessary to save the vision and not a total ablation of the lesion which might damage the vital structures which may not be easily identifiable in presence of the lesion but have the full potential of recovery following the involution.

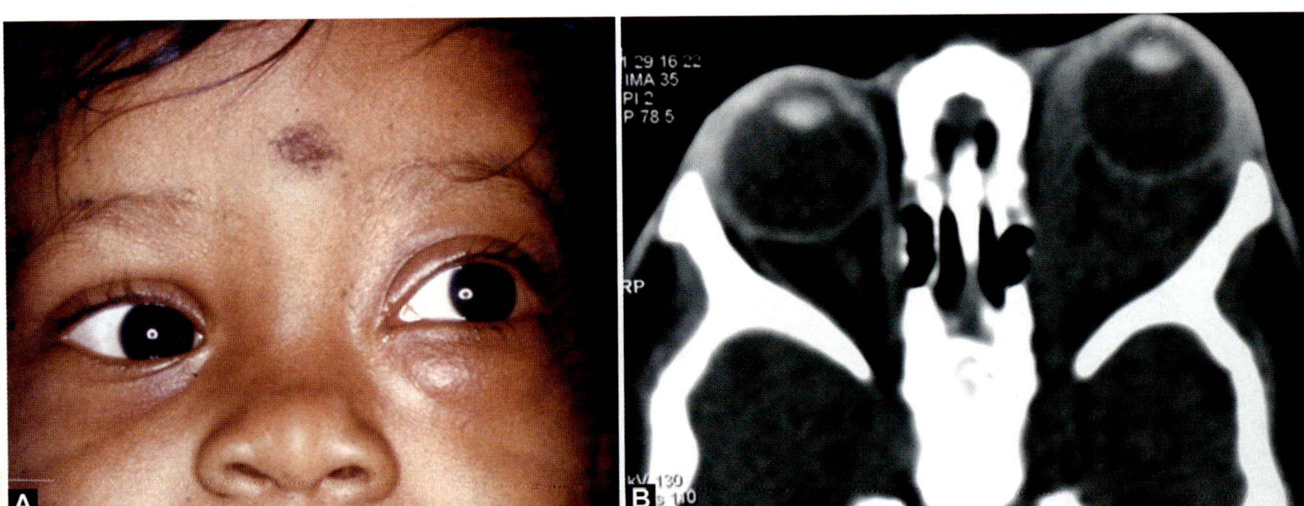

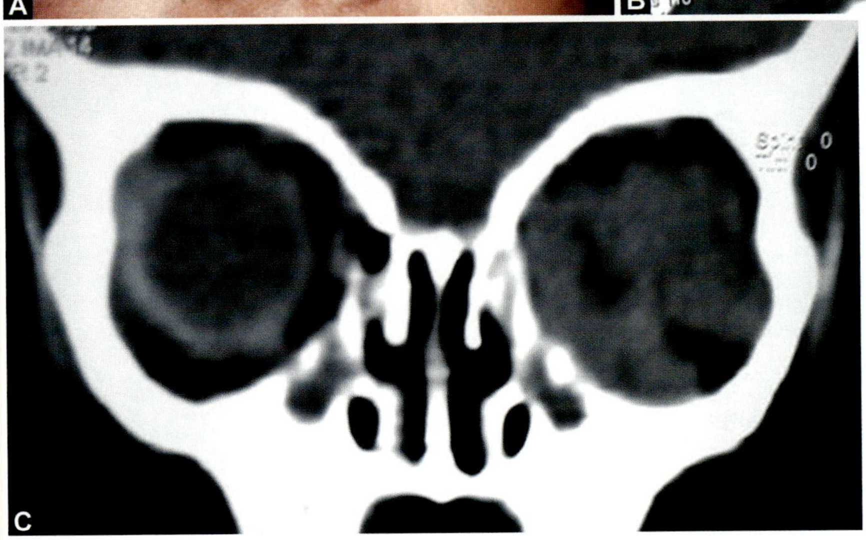

FIGURES 5.5A to C

The Debulking of the Orbital CHI—A five year study: (A) A 11months old with proptosis and upward displacement of globe; (B and C) CT Scan-shows an ill defined multilobulated intra and extraconal soft tissue lesion causing mild proptosis and remodeling of the floor. The inferior rectus muscle cannot be identified separately. The medial rectus and the lateral rectus are identifiable with the former minimally thickened. Optic nerve is displaced superiorly with its anterior part encased by the lesion

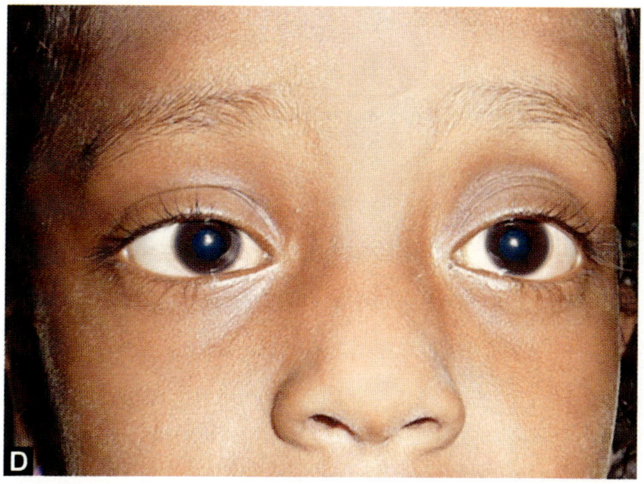

FIGURE 5.5D
The clinical improvement seven months after surgery

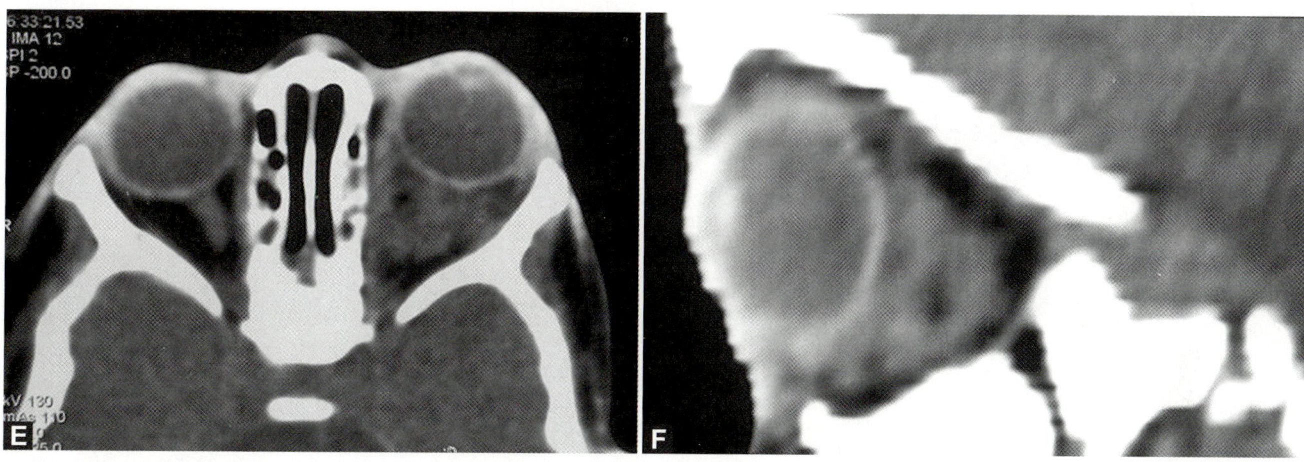

FIGURES 5.5E and F
The postoperative CTs show a significant reduction of the mass. Proptosis has reduced. The inferior rectus muscle cannot still be identified separately. The medial and lateral recti are now seen separately. The optic nerve continues to be displaced superiorly

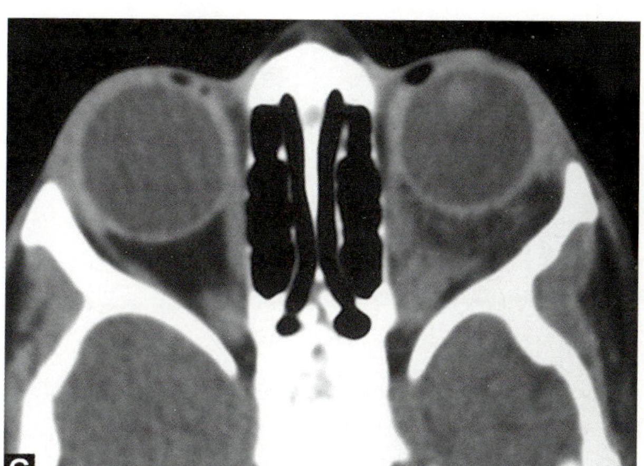

FIGURE 5.5G
Shows the status three and a half years later with the proptosis very much reduced, but the ill defined soft tissue lesion still seen in intraconal and extraconal space

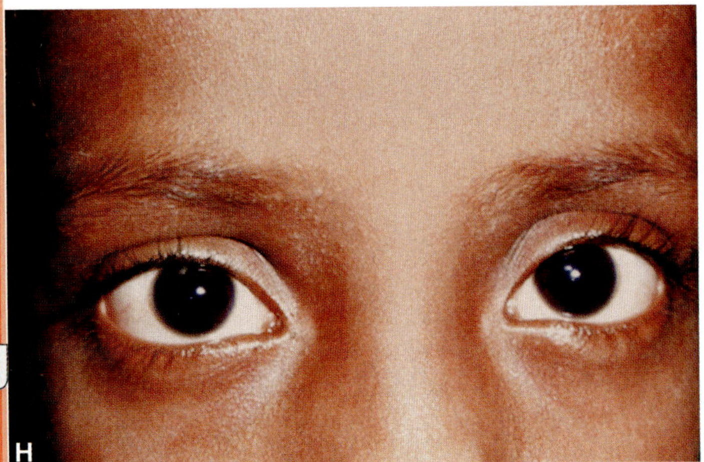

FIGURE 5.5H
Five years after surgery: no proptosis, the balanced face and normal vision

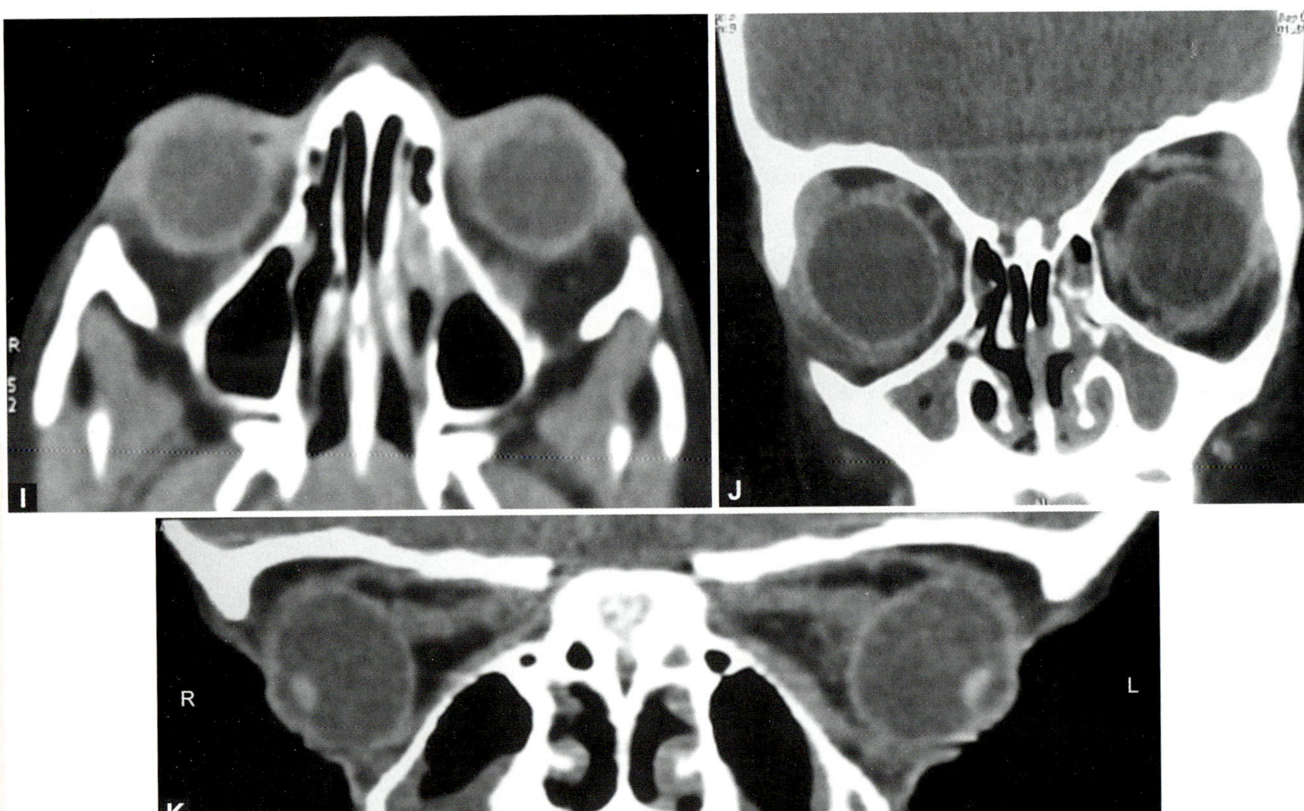

FIGURES 5.5 I to K
The axial, the coronal CT Scans and the saggital CT study shows no soft tissue lesion in the orbit and a resolution of the proptosis, reversal of the orbital expansion and a complete involution of the CHI

HISTOPATHOLOGY

It is a lobulated tumor in which the capillary sized blood channels are closely packed with proliferating endothelial cells. With involution, the connective tissue septae thicken, the endothelial cells flatten, the vascular channels decrease in number. Inflammatory and fat cells replace the vascular channels.

The Management of Infantile Hemangiomas

The certain biological involution, demands masterly inaction, except for the use of emollients on the skin surface to prevent drying and ulceration. Parents have to be counseled about the natural history of these lesions and convinced with the help of the photographs of other patients, about the progressive involution and the total resolution that is to follow. This would build up the parent's confidence and prevent uninformed advice which may lead to unnecessary and sometimes harmful intervention. The patient should also be advised to have periodic photographs in a standardized view, to monitor the involution. Ultrasound of the orbit is a very simple and economical investigation to monitor the involution. The radiation due to CT Scan and the cost factor can be avoided. But it needs an experienced sonologist to do it and interpret it. Beside this it does not give a picture to appreciate the anatomy of the orbit to plan surgery.

It is important to note the stage of the hemangioma, when the child is brought in. In the proliferating stage, it is important to correct the visual or the respiratory obstruction urgently. The systemic use of the steroids usually becomes necessary.

Systemic Steroids

The role of systemic steroids was noticed by Zarem HA and Edgerton M, 1967[18], when regression of Hemangioma was noticed incidentally while treating a case of Idiopathic Thrombocytopenic Purpura. The steroids are believed to inhibit angiogenesis and increase circulating vasoconstrictors. The dosage is 1.5 to 2.5 mgs/kg for six weeks. It should be given under the direct supervision of a Pediatrician.

The complications which are occasionally seen, are Cushinoid facies and gastrointestinal disturbances, e.g. diarrhea, constipation.

During the proliferative phase, it is equally important to prevent the secondary problems arising from it and the bleeding episodes or ulceration. As the epidermis covering the lesion is very thin, chances of injury are high. Hence, at the time of the first consultation itself, parents must be informed of the chances of bleeding and ulceration and of the first aid which needs to be administered. As a first aid, cotton or gauze dipped in cold water should be placed over the area and pressure applied with the hands for five to ten minutes. I believe, that the bare finger is the most readily available appliance which can be instantly applied as a pressure appliance in the same way as above. This helps the bleeding to stop. If it persists, the bleeders can be cauterized or mattress sutures can be taken. Emmolients or moisturizers must be used to prevent the skin from drying. Once ulceration has occurred, protective dressing with antibiotic ointment should be recommended. Ulceration produces severe pain. Depending on the other symptoms, appropriate antibiotics and analgesics should be given.

The first line of treatment is conservative as involution is natural to CHI. Small isolated lesions, which can be easily closed after excision without any problematic secondary defect, should have excision as the first choice. Larger lesions even if they are refractory to Triamcinalone Injections, are amenable to excision. Figure 5.6A shows a three month baby with a microcornea and nystagmus, who has a large CHI which covers the left eye and did not respond to injection of Triamcinalone (Fig. 5.6B). To reduce mechanical ptosis and to prevent amblyopia, an early surgical excision and resurfacing with a split skin graft was indicated (Fig. 5.6C). Figure 5.6D shows the follow-up three years later. Child also had lensectomies in both eyes. The vision is poor and child has to wear spectacles to correct the refractive error but there is no amblyopia in left eye.

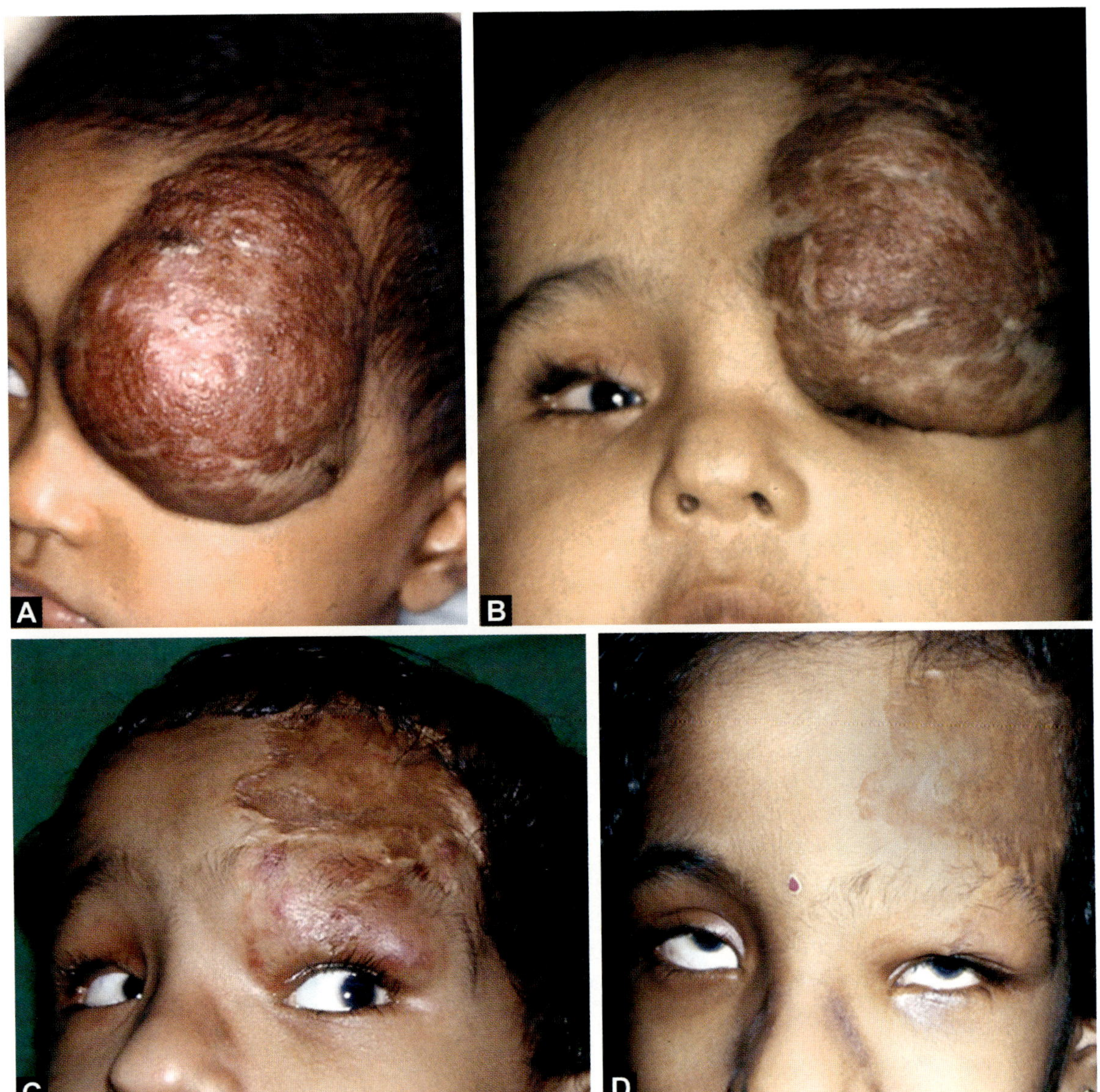

FIGURES 5.6A to D

Treatment with Injection Triamcinalone and Surgery: (A) A large CHI forehead and upper eyelid producing ptosis with an associated microcornea and nystagmus; (B) Triamcinalone injection did not produce any regression; (C) The lesion over the forehead was excised and grafted with split thickness skin graft; (D) A follow-up three years later—except for fullness of sub-brow region good involution of hemangioma is noted

For large lesions, which are growing rapidly and which may obstruct the visual axis, Intralesional Triamcinalone Injection is recommended as the first choice.[11,22] (Kushner BJ, 1979 and Ranchod TM, et al 2005). A complete workup of the coagulation profile is to be done before the injection is given. The child should be free of upper respiratory infection and under pediatric care. No vaccination should be given two weeks prior to or after the injection.

Triamcinalone Injection Administration

Triamcinalone injection is given under sedation or general anesthesia. A tuberculin or Insulin Syringe is ideal. While injecting, ensure that the needle has not entered a vessel and it is not given too superficially. Administer the injection very slowly at three or four different sites. About 0.2 ml to 0.3 ml is given at each site. For smaller lesions, only 10 mgs is needed to be given. For larger lesions, more than 2 cms in size upto 40 mg can be given. It is better, not to give more than 40 mgs per sitting . Record the area of injection, to avoid repeating in the same area again. The second injection should be given after four to six weeks at different sites. This is to ensure, that the drug is uniformly distributed. Depending on the response, only three to five injections are required. A combination of Betamethasone with Triamcinalone is recommended by some authors. Triamcinalone was used in the patient shown in Figure 5.7, who had a rapidly growing lesion with episodes of bleeding. The response to the Injection of Triamcinalone was not dramatic but as seen in Figure 5.7B the involution was complete without any functional impairment.

The fundus needs to be examined after the injection has been given. This is done to rule out any compression to the optic nerve due to the pressure caused by the injection.

In small lesions, the regression is noticed dramatically after one or two injections as seen in Figures 5.8A and B.

Complications of Triamcinalone Injections

The various complications noticed following triamcinalone injections may be local and general. If the injection is too superficial, skin necrosis can occur or white deposits can be seen in the subdermal plane. Subcutaneous atrophy is noticed, if the injection has been given in the normal skin.

Systemic Complications of Steroid Therapy

Systemic complications are Cushinoid facies and excessive hair growth, as shown in Figure 5.9A which shows a six weeks old neonate with rapidly growing OCHI covering the left eyelid and periocular area , extending to the temporal region with a small lesion in the lower eyelid too, who showed an excellent response to intralesional injections of Triamcinalone Figure 5.9B. With only three injections of intralesional Triamcinalone, systemic side effects were seen Figure 5.9C. These are usually reversible as in this case, where they disappeared once the treatment was over, as seen in Figure 5.9D below. In a couple of areas, white deposit under the skin were seen due to a very superficial injection.

A rare complication of central retinal artery occlusion has been reported and is attributed to a too rapid infusion. Growth retardation has been reported but is very rare.

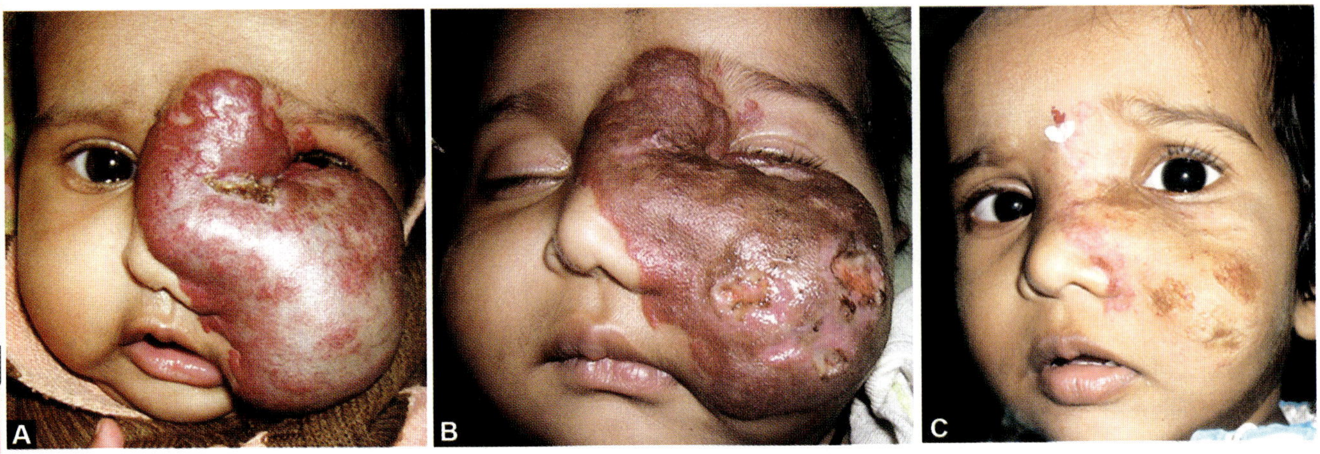

FIGURES 5.7A to C

Response to injection triamcinalone: A rapidly increasing CHI in a six weeks old child: (A) Six weeks old with a rapidly increasing CHI. Ulceration with bleeding episodes; (B) After two injections of triamcinalone, a month apart, some involution, new ulcerations; (C) Two years later. Complete involution and mild telangiectasia over the nose and scar over areas of ulceration and no visual impairment

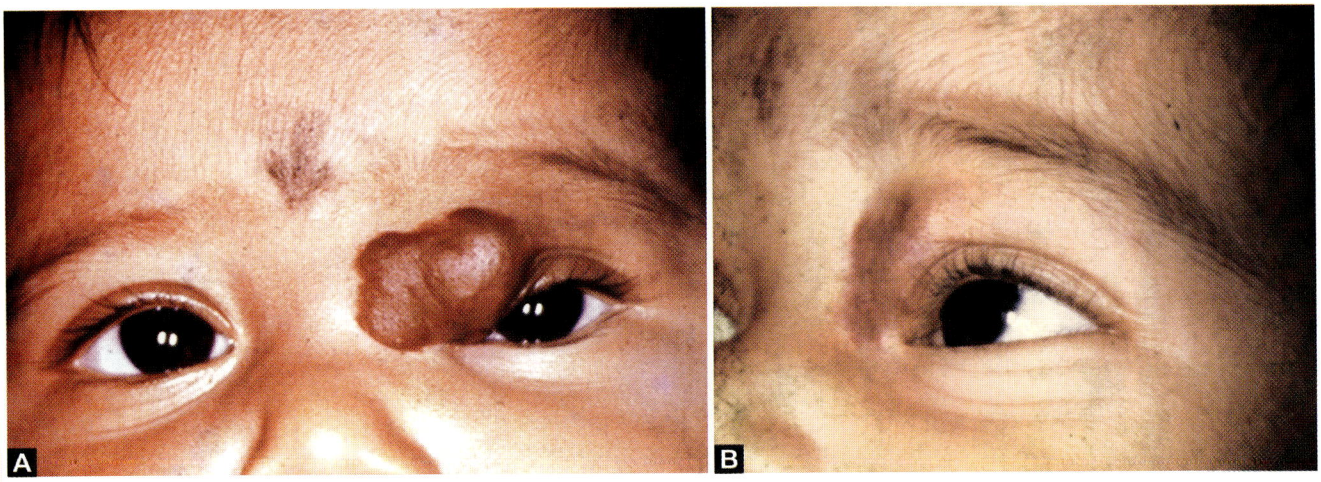

FIGURES 5.8A and B

Dramatic response to triamcinalone: (A and B) Superficial CHI showing involution after an intralesional triamcinalone injection

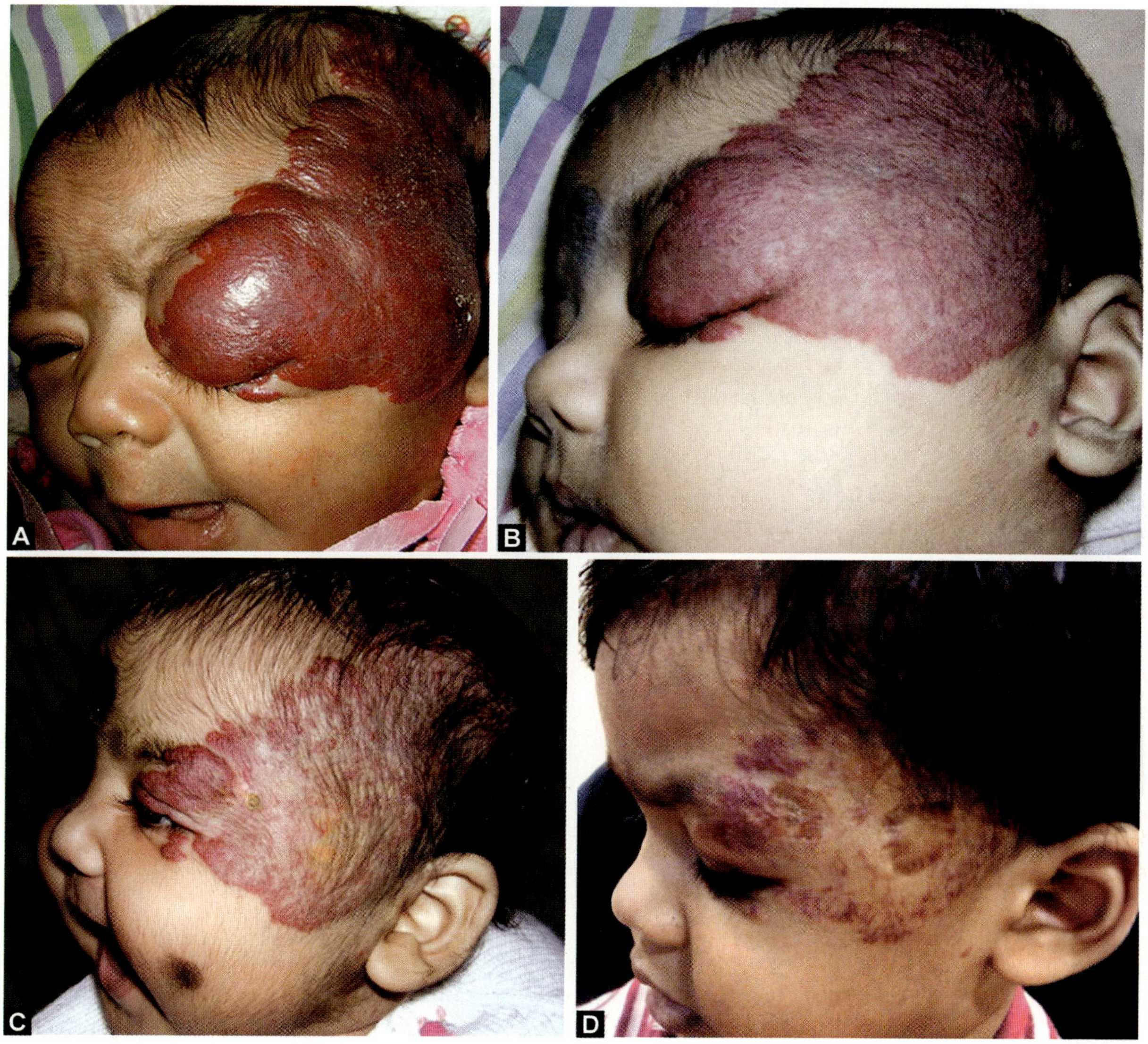

FIGURES 5.9A to D

Intralesional steroid with occasional Systemic Complications: (A) Six weeks old neonate with rapidly growing CHI; (B) Very good response to intralesional triamcinalone injection; (C) After three injections: good involution, Cushinoid facies, and extra growth of hair; (D) 18 weeks later: good involution. Telangiectasia at the margins, Cushinoid facies, and extra hair growth have cleared up

Interferon Alfa (INF)

Interferon alfa has been tried in Hemangiomas which do not respond to steroids, or show recurrence. It acts by inhibiting angiogenesis and by reducing endothelial cell proliferation. Especially in Kasabach-Merrit syndrome, it is supposed to have an additional beneficial effect of reducing the platelet adherence. But the side effects of fever, neutropenia and neurotoxicity restricts the use of Interferon. It is advisable to leave the choice of using INF in Kasabach-Merrit syndrome or refractory CHI to the Pediatrician from the beginning.

Vincristine and Bleomycin are being tried in large Hemangiomas especially associated with PHACES. Neurotoxicity of Vincristine and Interferon make their use limited. Bleomycin is still in the trial phase.

It has been suggested, that the appearance of blanched skin or scarring, before involution commences is possibly due to hypoxia. This prompts one to think whether Bevacizumab (Avastin) can be tried in CHI[12] (North PE and Waner H).

Recent reports on use of topical Imiquimod are interesting. But it can only be used in small size Hemangiomas. Recently there are some reports on use of Propranolol in very large Hemangiomas[24] (Le'aute'-Labreze C, et al 2008).

Lasers

Lasers have been used in the treatment of infantile Hemangiomas. Carbon dioxide laser has been used for surgical excision as it is hemostatic. Pulsed dye laser is not useful for infantile Hemangiomas as it cannot penetrate the dermal layer. It is useful in capillary malformations and for removing the telangiectasia of skin after the Hemangioma has involuted.

Management of Post Involutional Sequelae of the Hemangiomas

The sequelae which are left behind after the Hemangiomas have involuted, are functional and esthetic. The visual function disturbances are dystopia, ptosis, amblyopia and strabismus. The esthetic sequelae are mainly due to the scars left behind after the involution of the Hemangioma. There may be distortion or destruction of the anatomical features. The size and site determine the age and stage when corrective surgery should be done as shown in Figures 5.10A to C.

Significant deformities may need multiple reconstructive procedures and the resultant psychosocial complications due to them can become major problems. Therefore, the reconstructive procedures have to be started early and may need to be continued till the teenage period[21].

Occasionally, extensive scarring and deformities are seen after involution of a CHI. These patients need multiple surgeries to resurface the disfigurements, both primary and secondary—related to growth. These need correction of deformities and resurfacing to restore color and harmony.

All the basic concepts and approaches used in Plastic Surgery come in handy to give a cosmetically acceptable result viz. the concept of aesthetic units, the technique of serial excision, the selective use of skin expansion, local flaps and full thickness skin grafts.

Amblyopia is seen due to 'deprivation' because of partial or complete lid closure. Ptosis correction at an early stage can prevent amblyopia. The other methods are occlusion of the normal eye by patching it or using Atropine or Cyclopentolate to produce pharmacological patching. This would make the child to use the affected eye and improve its function.

Strabismus is corrected by squint surgery.

Dystopia and enophthalmos need imaging to evaluate the amount of orbital volume deficit and orbital floor anatomy. The expansion of the orbit caused by CHI which has not regressed, produces enophthalmos due to the increased orbital volume. This may need reducing the orbital volume and mainly the elevation of the floor, by placing an

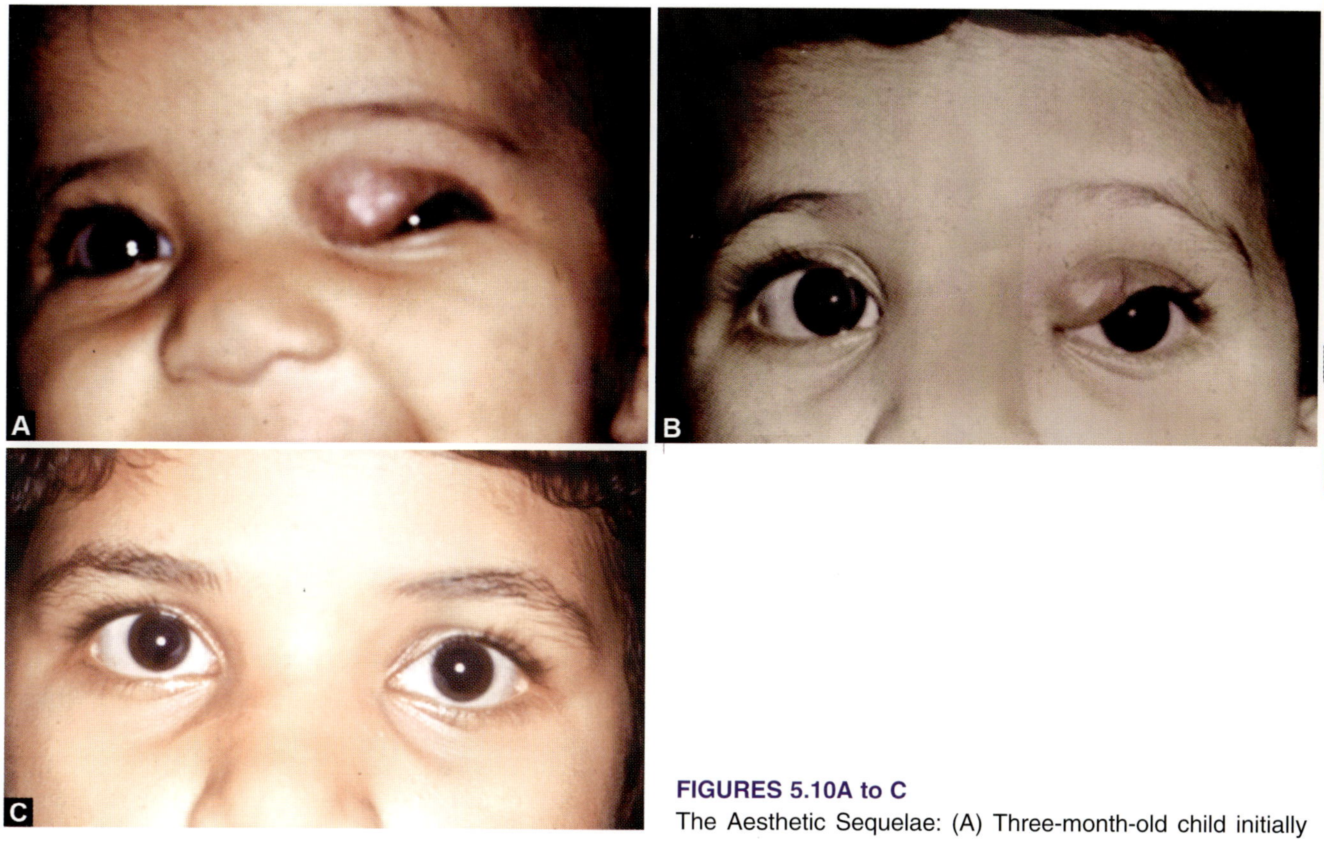

FIGURES 5.10A to C

The Aesthetic Sequelae: (A) Three-month-old child initially treated with triamcinalone injection; (B) Excision of lesion done to get full correction of ptosis; (C) Seven years later: A very natural eyelid. The CHI can be forgotten

autologus bone or cartilage or a synthetic implant to raise the level of the floor of the orbit. Illustrated in Figure 5.11A, which shows a patient who has dystopia of the left orbit, hypertropia due to the involvement of extraocular muscles, expansion of the eye brow and brow ptosis. Elevation of floor of the orbit with implant was done to correct the dystopia and browpexy was carried out by revision of the forehead scar (Fig. 5.11B). The squint too was corrected. However, the vision was impaired.

SYNDROMIC HEMANGIOMAS

PHACE Syndrome or Neurocutaneous Syndrome

The Facial Hemangiomas are the most striking feature of this syndrome and may be the first presentation. The term PHACE or the neurocutaneous syndrome has the following features, (P) posterior fossa malformation, (H) large and/or extensive Facial Hemangiomas, (A) arterial malformations, (C) cardiac anomalies and aortic coarctation and (E) eye abnormalities. Hemangiomas that occur in the PHACE syndrome are treated similar to CHI elsewhere. The options include systemic or local steroid administration for Hemangioma besides treatment for other anomalies. For ophthalmologic complications their detection and prevention are most important.

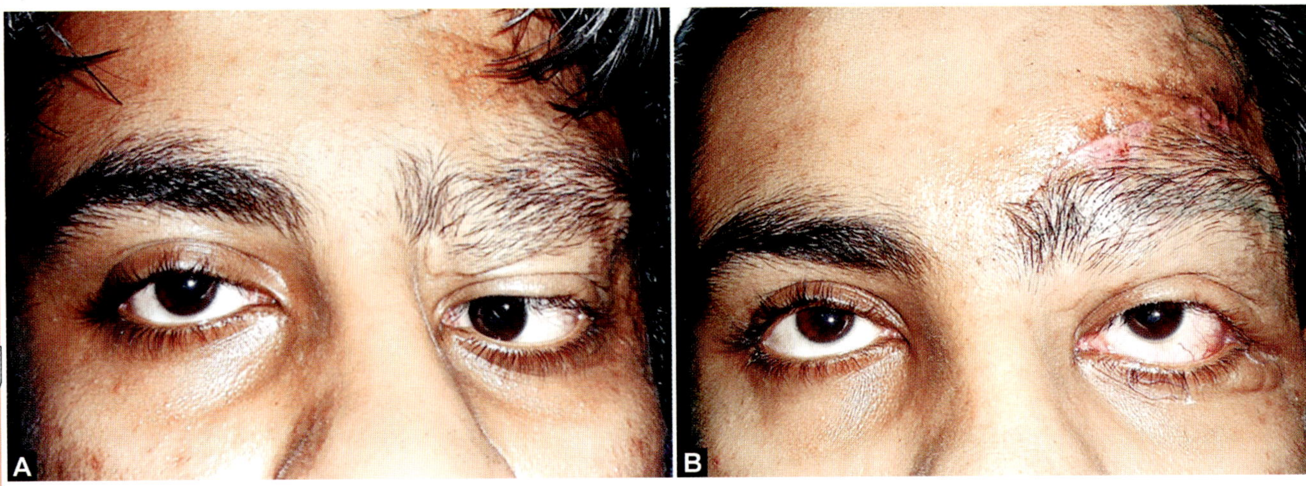

FIGURES 5.11A and B
Post CHI involution sequelae: (A) Dystopia, hypertropia, expansion of brow, brow ptosis and post involution scar over forhead; (B) Following correction of the orbit floor, browpexy with revision of forehead scar and correction of the squint

Kasabach-Merritt Syndrome

Large hemangiomas with a high flow, may be associated with platelet trapping and thrombocytopenia, a condition called the Kasabach-Merritt syndrome. This condition has to be treated with Systemic steroids. Interferon has been tried in Hemangiomas which do not respond to steroids, or show recurrence. It acts by inhibiting angiogenesis and by reducing endothelial cell proliferation. It has an additional beneficial effect of reducing the platelet adherence.

MALIGNANT VASCULAR NEOPLASMS

- Hemangiopericytoma
- Hemangioendothelioma
- Kaposi sarcoma.

Hemangiopericytoma

Hemangiopericytoma is a rare slow growing but potentially malignant vascular neoplasm. Its occurrence in the orbit is quite rare. They have been shown to occur in conjunctiva, ciliary body and lacrimal gland. They arise from pericytes covering the capillaries and venules. Telengiectasia of the adenexal tissue overlying the lesion is sometimes seen. Secondary involvement of orbit can occur from a primary lesion of the ethmoid or the maxillary sinus. Nearly half of the cases are malignant. They tend to recur if incompletely excised. Wide excision is recommended. Recurrence can occur anytime between four months to a few years. Clinically, it is difficult to identify as it can show a variety of clinical features in different locations and exhibit an equally unpredictable malignant behavior[13, 16] (Karcioglu ZA et al, 1997 and Mahesh Lakshmi and Subramanian N, 2000). Their presentation is quite similar to Cavernous Hemangioma. CT Scan shows features of a vascular tumor and can be misdiagnosed as Cavernous Hemangioma.

Figure 5.12A shows a middle aged man who presented with a right sided eccentric proptosis with epiphora and pain. He gave a history of orbital biopsy done elsewhere, but no details were available. The CT Scan showed a well circumscribed, extraconal, rounded, enhancing mass in the right superior orbit diagnosed as a Cavernous Hemangioma (Figs 5.12B and C). Lateral orbitotomy is done to excise the lesion. Histopathology showed it to be a Hemangiopericytoma (Fig. 5.12D).

It usually shows a well defined homogenous mass. It may show infiltration. MRI angiography shows a significant blush in all three phases. It is important to include hemangiopericytoma as a possible differential diagnosis in cases which show characteristics of a vascular mass lesion.

Histopathology reveals a more solid tumor, compared to a Cavernous Hemangioma. There is a uniform cellular and vascular pattern with reticulin fibers that surround pericytes. Plump cell and spindle shaped cells are seen. Sinusoidal vascular compartment has the staghorn configuration. The number of mitotic figures differentiate the benign from malignant.

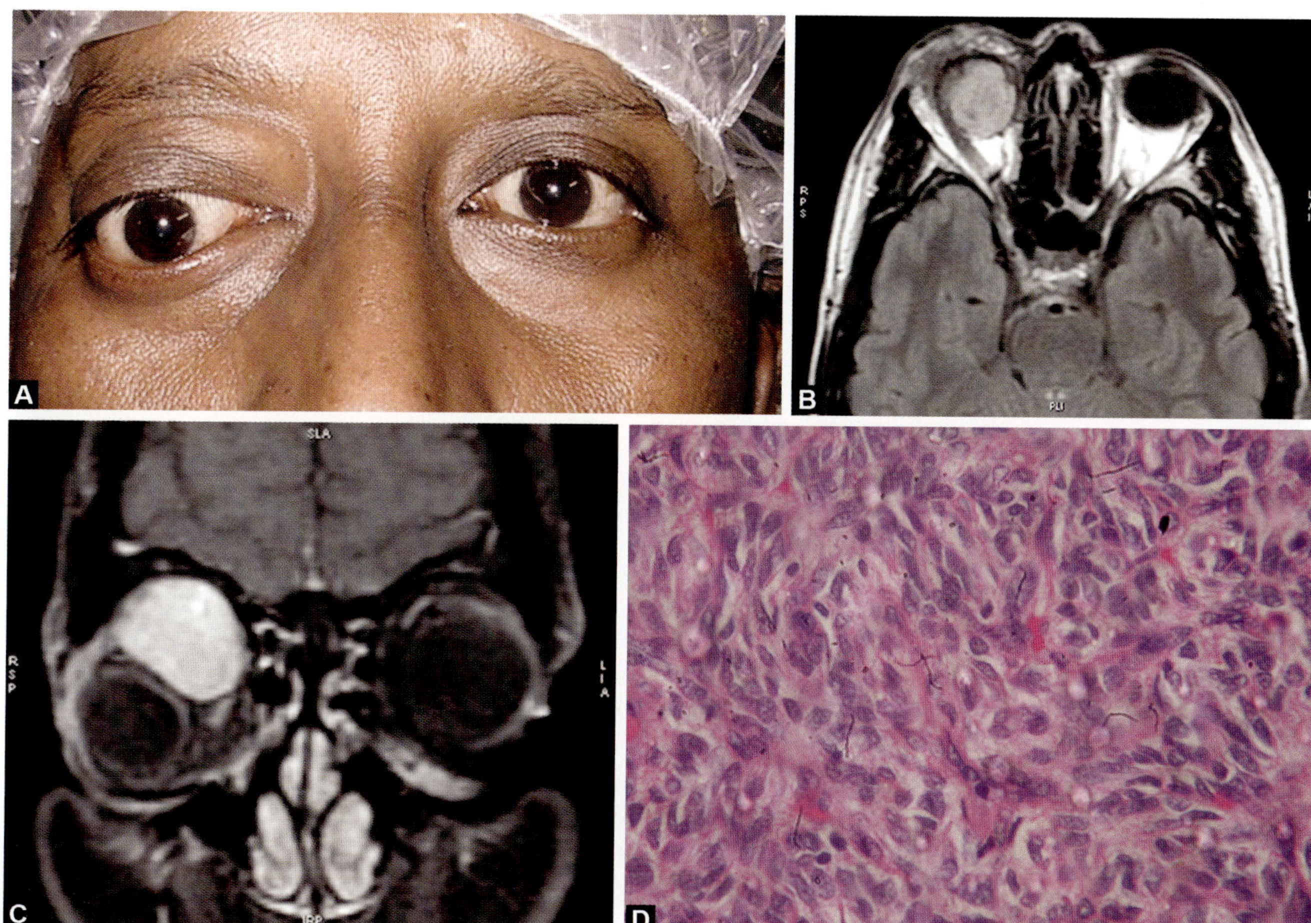

FIGURES 5.12A to D

A case of Hemangiopericytoma: (A) Middle aged man presented with eccentric proptosis, watering and pain; (B and C) Well circumscribed, extraconal, rounded, enhancing mass lesion of the right superior orbit. Preoperative diagnosis of cavernous hemangioma; (D) Histopathology showed it to be hemangiopericytoma showing the spindle cell tumor cells with numerous tiny blood vessels

Treatment

Complete surgical excision of the mass is recommended. Recurrence occurs, if any residual tumor is left behind. For recurrence and malignant transformation of the tumor, exenteration is advised. This has to be followed by radiotherapy.
Due to the rarity of the lesion, no definitive therapeutic regime has been developed.

Vascular Malformations

Vascular malformations of the orbit are quite rare. Depending on the hemodynamic flow, they are classified by Rootman into, no flow, venous flow and arterial flow lesions.

The biological behavior of vascular malformations is distinctly different from the CHIs. These too are also present at birth but are noticed later. They continue to grow in proportion to the growth of the child and do not involute. Here the growth is not due to the endothelial proliferation but due to the effect of hemodynamics of the pre-existing network of dysplastic vessels. The skeleton of the orbit responds to this hemodynamics by hypertrophy, remodeling or bone destruction. The increasing volume of contents sometimes expands the orbits and depending on their location, displaces the globe.

SMALL CHANNEL NO FLOW VASCULAR MALFORMATIONS

A. Lymphangiomas
B. Capillary malformations.

Lymphangiomas

Lymphangiomas of the orbit are poorly defined diffuse lesions, seen in children and young adults. The lack of clear cut margins, makes their surgery very difficult. They produce impairment of vision besides causing significant disfigurement.

The word 'Lymphangioma' was originally coined by Jones in 1959 to describe vascular malformations in the orbit. 'Oma' is typically reserved for neoplasm whereas Lymphangioma is considered to arise from the pluripotent venous analoge which may develop into both venous and lymphatic structures.[4,15] During the development of the vascular system at the stage of undifferentiated capillaries, defective blood flow in the capillaries can form an isolated infiltrative lymphatic or combined venolymphatic malformation.[14] They are also called Hamartomas or choristomas depending on the histology which may show true lymphatic or dysplastic blood vessels.[4]

Classification

As mentioned earlier, Rootman has classified them as no flow vascular malformations. Lymphangioma channels are isolated from orbital vascular channels. Hence, there is no change due to the posture—a phenomenon seen in the orbital varix. According to Rootman, many of them are in fact mixed venolymphatic malformations. This, he claims, is due to the fact that lymphatics are absent in the orbit. Hemorrhage occurs frequently in the cyst after a minor trauma or infection. It can also be spontaneous.

Histopathologically, it is sometimes very difficult to differentiate between a Lymphangioma and a venous malformation.

As described by Rootman,[3] the Vascular Malformations of the orbitopalpebral lesion are also grouped, as for CHIs, into four types, depending on their anatomical location as Superficial, Deep, Combined and Complex.

A. Superficial involve only the skin or conjunctiva.
B. Deep are located in the orbit.
C. Combined involve both the superficial and the orbital regions and
D. Complex involve other areas besides periorbital and orbital.

They are further classified into microcystic or macrocystic, depending on the size of the cystic channels.

They may be evident at birth or manifest in childhood or teens. They are unilateral, rarely bilateral. A superficial lymphangioma may present as small bubble like lesions in the conjunctiva or lid, filled with clear serous fluid as seen in Figure 5.13A. These cysts may suddenly increase in size and become reddish due to hemorrhage. As seen here, they may be associated with a deep component.

Sometimes these may show a sudden increase in size due to a hemorrhage, usually in association with an upper respiratory tract infection as seen in Figures 5.14A and B where blood is seen coming from the conjunctival sac. A subconjunctival hemorrhage retains its bright red color and takes a longer period to clear.

Very occasionally a lymphangiomatous conjunctiva may need an excision and replacement with a mucosal graft as shown in Figures 5.15A to C.

Occasionally a preseptal lesion may be almost independent of a retroseptal lesion as seen in Figure 5.16A where a cystic swelling in the medial side of the upper eyelid — a cystic lymphangioma had no obvious connection to the lesion seen in the retrobulbar space — both intraconal and extraconal Figure 5.16B seen in the CT scan. Only the preseptal lesion was removed Figure 5.16C.

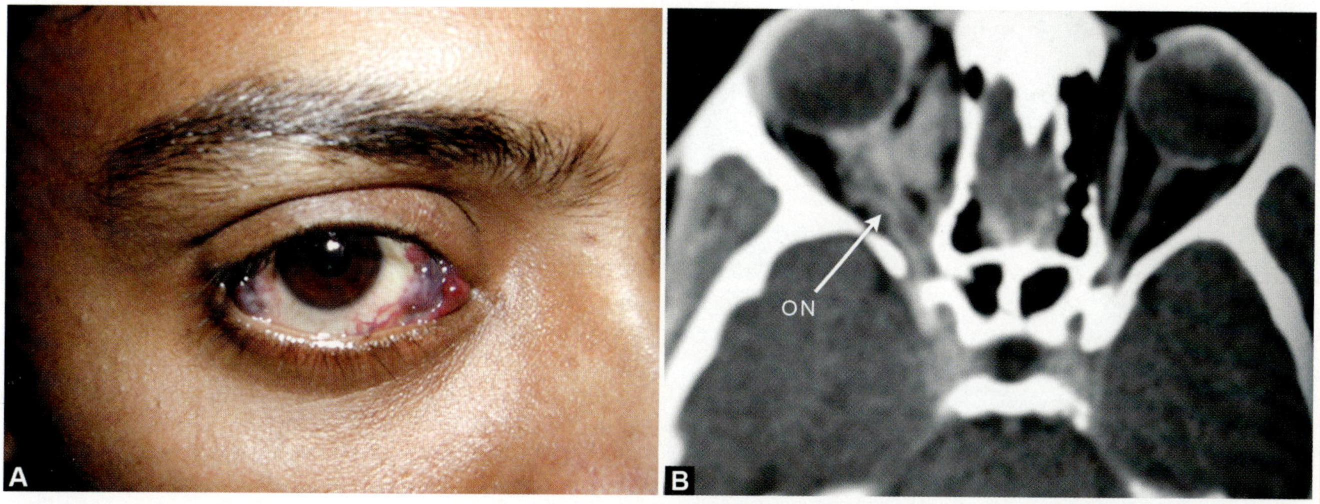

FIGURES 5.13A and B

A Conjunctival Lymphangioma associated with a deep component: (A) Lymphangioma seen in the conjunctiva as red and blue cyst; (B) Ill defined infiltrative lesion surrounding the optic nerve

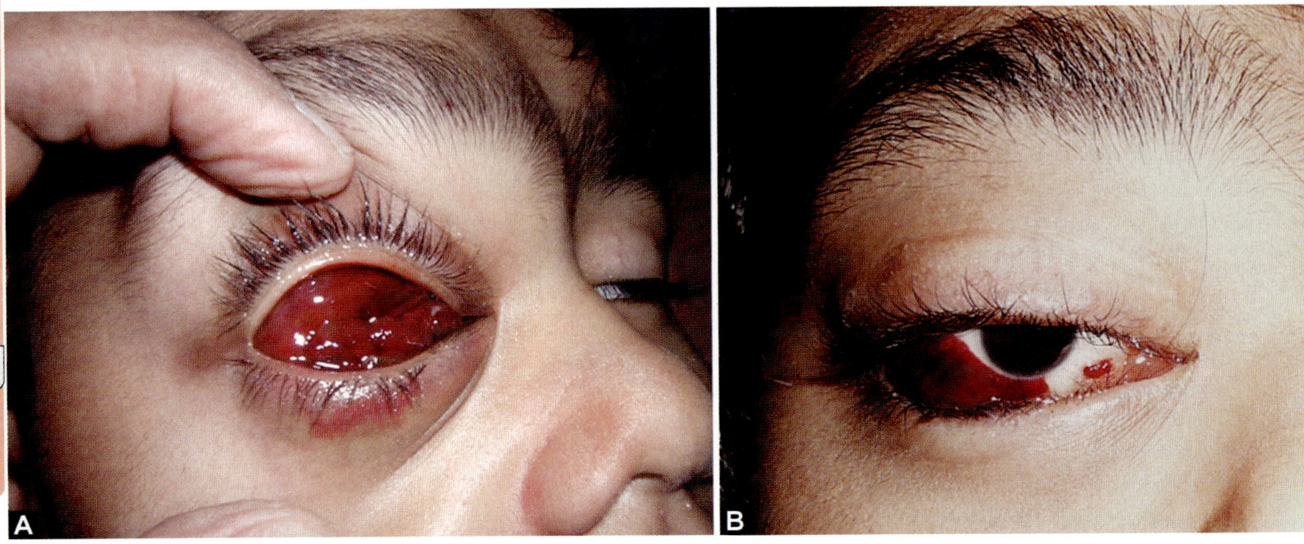

FIGURES 5.14A and B

Conjunctival Lymphangioma — Bleeding: (A) Increase in the swelling and bleeding during an episode of upper respiratory tract infection; (B) Reduction of chemosis after clearing of URTI

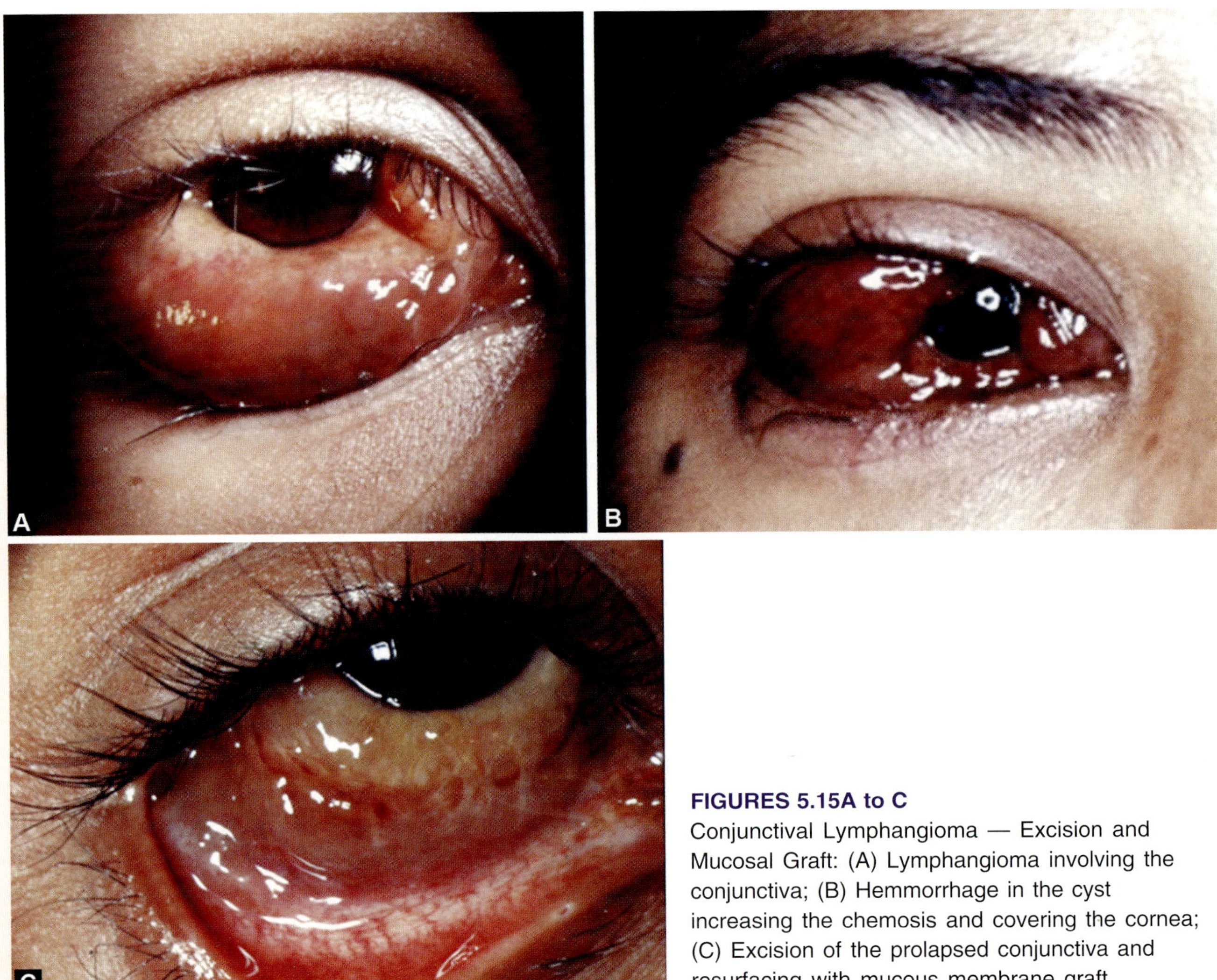

FIGURES 5.15A to C

Conjunctival Lymphangioma — Excision and Mucosal Graft: (A) Lymphangioma involving the conjunctiva; (B) Hemmorrhage in the cyst increasing the chemosis and covering the cornea; (C) Excision of the prolapsed conjunctiva and resurfacing with mucous membrane graft

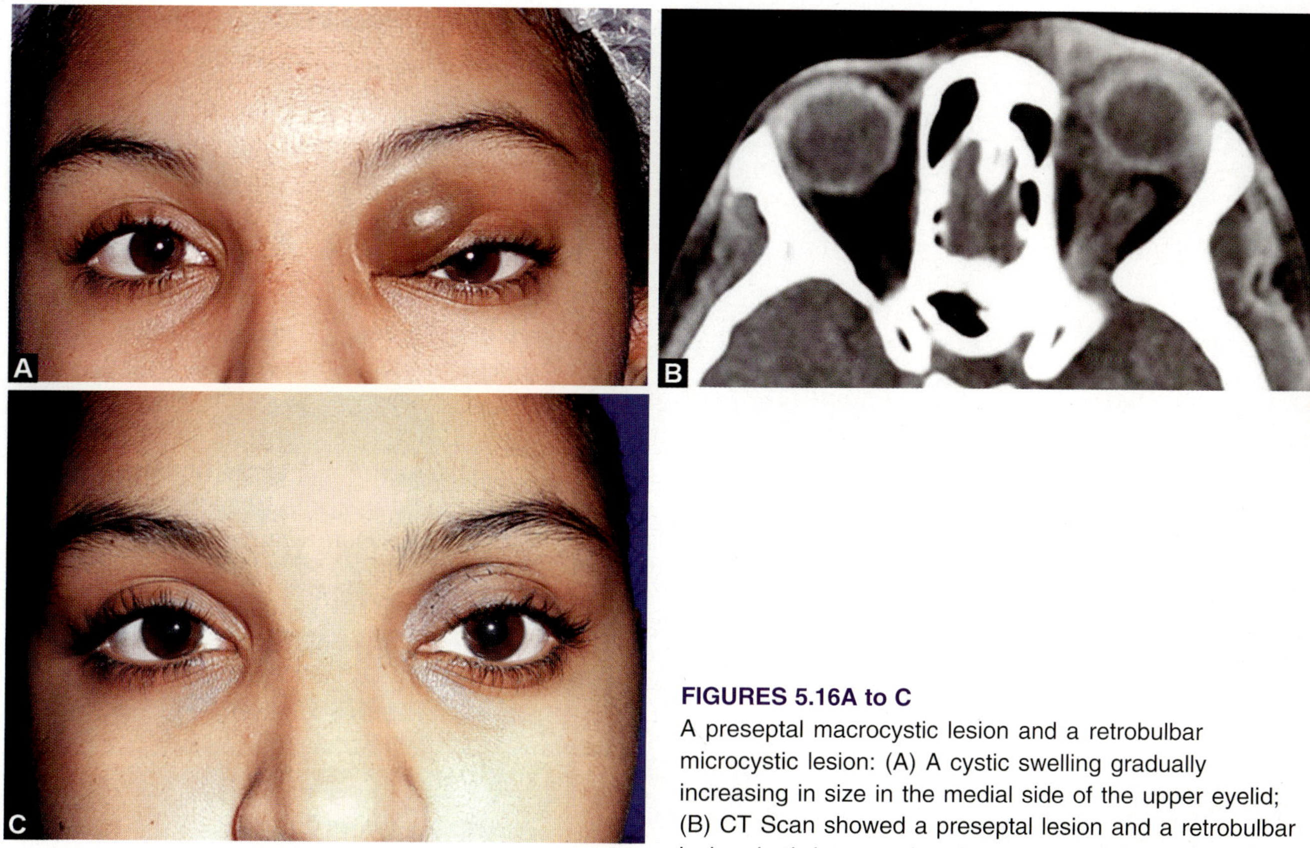

FIGURES 5.16A to C
A preseptal macrocystic lesion and a retrobulbar microcystic lesion: (A) A cystic swelling gradually increasing in size in the medial side of the upper eyelid; (B) CT Scan showed a preseptal lesion and a retrobulbar lesion, both intraconal and extraconal; (C) Through a supratarsal fold incision, the preseptal cystic lesion was removed and no deeper connection was found

Displacement of the Globe

Displacement of the globe occurs depending on the location of the lesion in the orbit. Proptosis may be the first presenting symptom in a patient, and can be severe as seen in Figure 5.17A where a lesion in the inferomedial part of the orbital cavity has severely displaced the eyeball upwards, laterally and outwards producing a loss of vision, in fact even a loss of perception of light.

In the early stages, the ocular movements are not affected, but due to the diffuse nature of the lesion, the extraocular muscles get involved and the ocular movements get restricted. Vision gets affected due to the stretch and pressure on the nerve or aggravated by the bleeding episodes. Exposure keratitis and corneal ulceration can occur due to gross proptosis.

Effects on the Skeleton

Secondary effects on the surrounding bony skeleton may result in the expansion of the orbit as seen in Figure 5.13B and occasionally the hypertrophy of the adjacent cranial skeleton as seen in Figure 5.16B. Generally, these lesions are painless, but due to spontaneous hemorrhage, pain may be the principal presenting symptom.

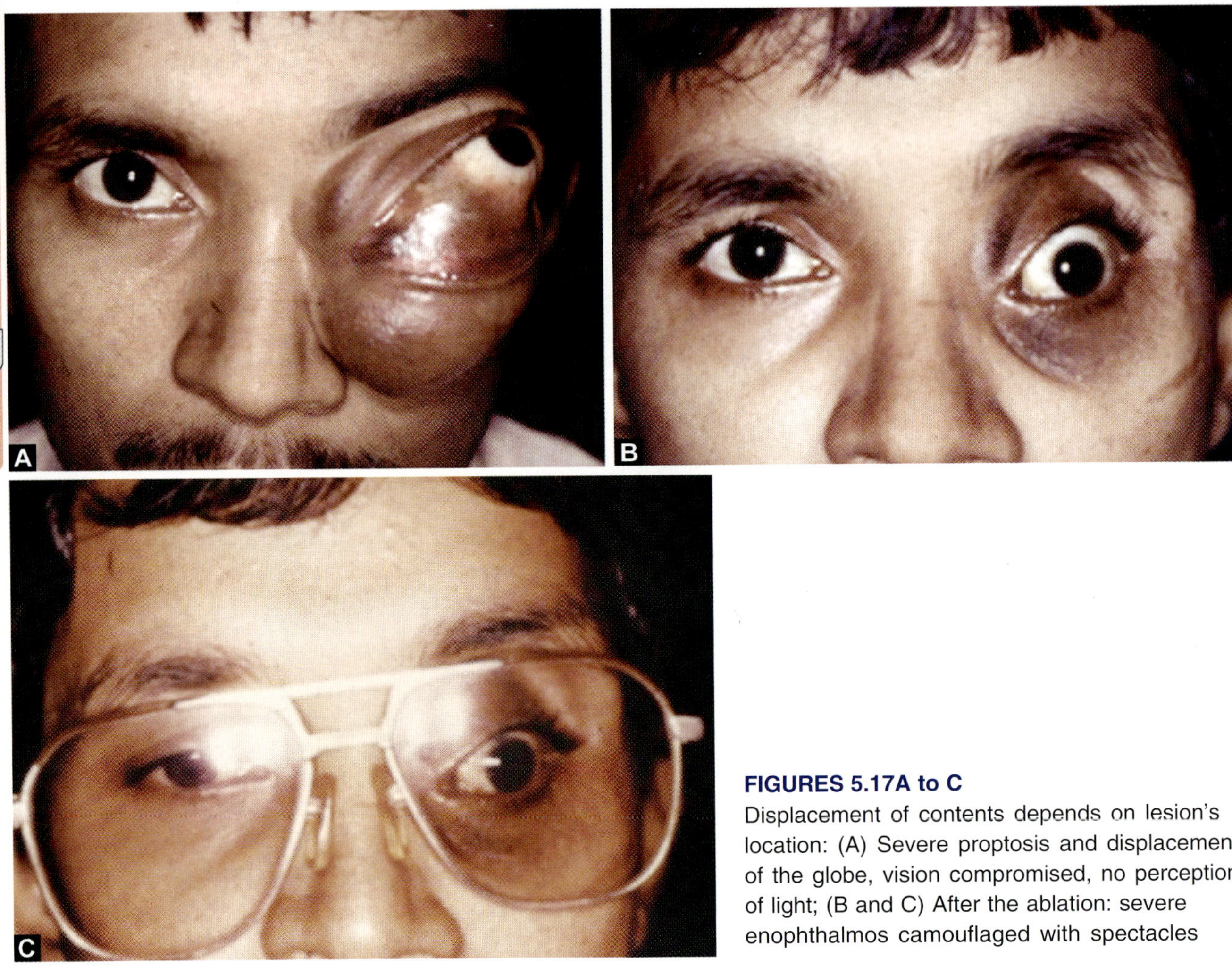

FIGURES 5.17A to C
Displacement of contents depends on lesion's location: (A) Severe proptosis and displacement of the globe, vision compromised, no perception of light; (B and C) After the ablation: severe enophthalmos camouflaged with spectacles

LYMPHANGIOMA IMAGING

Ultrasonography (USG)

Lymphangiomas are generally diffuse and do not show well defined borders in the USG. They can be quite extensive and involve the orbit, periocular areas and other parts of the face. In A-scan the ultrasonographic structure is irregular with low reflective spaces divided by high reflective septae. This is due to the multiple cystic lesion of the lymophangioma.

B-scan shows several low reflective spaces combined to form a mass. Lymphangiomas can bleed into the cysts spontaneously or following trauma. Ultrasonography will show a marked dilatation of the spaces. The blood within, usually does not clot and internal reflectivity is slightly higher than lymph. Fluid-level can be demonstrated.

CT Scan

An ill defined unencapsulated lesion is seen in the intraconal and/or extraconal compartments of the orbit. It may show multiple cystic spaces of varying sizes as seen in Figures 5.20D and E. It crosses anatomic boundaries and insinuates around normal structures. Little or no enhancement is seen on post contrast administration. Dilatation of the venous component may be seen on Valsalva's maneuver, which shows enhancement on postcontrast scans. Lack of communication with systemic circulation is utilized as a criterion for differentiation from orbital varices. Phleboliths are some times seen. Fluid levels are diagnostic of lymphangioma. Bony orbital enlargement may be present. Sometimes hyperostosis of bone is also seen as in Figure 5.23F.

MRI Imaging

MRI delineates the various components of the lesion very well. Cysts of varying sizes, filled with serous fluid or blood, are well demonstrated in Figures 5.21D to F. The relationship of lesion to optic nerve is well demonstrated and helps in planning the surgical treatment. MRI is helpful in detecting the age of the hemorrhage. Signal intensity depends on the type of the fluid in the cyst.

The lesion appears heterogenous, with the lymph containing areas being hypointense in T1 weighted images and hyperintense on T2 weighted images. Areas of subacute hemorrhage may appear hyperintense in to confirm T1 weighted images. Chronic cysts have high signals due to hemosiderin and ferritin (well illustrated in Fig. 5.21).

Histology

These malformations consist of irregular vascular channels of varying size. They are thin walled and lined by flat endothelium. The channels are filled with serous fluid or blood. The size of channels varies from very large cyst to microcystic cyst like a honeycomb. In between the channels, poorly developed muscle fibers and lymphoid aggregates are seen. Old and new blood products are seen in the cysts.

Management

The management of orbital lymphangiomas is quite problematic. The lesion being un-encapsulated and diffuse in nature, it is difficult to completely excise it. The chances of damage to optic nerve, either directly or indirectly, are very high. Surgery is indicated mainly for cosmetic reason or decompression for hemorrhage in the lesion. Surgery may have to be repeated.

The treatment is based on the size, the location, the possible secondary problems and the amount of vision compromise already present. The Macrocystic lymphangiomas generally do not recur after ablation. The microcystic lesion are far more prone to recur.

The superficial cystic lesions, which are present anteriorly, can be punctured and cauterized. The localized cysts can be excised.

The deeper macrocystic ones, which are preseptal, can also be excised completely. Cysts which are posterior can be decompressed and removed. Some authors have advocated use of Cyanoacrylate glue or Fibrin[7] glue to fill the cyst after aspiration to help in the removal of the cyst with fragile wall. This is a useful technique.[17]

Sclerosants like sodium tetradecylsulfate, ethanol have been used besides triamcinalone injections. A Japanese formulation called OK 432 (a deactivated strain of group A *Streptococcus*) has been tried. The results have neither been consistent nor encouraging. The drug is also not freely available and does not have FDA approval.

The microcystic lesions are most difficult to remove. There is generally no plane of cleavage for dissection. Carbon dioxide lasers have been recommended for ablation.[5] With large intraorbital lesions, the vision is already badly affected and the patient mainly wants a cosmetic correction. Sometimes, they are unable to even wear a spectacle which may be necessary for the vision of the other eye (Fig. 5.21). Hence, they are prepared to accept a further compromise of the vision of the affected eye.

The Surgical Approach

The approach to a lesion depends on its location and size. The approaches that follow can be transconjunctival, paraciliary or through a natural fold, viz. supratarsal fold in as shown in Figure 5.16A.

The Anterior Superior Orbitotomy

When the lesion is situated deeper, anterior superior orbitotomy is a useful route. Figure 5.18A shows a one year old child with a superior intraconal well defined mass which has displaced the eyeball downwards and forwards and illustrates its evaluation, the adequacy of the exposure and the result (Figs 5.18 B to E).

The Anterior Superior Orbitotomy, can also access the medial part of the orbit (Figs 5.19A and B). The increasing proptosis seen was first noticed a few weeks after birth. A fullness also developed over the medial part of the eyebrow. The exposure through an Anterior Superior Orbitotomy enabled the delivery of a large mass from the superior orbit, smaller lesions from medial orbit. The pupils were monitored throughout the surgery.

A *coronal approach* is chosen when the forehead skeleton has to be contoured and/ or bone has to be harvested to build up the orbital floor for correction of dystopia. An Anterior Superior Orbitotomy can be combined through this incision.

As seen in the four year girl seen in Figure 5.20A who had an asymmetry of face, proptosis right eye, prominence of the adjacent forehead and the adjacent paraorbital skeleton and very poor vision. The skull was contoured through a bicoronal incision Figure 5.20B. A large multicystic mass removed from the inferior orbit Figure 5.20C. There was marked dystopia. Cranial bone graft harvested and used to elevate the floor of the orbit. Histopathology report confirmed it to be Lymphangioma.

A Lateral orbitotomy provides the best approach for the very large lesions in the inferiolateral part of the orbit and can be combined with an inferior orbitotomy — a panorbitotomy.

Figures 5.21A to C shows a twenty-two years old girl with a gross proptosis and chemosis of conjunctiva of the right eye and a loss of vision. Her immediate concern was an inability to wear spectacles to correct the vision of the opposite eye. The proptosis was present since childhood and was painless. She had recently started having heaviness on right side of face and headache, especially on bending down. The vision was very poor with mere perception of light.The MRI study (Figs 5.21D to H) defines the extent of the lesion. Through a Lateral Orbitotomy the orbital lesion was removed. Simultaneously, the lesion going into the infratemporal fossa could also be removed. Postoperatively (Fig. 5.21I) proptosis, headaches and heaviness had cleared. The vision remained unchanged and she had a partial ptosis.

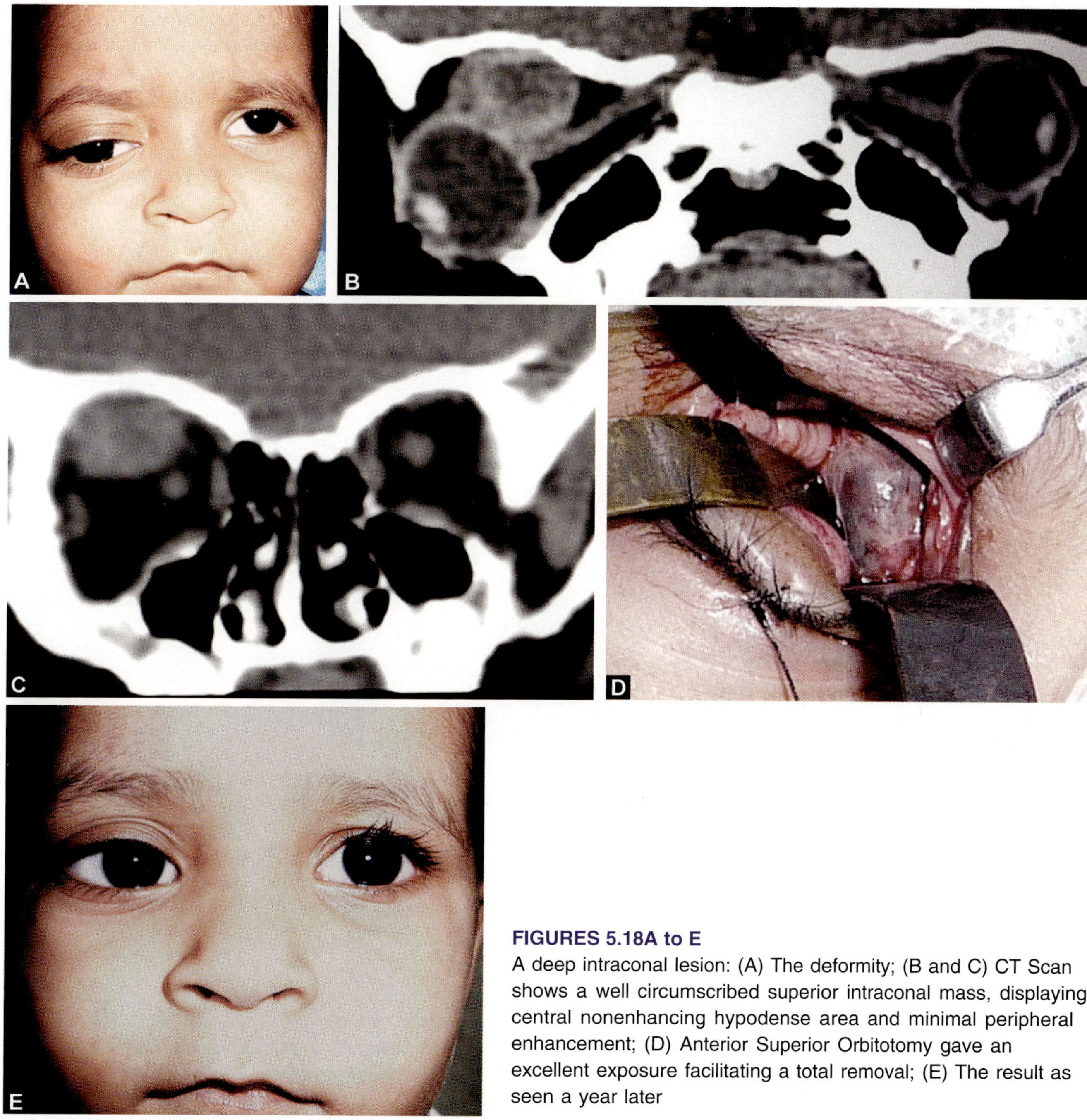

FIGURES 5.18A to E

A deep intraconal lesion: (A) The deformity; (B and C) CT Scan shows a well circumscribed superior intraconal mass, displaying central nonenhancing hypodense area and minimal peripheral enhancement; (D) Anterior Superior Orbitotomy gave an excellent exposure facilitating a total removal; (E) The result as seen a year later

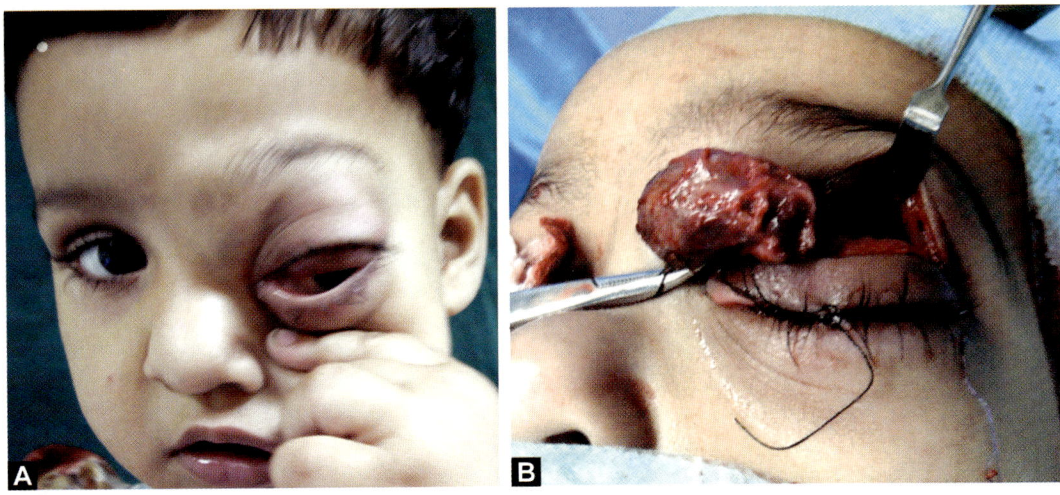

FIGURES 5.19A and B
The anterior superior orbitotomy for a medially located lesion: (A) The deformity at 18 months; (B) The exposure through an Anterior Superior Orbitotomy done. Note the lesions being removed from under the medial end of eyebrow

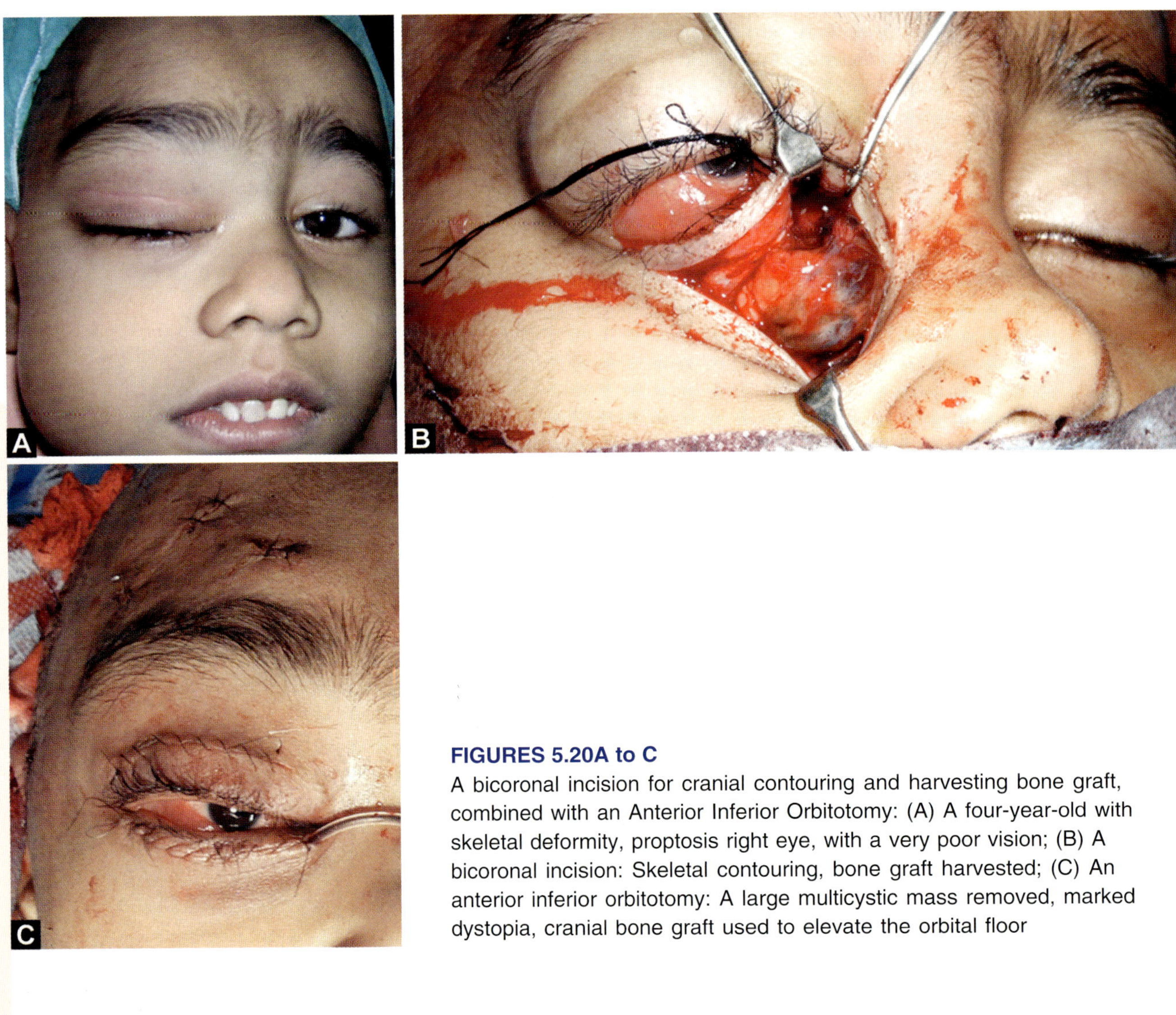

FIGURES 5.20A to C
A bicoronal incision for cranial contouring and harvesting bone graft, combined with an Anterior Inferior Orbitotomy: (A) A four-year-old with skeletal deformity, proptosis right eye, with a very poor vision; (B) A bicoronal incision: Skeletal contouring, bone graft harvested; (C) An anterior inferior orbitotomy: A large multicystic mass removed, marked dystopia, cranial bone graft used to elevate the orbital floor

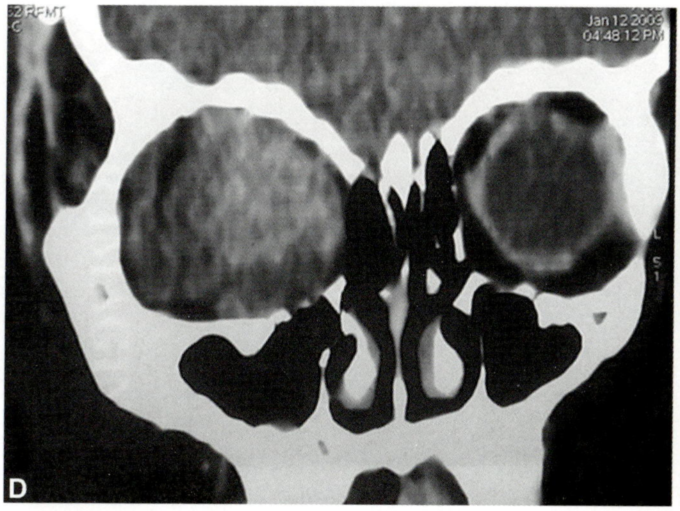

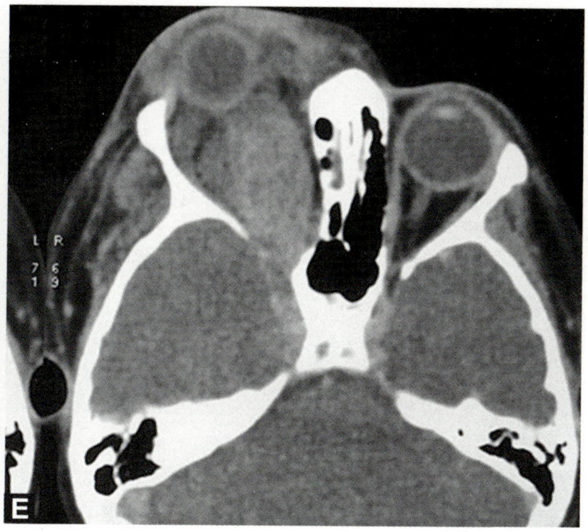

FIGURES 5.20D and E

CT Scan: Coronal and axial views show multicystic lesions occupying the entire orbit. Enlargement of orbit and soft tissue swelling in the forehead and nose is seen

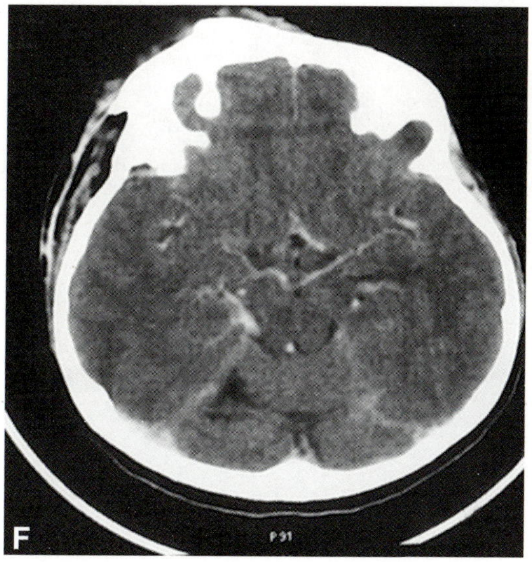

FIGURE 5.20F

Note the hypertrophy of frontal bone

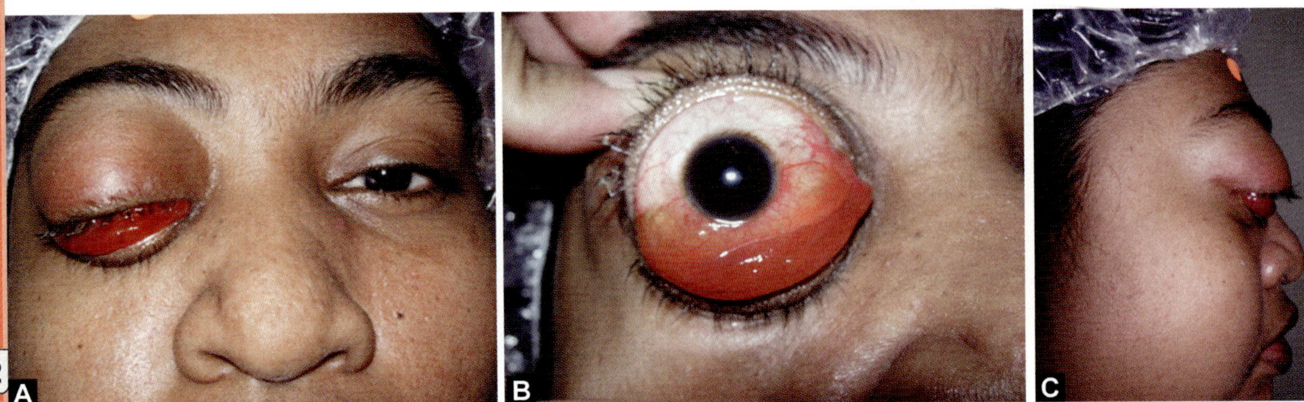

FIGURES 5.21A to C
A massive intraorbital lymphatic malformation, severe proptosis and loss of vision: (A to C) A twenty-two years old girl with gross proptosis, chemosis, loss of vision and inability to wear glasses

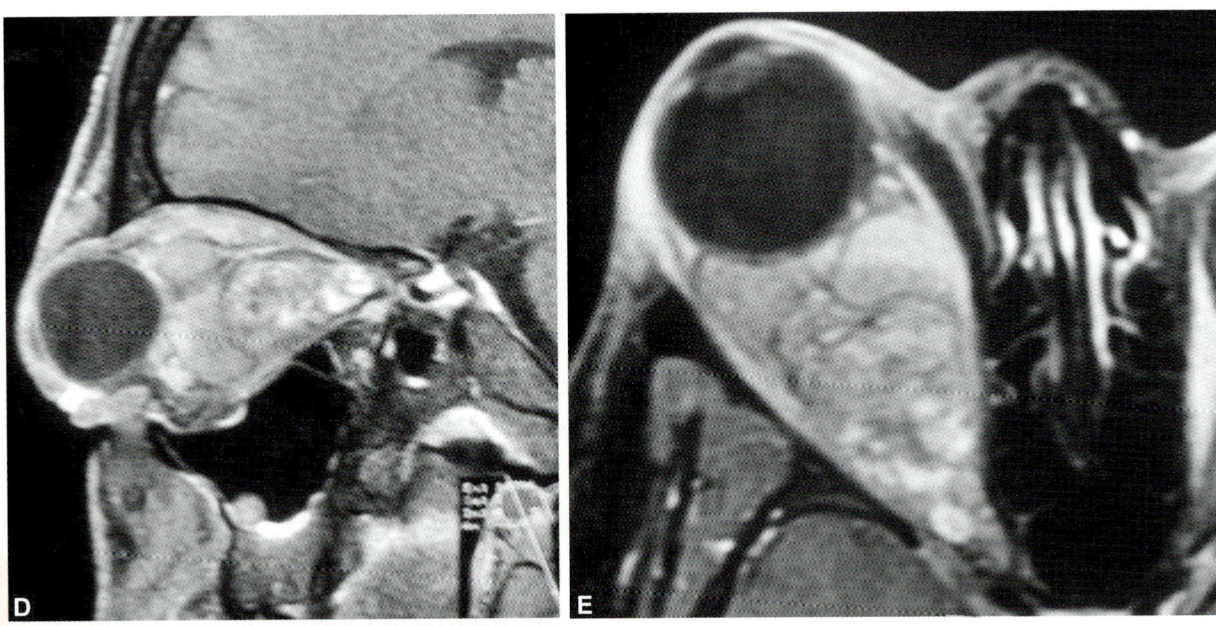

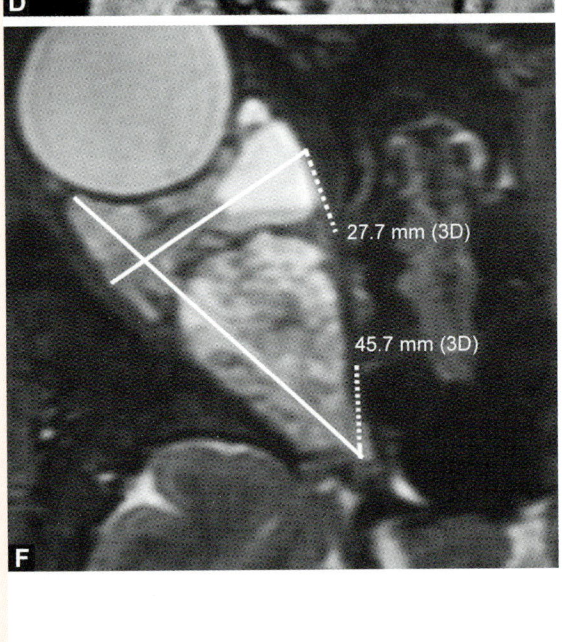

FIGURES 5.21D to F
MRI studies show a diffuse, ill defined, heterogeneous, retrobulbar mass in the intraconal and extraconal space. T1 and T2 weighted images show homogeneously hyperintense patches, suggestive of hemorrhagic areas. The extraocular muscles are not well delineated. The optic nerve is completely encased by the lesion. The lesion extends up to the orbital apex with no evidence of intracranial extension

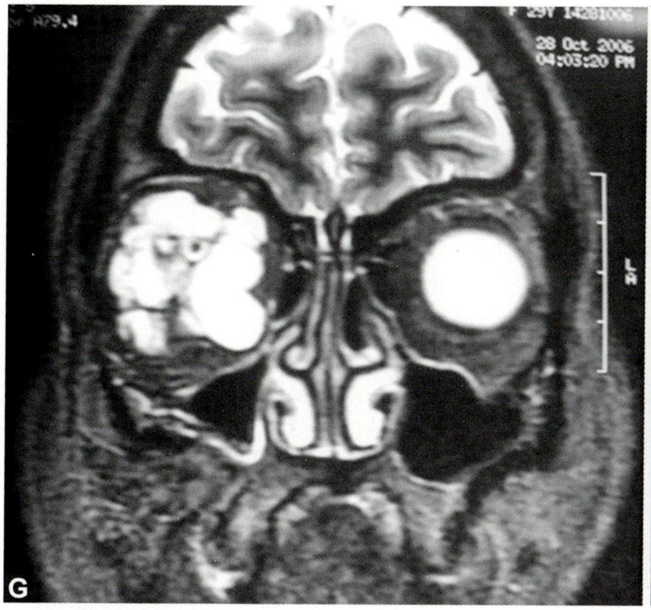

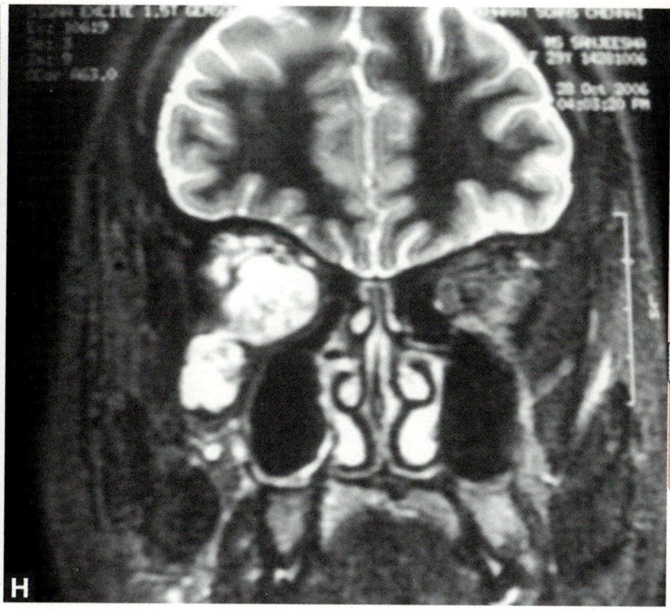

FIGURES 5.21G and H

Show extension of the lesion through the inferior orbital fissure into the infratemporal fossa. Soft tissue thickening is seen in the cheek area and also in the masseter and buccinator muscle. The lesion measures 27.7 mm × 45.7 mm

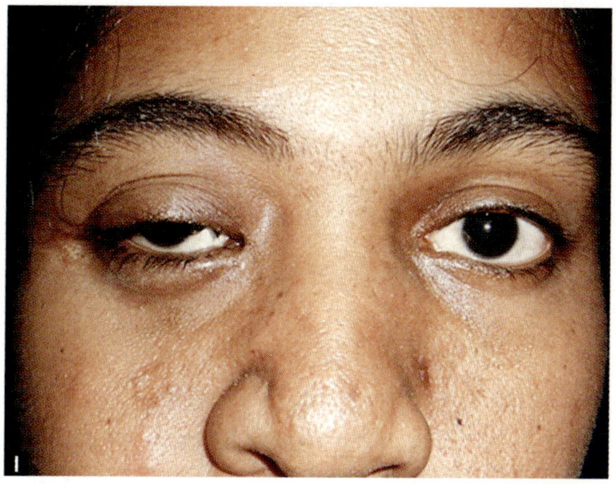

FIGURE 5.21 I

The patient seen six weeks postoperatively with no proptosis and a partial ptosis

Anterior Inferior Orbitotomy is the choice for the lesions located in the inferior orbit. The patient shown in Figure 5.22A is a middle aged lady with gradually increasing painless swelling elevating the globe but not affecting her vision. It was excised by an inferior orbitotomy through a subciliary incision (Fig. 5.22B). Histopathology diagnosis was a hemangiolymphangioma and the postoperative status six weeks later is shown in Figure 5.22C.

Multiple debulking procedures may be required to control the volume of the lymphangiomatous mass as illustrated in Figure 5.23. The four-year-old child shown there, presented with sudden onset of proptosis and pain in the left eye, Figures 5.23A and B. The parents were not committal on the existence of a prior proptosis. However, the vision was poor, there was a gross proptosis, conjunctival chemosis and exposure keratitis. The ocular movements were restricted. The extensive lymphangioma is well illustrated in the CT studies (Figs 5.23C and D). Most of the lesion was ablated through a lateral orbitotomy. Histopathology confirmed the diagnosis of a Lymphangioma. The benefit as seen seven months later is seen in Figure 5.23E. The CT study shown in Figures 5.23F and G show the residual lesion at this time, particularly the encasement of the optic nerve and some infiltration of the extraocular muscles. Five months later, a year after the first operation, the child was brought with severe proptosis, possibly following a mild injury, Figures 5.23H and I. A second debulking was carried out after seven months. The appearance has considerably improved, debulking has been adequate but the vision continues to be poor, Figures 5.23J and K.

Dystopia results when the enhanced orbital volume caused by the lymphatic malformation becomes associated with reduction of contents following ablative surgery. The result is a significant enophthalmos requiring secondary corrections to help to adjust the position and the level of the eyeball of the orbit, bringing the two eye balls to the same level, using auto grafts or implants. The use of cranial bone graft has been demonstrated in Figure 5.20. A dermolipomatous autograft harvested from the gluteal region is another useful filler.

Limitations and Complications

If the lymphangioma is not removed, it continues to grow and produces vision compromise.

As the lesion is not encapsulated, chances of injury to the optic nerve indirectly or directly are more.

A total removal is not always possible. Carbon dioxide laser has been used by some authors successfully.[5] But we have not tried it.

Recurrence is more common in children as the lesion continues to grow and rapid increase seems to be initiated by bleeding or following the URTI. For recurrence, repeated surgery is usually needed (see Fig. 5.23).

The secondary deformities may be quite severe and may need repeated debulking. A restoration of a perfectly normal appearance is very difficult to achieve.

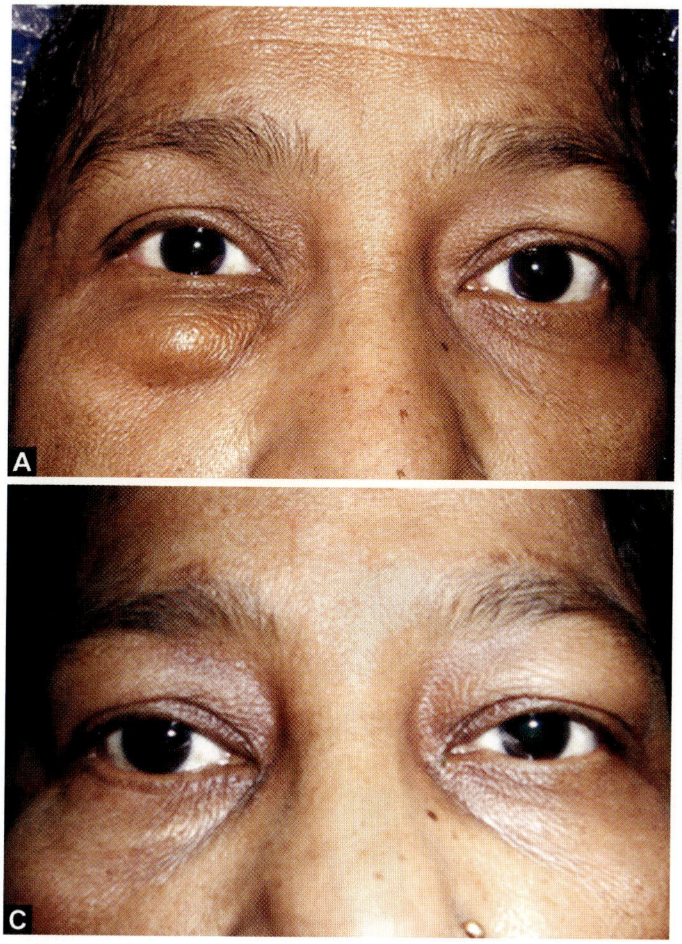

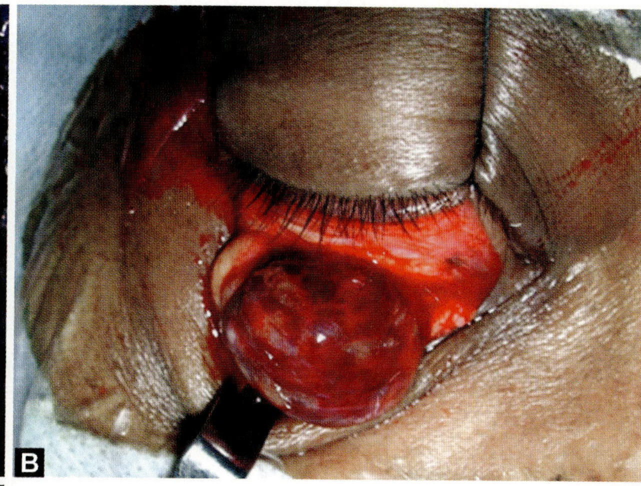

FIGURES 5.22A to C

Anterior Inferior orbitotomy for lesions placed inferiorly: (A) Gradually increasing proptosis with elevation of the globe. Vision normal; (B) An Inferior Orbitotomy through a subciliary incision. A well defined reddish mass removed; (C) Result six weeks post operative

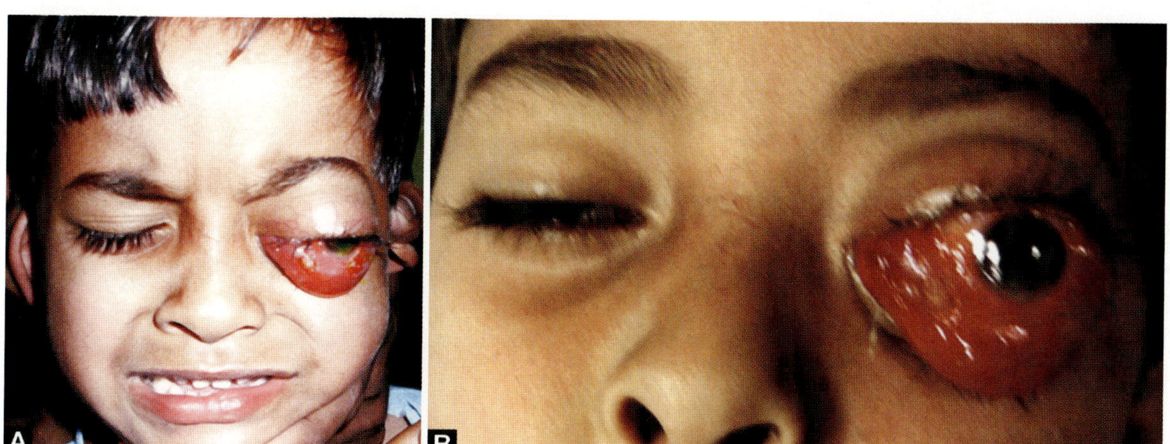

FIGURES 5.23A and B

Multiple Decompressions: (A and B) A four-year-old presented with sudden proptosis, pain, chemosis, and exposure keratitis

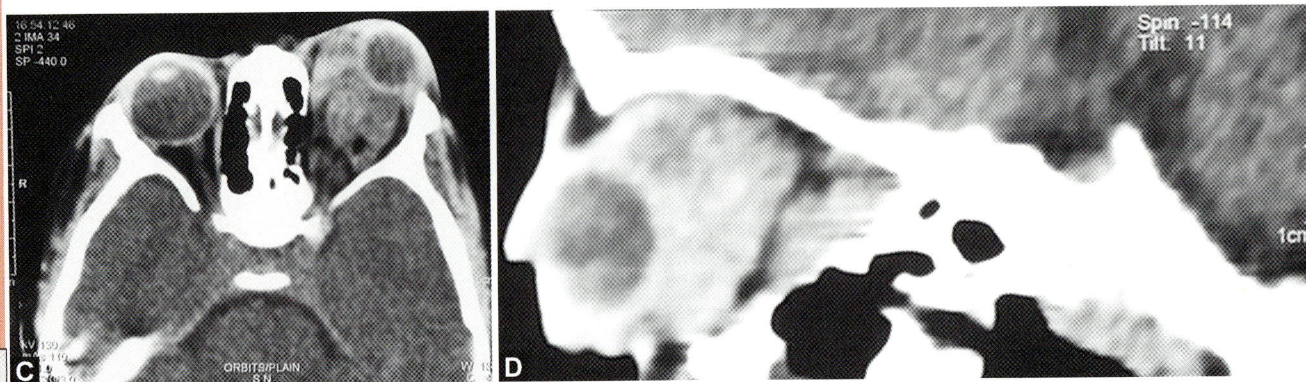

FIGURES 5.23C and D
Axial CT Scan shows a multilobulated ill defined, intraconal and extraconal mass going around the optic nerve and the globe

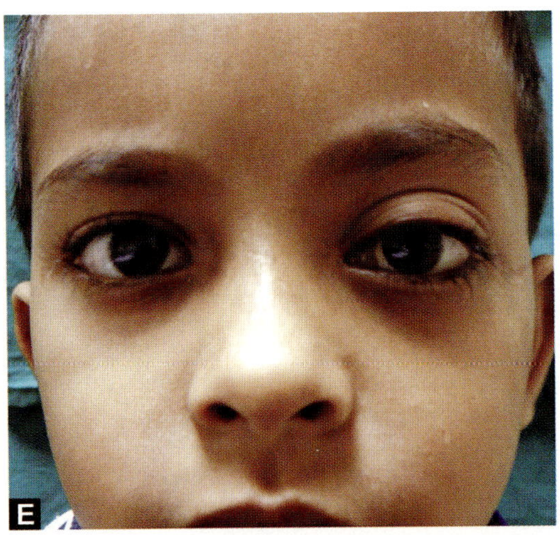

FIGURE 5.23E
Seven months after debulking through a lateral orbitotomy, Considerable benefit, Mild proptosis persists

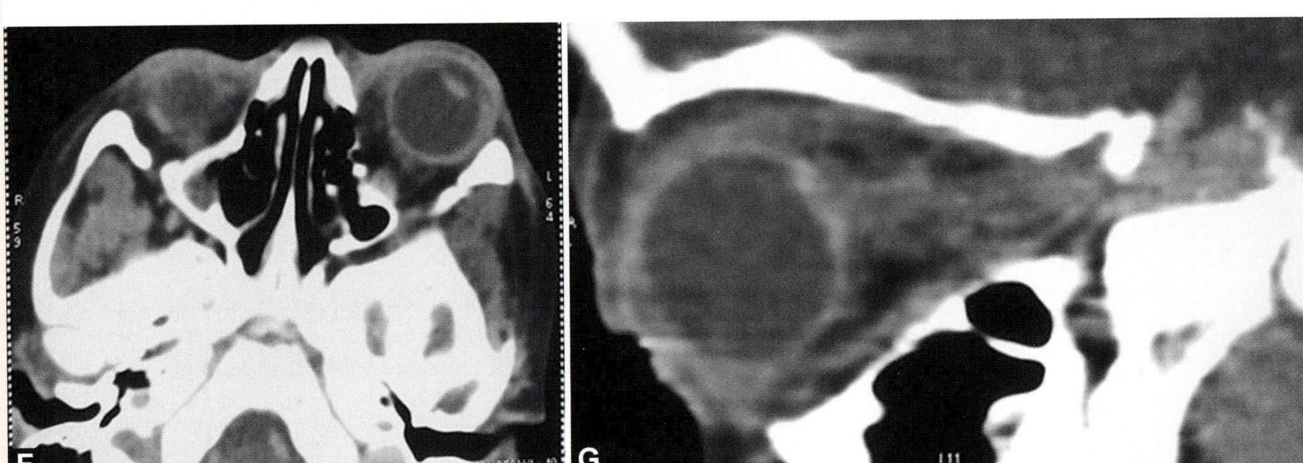

FIGURES 5.23F and G
The CT Scans show a diffuse residual intra and extraconal lesion, partly encasing the optic nerve and partly infiltrating the extraocular muscles

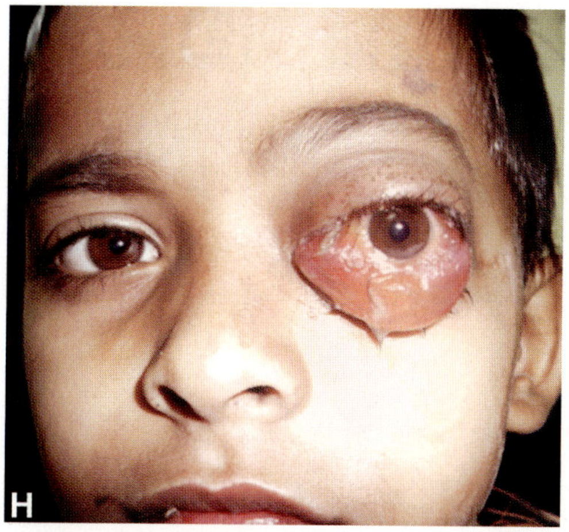

FIGURE 5.23H
Five months later, brought with severe proptosis, possibly following a mild injury

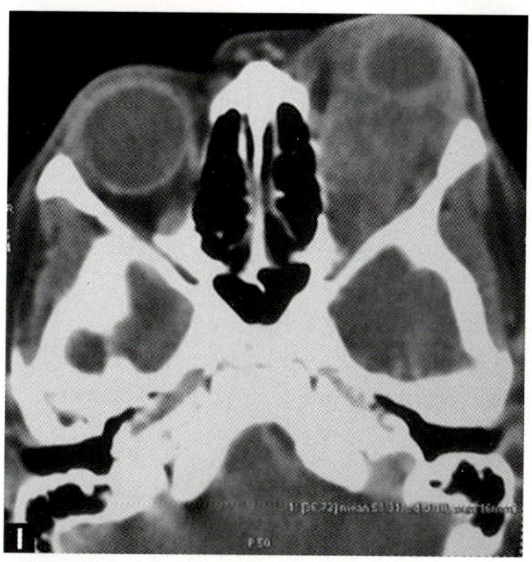

FIGURE 5.23I
The axial CT Scan shows a diffuse ill defined, infiltrating lesion, having a few cysts with a fluid level

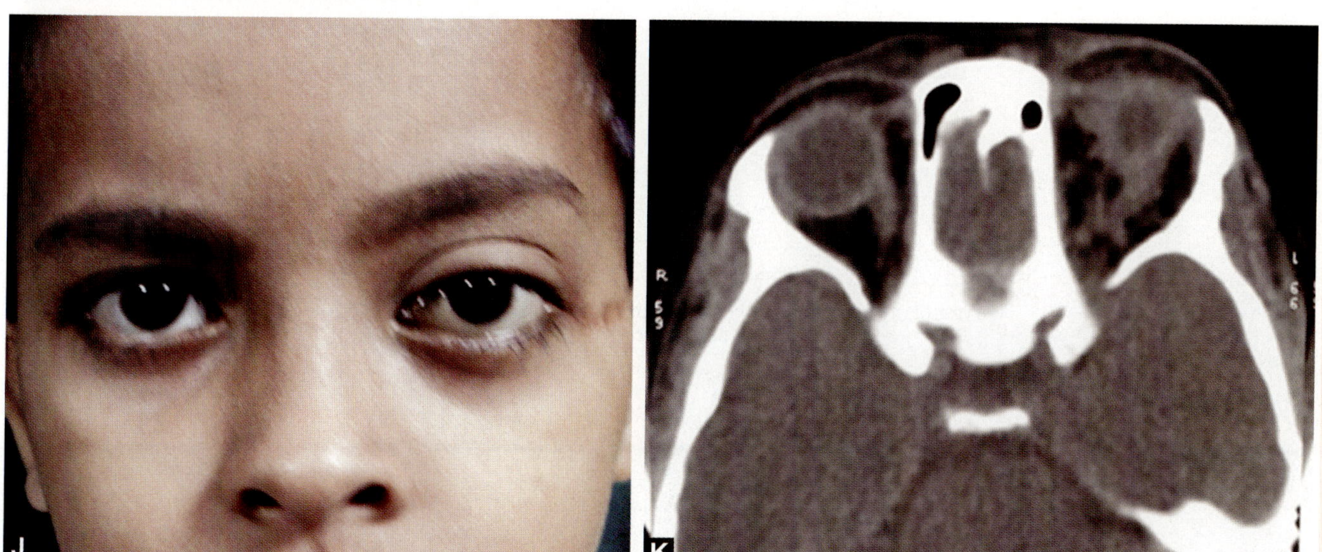

FIGURES 5.23J and K
The appearance seven months after the second orbitotomy. Proptosis has reduced, vision is poor. CT Scan shows significant reduction in the the lesion

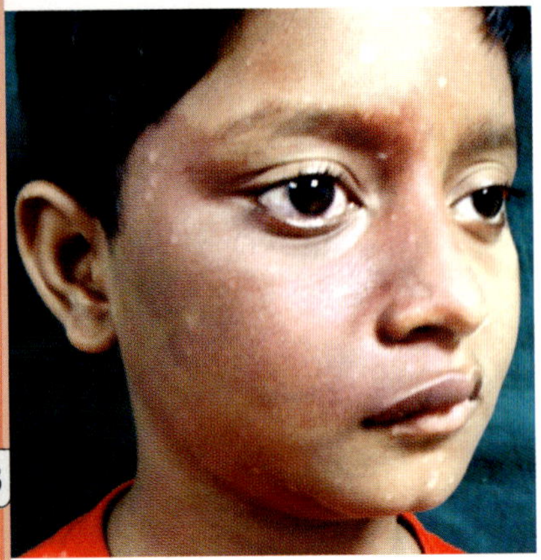

FIGURE 5.24
Capillary malformation involving the maxillary division (V2) of the trigeminal nerve

CAPILLARY MALFORMATIONS

Capillary malformations, also called port-wine stains, are present at birth and are seen as pink or violet, (depending on the complexion) well circumscribed patches on the skin (Fig. 5.30). On the face, they are usually distributed along the division of trigeminal nerve and are usually referred to as Sturge—Weber syndrome (Fig. 5.24), the facial localization being referred as V1, and V2 which involve the orbital area and VII which covers the mandibular area. Eyelids and periocular areas are often involved.

They do not grow beyond the areas seen at birth and do not involute. They are associated with episcleral telangiectasia, choroidal hemangiomas and leptomeningeal hemangiomas. Epileptic seizures are also seen. A complete ophthalmologic examination must be done to rule out glaucoma which is commonly associated with these lesions.

Local Management at this Stage

Before the advent of Lasers, the port-wine stains were covered with various creams going by the trade name 'COVERMARK' to camouflage the colour difference.

Pulsed dye laser is now being used to remove the port-wine stain (Refer Chapter 6 on Lasers).

With the passage of time (a few years), capillaries in the dermis show dilatation. The tissue between the blood vessels increase and may show hyperkeratinization and nodularity (Figs 5.25A and B). The hyperkeratotic skin, if it is cosmetically unacceptable, can be excised and resurfaced with skin graft.

Figure 5.26 shows a mechanical ptosis due to a hyper keratotic skin whose forehead had been treated earlier with a skin graft, Figures 5.26A and B. The thickened keratotic skin on the eyelid was excised and the ptosis corrected by appropriate resurfacing.

VENOUS MALFORMATIONS OF THE ORBIT[6]

Orbital venous malformations are presumed to result from the congenital weaknesses in the postcapillary venous wall[9] (Smoker RK et al, 2008). As there is continuous pressure in the veins, the venous elements proliferate and this leads to the dilation of

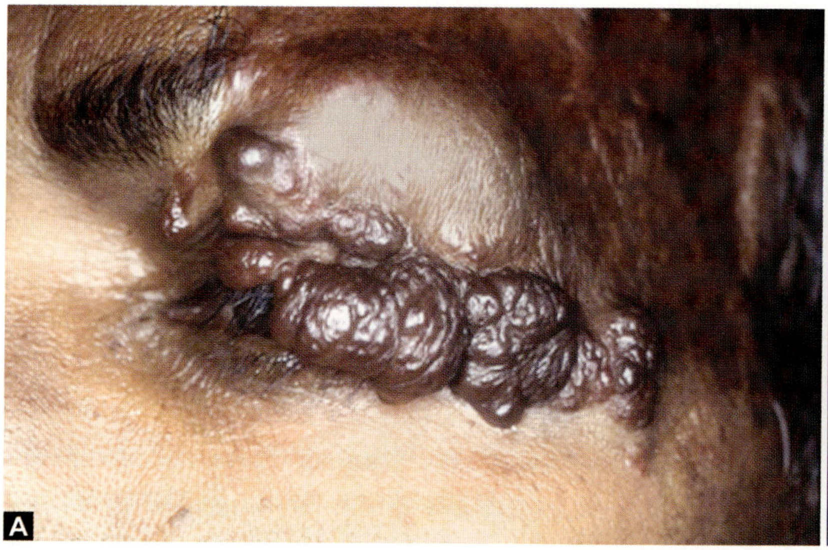

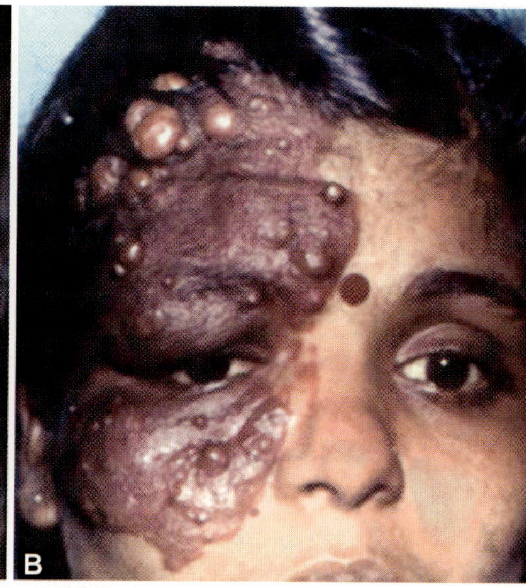

FIGURES 5.25A and B

Hyperkeratosis in capillary Malformations: (A) Localised V2 eyelid lesion with mechanical ptosis and nodularity; (B) Extensive V1 and V2 lesion producing hyperkeratosis and nodularity in that region and mechanical ptosis

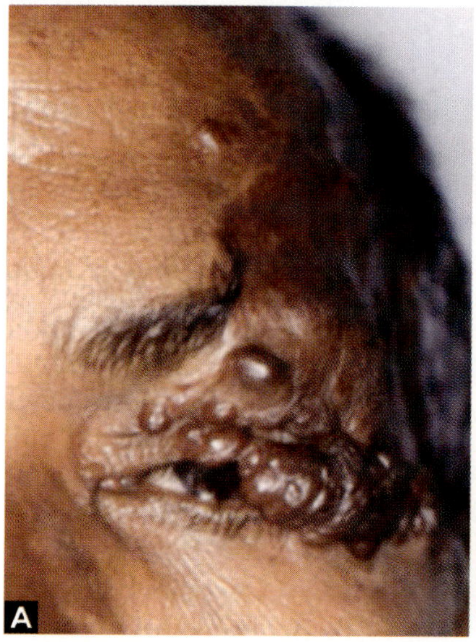

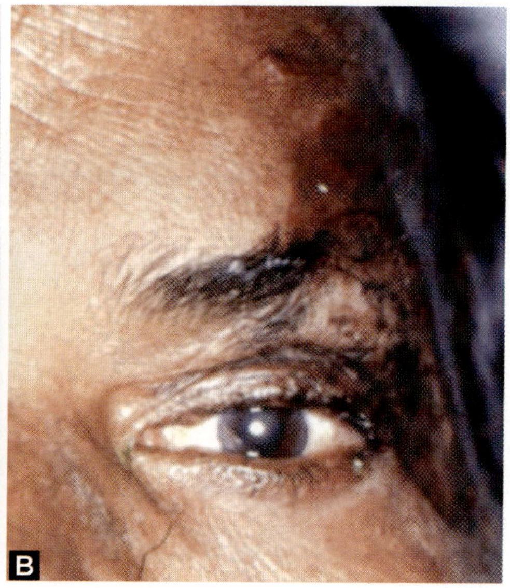

FIGURES 5.26A and B

Ptosis due to Hyperkeratotic skin: (A and B) Hyperkeratotic nodules producing mechanical ptosis. Excision and skin grafting to correct ptosis

the veins which are valveless in the orbit. These anomalies are quite rare. They are congenital but usually present in the second or third decades of life. The first symptom to be noticed is often intermittent proptosis of the eye, which may be associated with situations caused by increased venous pressure. Depending on the size of communication with the systemic venous system, they are divided into distensible and nondistensible orbital venous anomalies. Depeding on their anatomical location, like the Lymphangiomas, they too can also be categorized into four types as Superficial, Deep, Combined, and Complex.

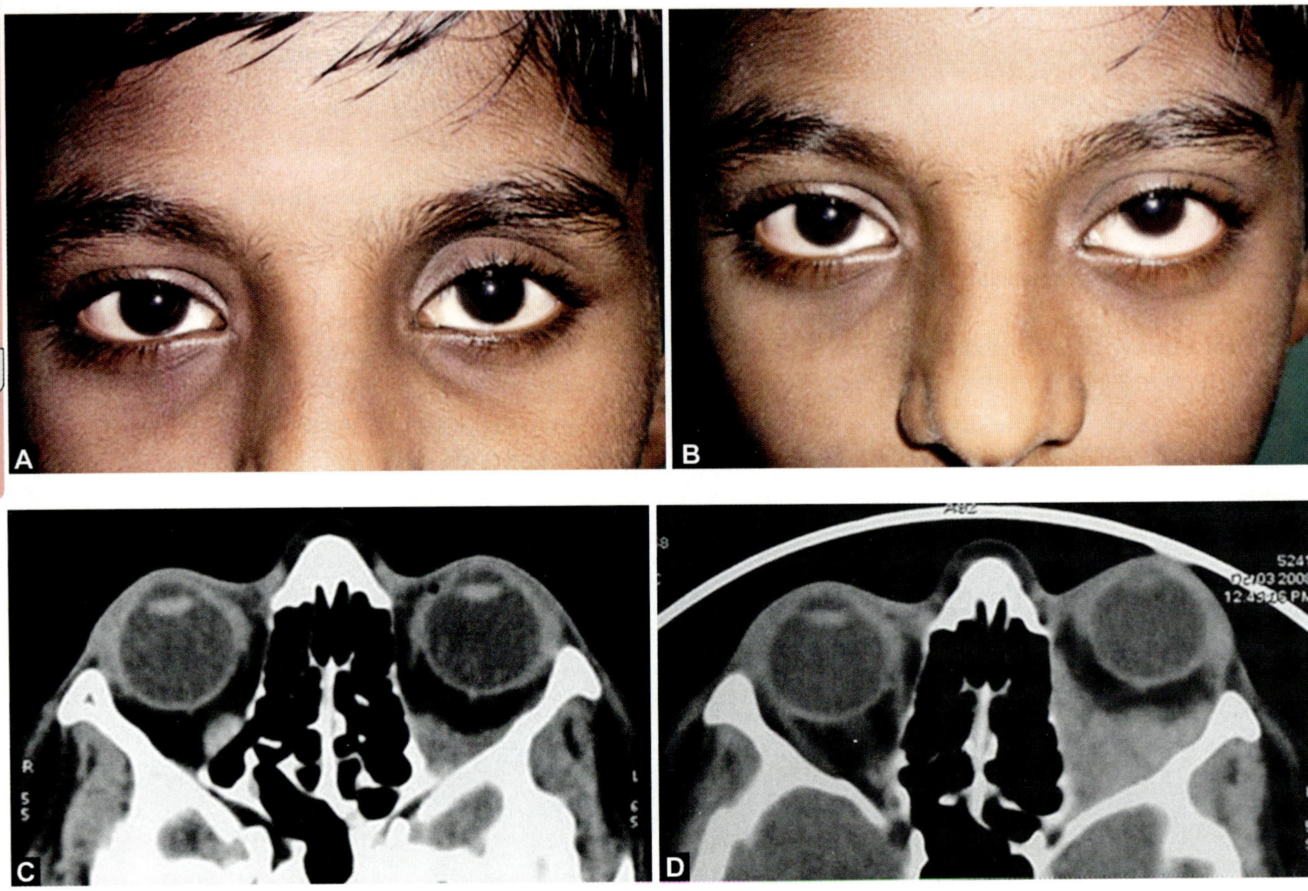

FIGURES 5.27A to D
Orbital Varix with a positive Valsalva test: (A) A young lad of fourteen years shows a mild proptosis; (B). In upright position only a deepening of the suprasulcus area is seen; (C) The axial CT Scan shows the lesion and the mild proptosis; (D) Following Valsalva maneuver, there is significant increase in the size of the lesion, causing proptosis

Orbital Varix—The Distensible Orbital Venous Malformation

The distensible venous malformation is commonly known as an Orbital Varix. It consists of irregular distension of segments of a vein and has a connection to the systemic venous system. The degree of distension depends on the size of the connecting vein. They may be first noticed when the person gets up from sleep but disappears when they sit up. Proptosis may be obvious when they cough or strain. The fourteen year young lad seen in Figure 5.27A complained of a swelling of the left eye on bending down or while coughing. In upright position, a deepening of the supra sulcus area of the upper eyelid was seen, Figure 5.27B. A CT study revealed a homogenous enhancing extraconal mass showing a significant increase accompanied by proptosis following a Valsalva maneuver, Figures 5.27 C and D.

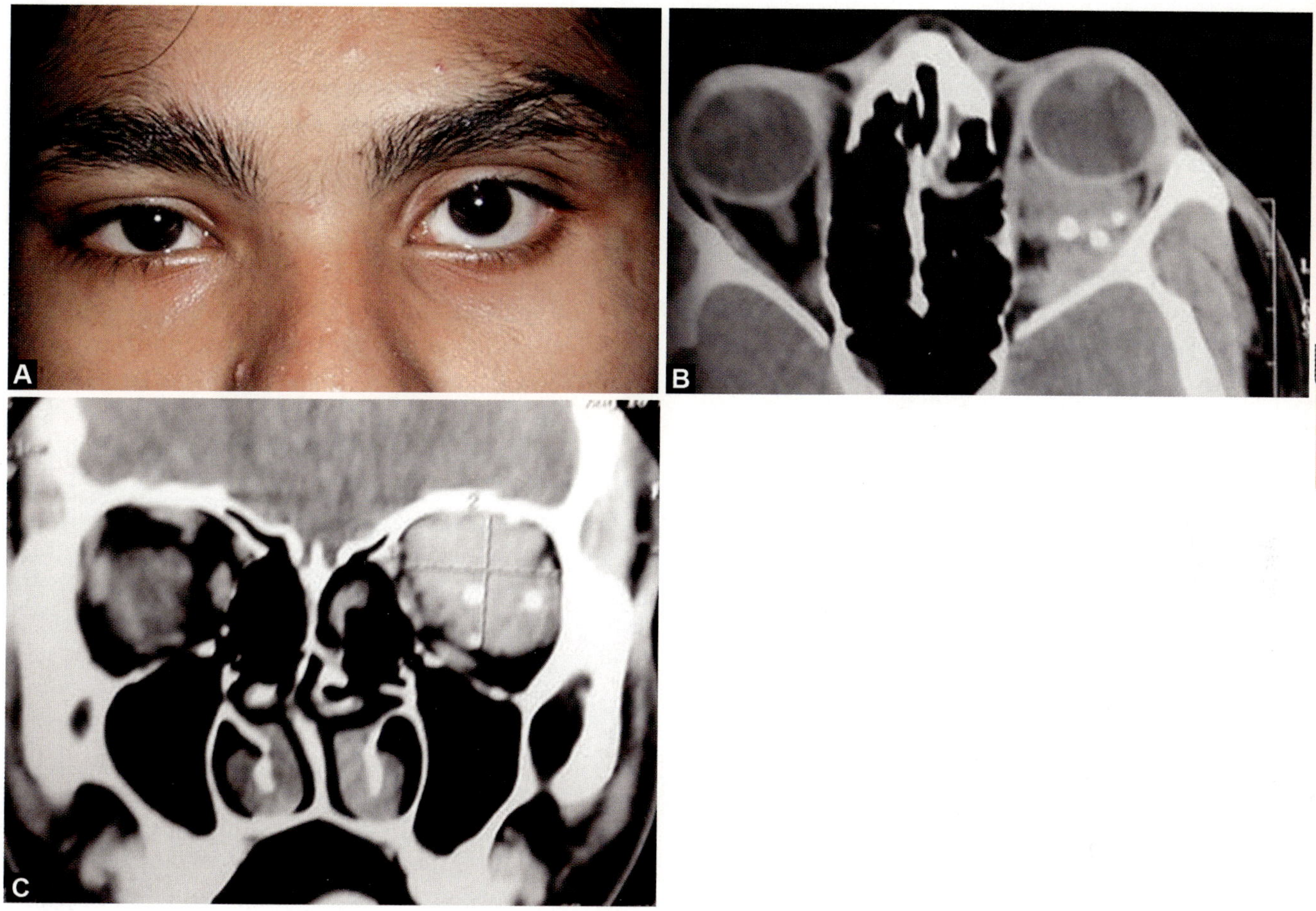

FIGURES 5.28A to C
An Intraconal Orbital Varix: (A) Patient with history of proptosis on bending down. No other symptoms; (B and C) CT Scans show a large lobulated enhancing mass lesion, retrobulbar area predominantly intraconal, multiple phleboliths, managed conservatively

An Intraconal Orbital Varix

Figure 5.28A shows a sixteen-year-old boy presented with history of proptosis on bending down of two years duration, with normal vision and no other symptoms. CT Scan shows a large lobulated enhancing mass in the left retrobulbar area predominantly in the intraconal space, with multiple phleboliths which was managed conservatively, Figures 5.28B and C.

There is no sex predilection. Generally, they are painless but when the intravenous pressure increases they may have mild to severe pain. There are no visual complaints. In long standing cases, enophthalmos is noticed as a deep superior sulcus deformity.

Women may complain that they are unable to do the household work due to proptosis.

If the patient complains of acute proptosis with severe pain, or the proptosis does not reduce, it usually implies that the varix has thrombosed. Severe pain and tenderness may also be noticed.

Orbital Varix Investigations

USG

Orbital varix is not detected by USG, if it is collapsed. The patient is asked to perform a Valsalva maneuver or put the head down. The venous spaces get filled and are seen as well outlined low to medium reflective lesions in the orbit. A varix can be in the shape of a blood vessel or resemble a mass. During examination, it has to be differentiated from the superior ophthalmic vein, which also distends slightly on increase in the venous pressure.

CT Scan

In the supine position, a CT scan may not show any positive findings. Hence, it is better to do it in a prone position or do a Valsalva maneuver or increase the venous pressure by pressing the neck to allow the varix to get filled.

An orbital varix appears as a well defined elongated mass lesion within the orbit, often with a club like configuration with a tapering end towards the orbital apex. Orbital enlargement and phleboliths are features of long standing cases.

The density and enhancement of the varices depends on the patency of its lumen. Thrombosis or hemorrhage will not show enhancement, whereas patent lumen will show brilliant enhancement.

MR Imaging

The MR signal will depend on the presence of flow within the varix. Patent lumen will appear as an area of flow void on both T1 and T2 weighted scans. Contrast enhancement is variable and may be absent. Slow flow or thrombus will give it a slight heterogeneous appearance. The use of fat saturation with contrast enhancement on MR imaging helps to delineate the varix better.

Intra cranial venous anomalies are associated with intraorbital venous anomalies. Hence, they should be looked for during evaluation by imaging.[9]

Direct venography will give a confirmative diagnosis. But with the advent of MRI, a noninvasive and yet a clear picture is available.

Histopathology

Congenital varix appears as a collection of blood filled channels of varying diameters and are seen lined with mature flattened endothelial cells. Disorganized smooth muscle fibers are seen in between. Phleboliths, inflammatory cell and thrombosis are seen in the channels.[20]

Management of Distensible Orbital Venous Malformations

Vascular anomaly of the orbit, which do not present with pain, episodes of hemorrhage or problems in vision can be managed conservatively. If there is any cosmetic disfigurement, a complete investigation must be done and depending on the degree of disfigurement, the treatment is planned. Sudden proptosis, or decrease in vision and pain are indications for surgical exploration.

Superficial and well circumscribed lesions which are well demonstrated by CT Scan and MRI, can be excised surgically with abundant precaution. The veins are thin walled and bleed excessively. If facilities are available, they can be sclerosed preoperatively and percutaneously after an angiogram and then excised.

Superficial and diffuse lesions are difficult to excise completely. They can be sclerosed prior to excision. However, the confines of the orbital space crowded with delicate structures possesses limitations and risks. Hence, alcohol or hypertonic saline, which can produce severe irritation, swelling, pain or congestion and pose a threat to vision, should not be used. The varix can be exposed and under vision it can be solidified with Cyanoacrylate glue and excised. Recently Tisseel fibrin glue has also been tried[8] (Boulos R Patric, 2005).

For deep lesion, embolization can be done prior to surgery or after exposing it surgically. Excision becomes a little easier after the lesion is thus embolized. The help of an interventional radiologist for percutaneous embolization is invaluable.

The major intraoperative complication is bleeding. Hence, blood should be available for the surgery.

The Nondistensible Orbital Venous Malformation

The nondistensible orbital venous malformations are a mass of ecstatic venous channels. They have a smaller communication with the venous system. Due to this smaller communication they do not increase during Valsalva maneuver. They may be present as a tangled mass of veins palpable in the upper or lower eyelids. Acute symptoms occur due to infection or thrombosis, and the presentation then would be pain and swelling in the lower or upper eyelids.

For nondistensible venous malformation, surgical excision is ideal.[10] Depending on the location, the exposure is planned. The mass is actually a cluster of veins which has already thrombosed. It may present as a tender mass in the upper or lower eyelid. Initially they can be excised but it is important to ligate the draining veins because the vein may retract and start bleeding which would then be quite difficult to control. In the orbit, it is very difficult to catch a bleeder and ligate it due to space constraints. Figures 5.29A and B illustrates the case of a thirty year old lady who complained of visible vessels on pulling the lower lid down and discomfort on bending down. CT Scan shows an ill defined isodense lobulated enhancing lesion in the left inferior periocular region, enveloping the inferior ocular surface with posterior extent just beyond globe, Figures 5.29C to F. Linear brilliant enhancing area is seen just posterior to the globe—a blood vessel. The excision of the convoluted mass of veins through conjunctival incision. The feeding vein was ligated. Figures 5.29G and H show the result six weeks later. The ill defined shadows appear to be a small residual lesion, Figure 5.29I.

ORBITAL HEMATOMA

Orbital hematoma though not a vascular lesion is a common complication seen after blunt trauma or in a pre-existing lesions like lymphangioma, hemangioma and orbital varix. Other causes are coagulation disorders, hypertensive disease, etc. These hematomas may be present in the subperiosteal space or in the intraorbital soft tissue.

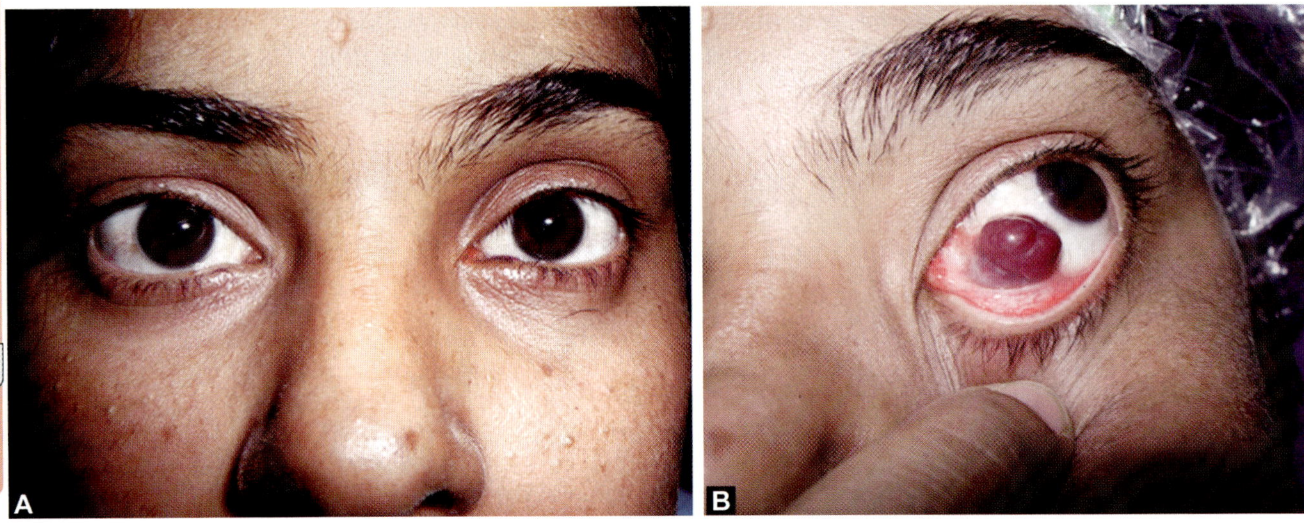

FIGURES 5.29A and B
A nondistensible orbital venous malformation: (A and B) A small lobulated vascular mass in the lower fornix seen on retracting the lower lid

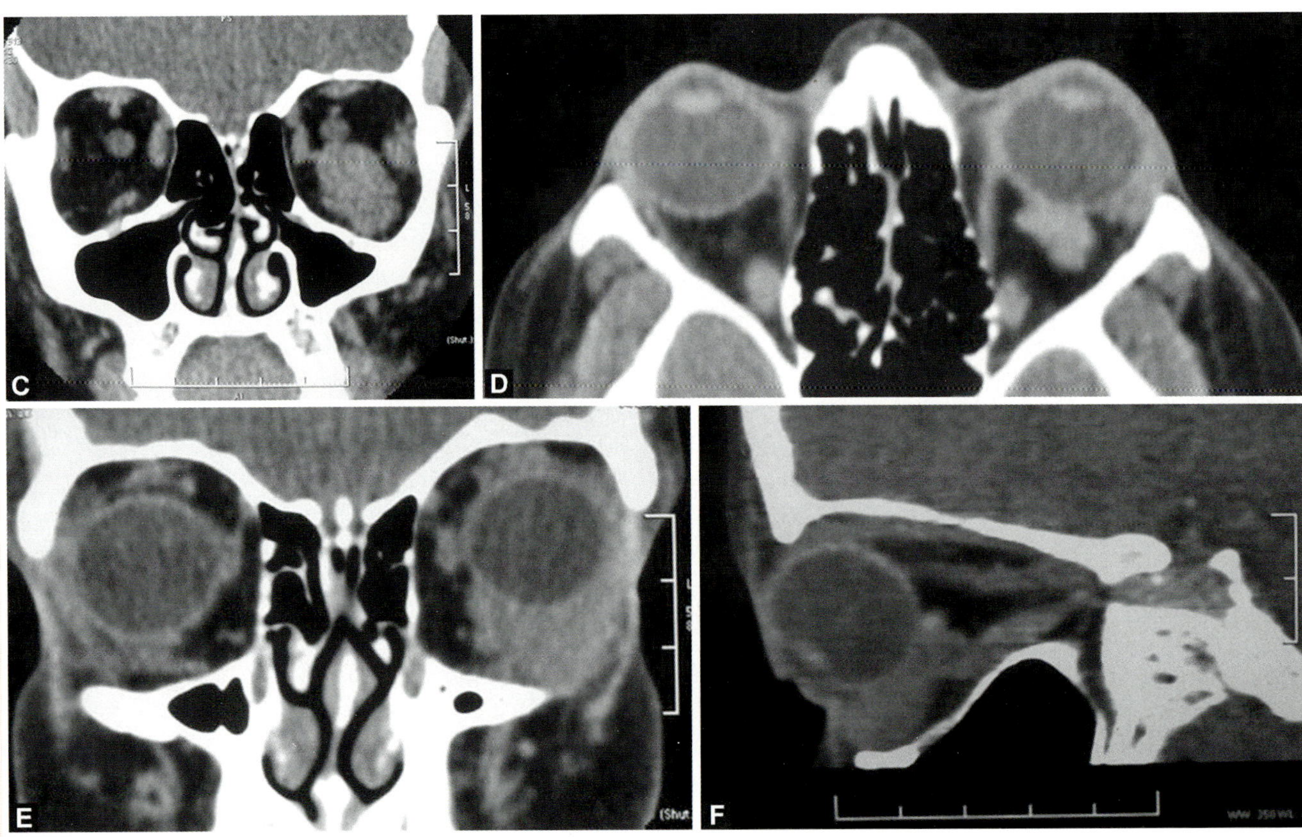

FIGURES 5.29C to F
CT Studies shows an ill defined isodense lobulated enhancing lesion in the left inferior periocular region

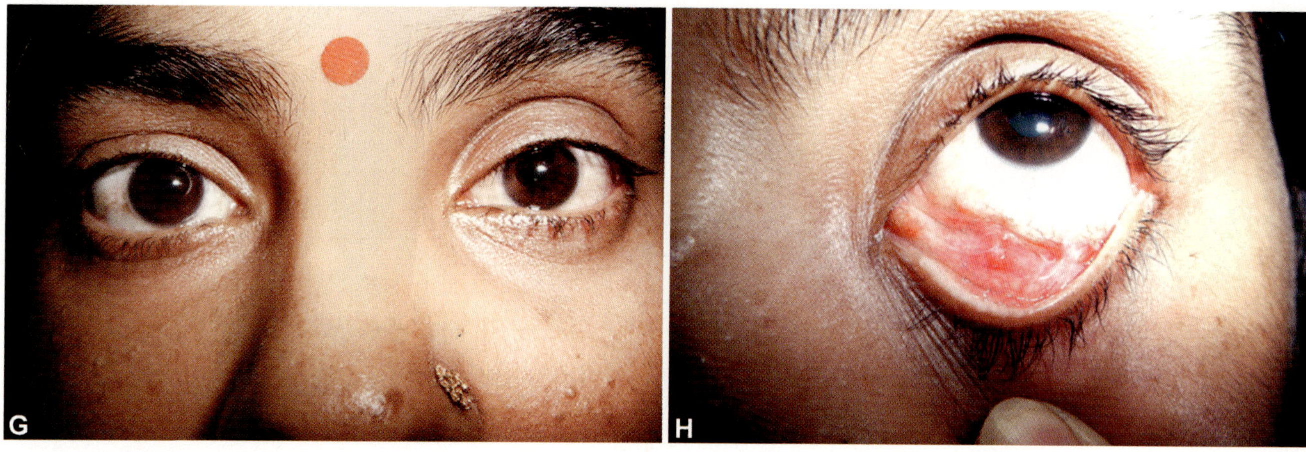

FIGURES 5.29G and H
The result six weeks after surgery through a conjunctiva incision in the lower fornix

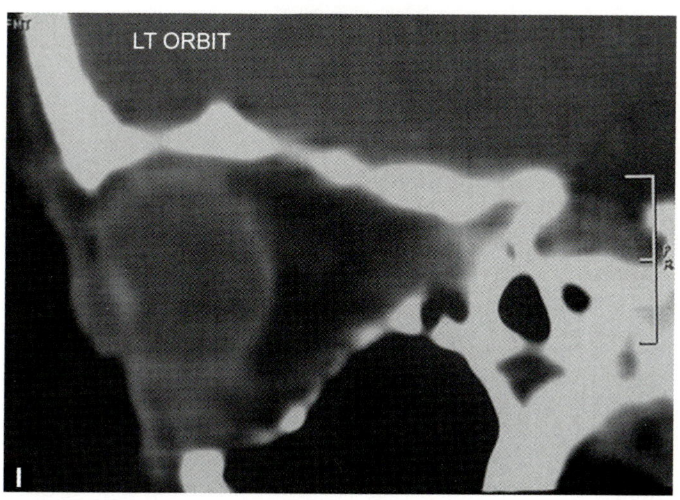

FIGURE 5.29 I
Postoperative CT Scan suggestive of an ill defined residual mass

Imaging

Imaging is the most valuable tool in the diagnosis and the localization of the lesion and in planning the surgical approach.

CT Scan localizes the anatomical location of the lesion in the orbit. The subperiosteal hematomas appear as sharply defined homogenous non-enhancing mass. Any skeletal injury, deformity or erosion are easily identified.

The MRI gives high signal on T1 and T2 weighted images showing characteristics of blood products.

Ultrasonographic guidance enhances the safety and precision of aspiration of an orbital hematoma.

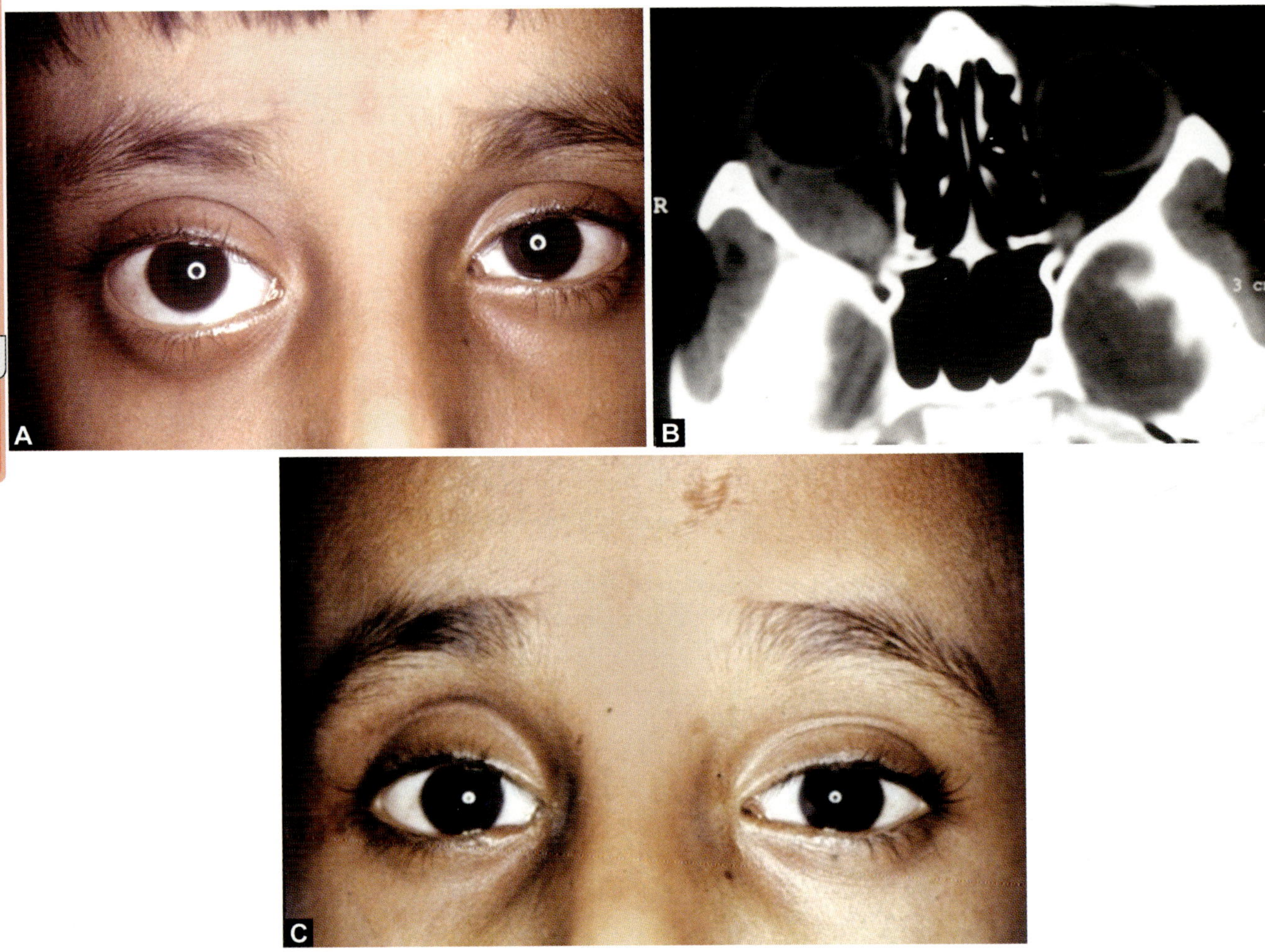

FIGURES 5.30A to C

Orbital hematoma following a Blunt Injury: (A) A twelve-year-old boy with proptosis following a blunt injury. No ecchymosis; (B) CT Scan showed a diffuse, laterally located mass in the lateral side of orbit; (C) After the hematoma was aspirated under ultrasound control

Clinical Presentation

Present as a sudden onset proptosis after a blunt trauma or as gradually increasing proptosis. There may be decrease in vision, diplopia, limitation of ocular movements or blepharptosis. There may be associated pain, swelling or erythema of eyelids or palpable orbital mass. Patient may present some years after trauma with swelling or displacement of globe with secondary pressure effects.

The 12-year-old boy shown in Figure 5.30A presented with a proptosis following a blunt injury. There was no ecchymosis. The CT Scan showed the intraorbital laterally located diffuse mass which was aspirated under ultrasound control, Figures 5.30B and C.

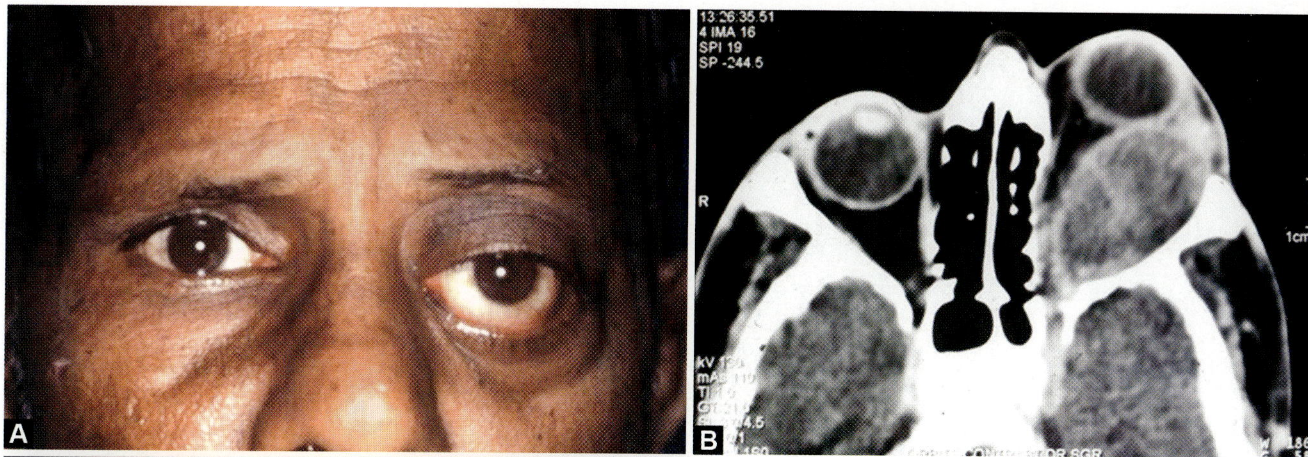

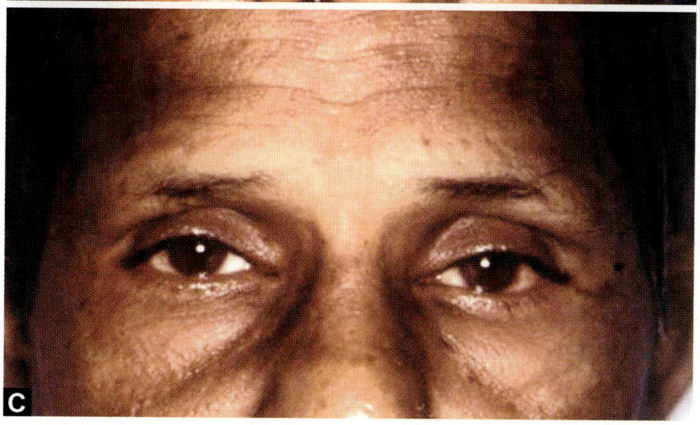

FIGURES 5.31A to C
Orbital Hematoma — A bleed from an Orbital Varix: (A) A middle aged male presented with sudden onset of proptosis with pain; (B) Axial CT Scan shows a large non enhancing hypodense lesion in the lateral orbit; (C) After a lateral Orbitotomy, control of a severe bleed, and an uneventful recovery. No disturbance in vision

Figure 5.31A shows a middle aged man who presented with a sudden development of proptosis and pain. A CT study revealed a large nonenhancing hypodense lesion in the lateral orbit, Figure 5.31B. A lateral orbitotomy was done. Severe bleeding was encountered and controlled. The recovery was uneventful and the vision totally undisturbed, Figure 5.31C. The whole event appeared to be a hematoma from a bleed in an orbital varix.

An organized hematoma needs a surgical evaluation.

CAVERNOUS VENOUS MALFORMATIONS (CAVERNOUS HEMANGIOMAS)

Cavernous VMs of the orbit are the most common benign noninfiltrative vascular lesions in adults. While removing a cavernous hemangioma hardly any vessel, which needs ligation or cauterization, is encountered They are generally seen in the third and fourth decades of life. In the western literature, they are seen more commonly in females but in our series no female preponderance was seen[19] (Subramaniam N and Selvarangan R, 1989).

Patients generally present with complaints of gradual onset of painless proptosis. Sometimes noticed incidentally in the imaging done for investigating a headache. The direction of the globe displacement is determined by the location of the lesion in the orbit. Generally the proptosis is axial, if the lesion is situated in the intraconal space. Proptosis is eccentric if the mass is situated in the extraconal space. They are generally solitary, rarely multiple, Figure 5.35E. They may be palpable under the lids if anteriorly placed.

Vision disturbance, diplopia can occur as the lesion increases in size. Exposure keratitis can occur in a severe proptosis. When the lesion is in the apex of the orbit, early changes in vision can occur due to the pressure on the optic nerve or artery.

Bone remodeling occurs due to long standing slow mass effect. Occasionally, pain along with chemosis of conjunctiva or swelling of the lid is seen.

Extraocular muscle involvement is due to the mass effect as the lesion does not infiltrate the muscle.

As the patient presents with proptosis, it is important to rule out other space occupying lesions of the orbit with investigations. A complete ophthalmological examination is very important.

INVESTIGATIONS

USG

A-scan: USG shows well defined borders due to the pseudocapsule. Moderate to high density internal reflectivity is observed due to large vascular spaces. There is acoustic alteration due to blood.

B-scan: It demonstrates a little compressible, well defined rounded lesion within the muscle cone. Doppler may show slow flow.

CT scan

CT scan shows a well circumscribed round or oval mass with well defined margins due to the pseudocapsule. It is also slightly hyperdense with marked contrast enhancement. The presence of phleboliths is pathognomonic of cavernous malformation and may be seen as small, round calcified deposits of varying sizes. Enlargement or indentation of orbital wall may be seen due to pressure. Optic nerve and extraocular muscle may be pushed due to the lesion.

The mass is usually intraconal in location, though it can be present anywhere in the orbit. They are usually single but can be multiple.

MRI Imaging

The mass is isointense on T1 weighted images and hyperintense on T2 weighted images. On heavily T2 weighted images, they are almost isointense to vitreous. On dynamic post contrast study, there will be a homogenous enhancement with slow filling towards the center. In large lesions, MRI will help to delineate the lesion from the optic nerve Figs 5.35B and C.

MANAGEMENT

Surgical Ablation

The management of cavernous hemangiomas depends upon the signs and symptoms with which they present. Very small cavernous hemangiomas, which do not produce any signs or symptoms and have been noticed during neuroimaging done for other conditions, need to be closely observed.

Lesions which show signs of visual compromise due to their location at the apex of the orbit or proximity to optic nerve need early intervention.

Patients who present for proptosis or exposure keratitis need an Orbitotomy to ablate them. The location of the lesion in the orbit, considerably influences the selection of the Surgical approach.

Surgical approaches to orbit are the same as detailed for the lymphatic malformations.

The choice depends on the location of the lesion. A CT scan is very useful in planning the approach as it gives a clear picture of the bony anatomical relationship of the lesion to the orbit.

For lesions which are situated very posteriorly at the apex of the orbit, very close to the optic nerve and with extension into the optic canal, the surgical approach is superior via a Craniotomy. This is done along with a neurosurgeon or by a craniofacial surgery team (see Fig. 7.7). Examples of the other approaches commonly used follow.

Anterior Superior Orbitotomy

Figure 5.32A shows a thirty-year-old man who presented with a gradual painless proptosis of the right eye. The globe was pushed down and out. Vision and ocular movements were normal. The CT (Figs 5.32B to D) studies precisely located the lesion which was removed through an anterior superior orbitotomy approach. The histopathology cofirmed the diagnosis of a cavernous hemangioma, Figure 5.32F.

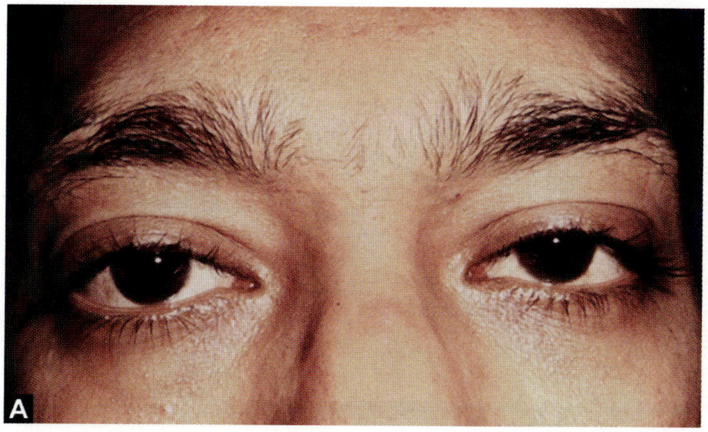

FIGURE 5.32A
A cavernous hemangioma in the roof of the orbit. A gradually increasing painless proptosis (Right eye)

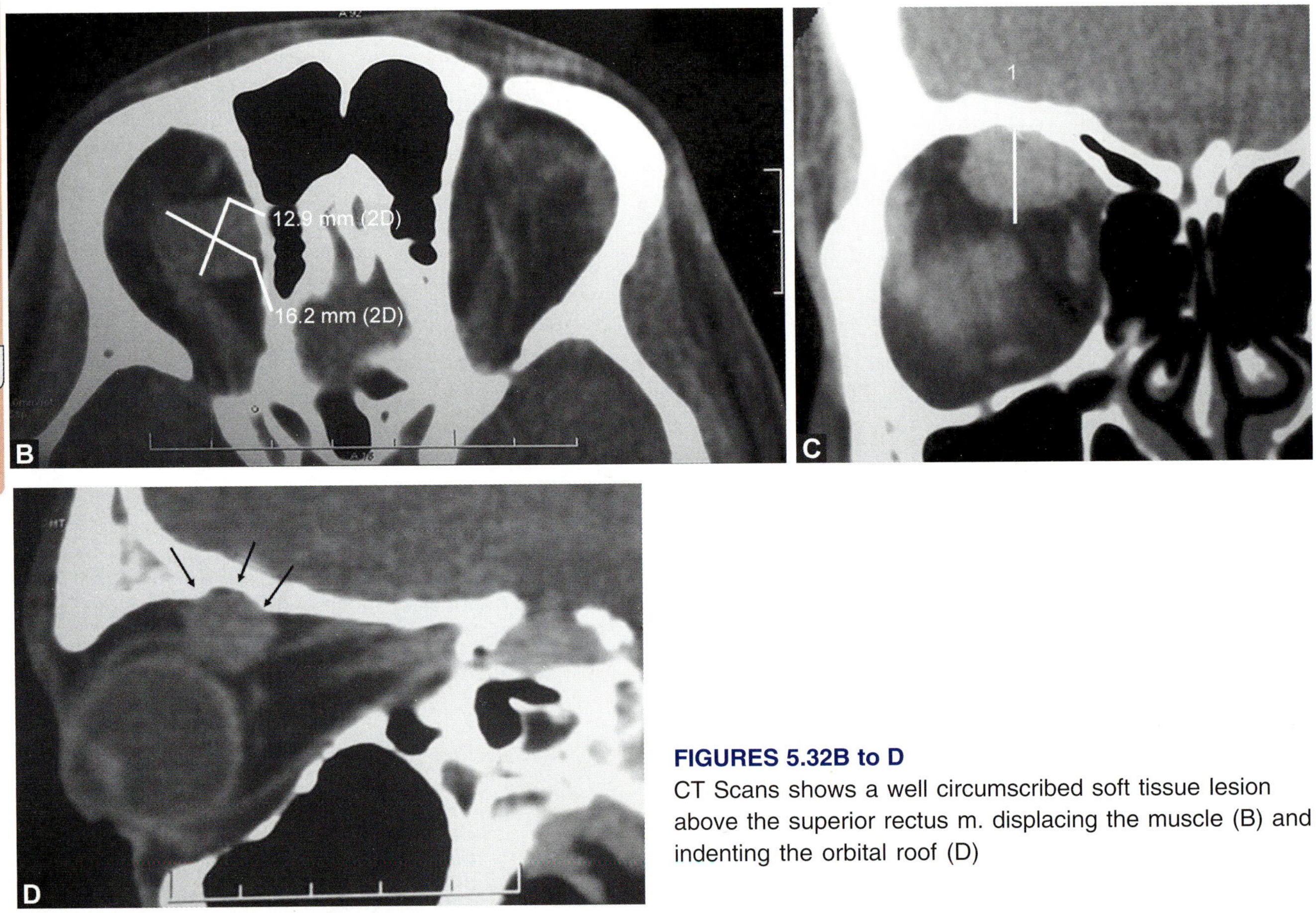

FIGURES 5.32B to D
CT Scans shows a well circumscribed soft tissue lesion above the superior rectus m. displacing the muscle (B) and indenting the orbital roof (D)

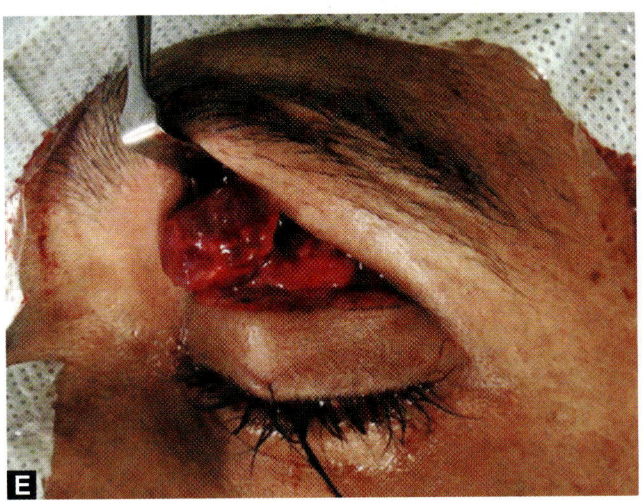

FIGURE 5.32E
Anterior Superior Orbitotomy through supratarsal fold incision showing the lesion being delivered

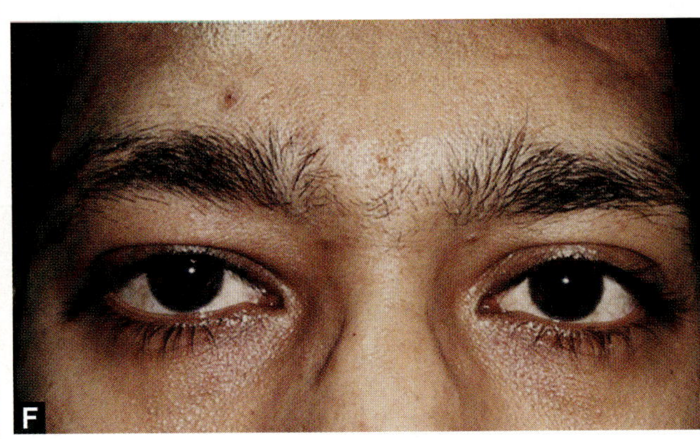

FIGURE 5.32F
Postoperative status: No proptosis, normal vision, no obvious scarring. Complete restoration of normalcy. Diagnosis confirmed by histopathology

Anterior Inferior Transconjunctival Orbitotomy

Figure 5.33A shows a cavernous hemangioma in the inferolateral part of the orbit as a painless mild proptosis and a mild swelling in the lateral part of the lower lid of 10 years duration Figure 5.33A. The vision was not affected. A change of posture or the Valsalva test did not change the size of the swelling. It was exposed through an anterior inferior transconjunctival orbitotomy. The result shows the restoration to a normal appearance. The vision too was normal.

Lateral Orbitotomy

Figures 5.34A and B depicts the story of a 34-years-male who presented with a painless and gradually increasing axial proptosis of 6 years duration with a gradual diminution of vision, more in the last few months. The MRI showed an infraconal mass displacing upwards the optic nerve. The lesion is filling the orbital cavity upto its apex and compressing the optic nerve, Figures 5.34C and D. The lateral orbitotomy showed a large, well encapsulated intraconal red mass. It was decompressed and removed, Figures 5.34E and F. The deformity was corrected but the vision continued to be poor.

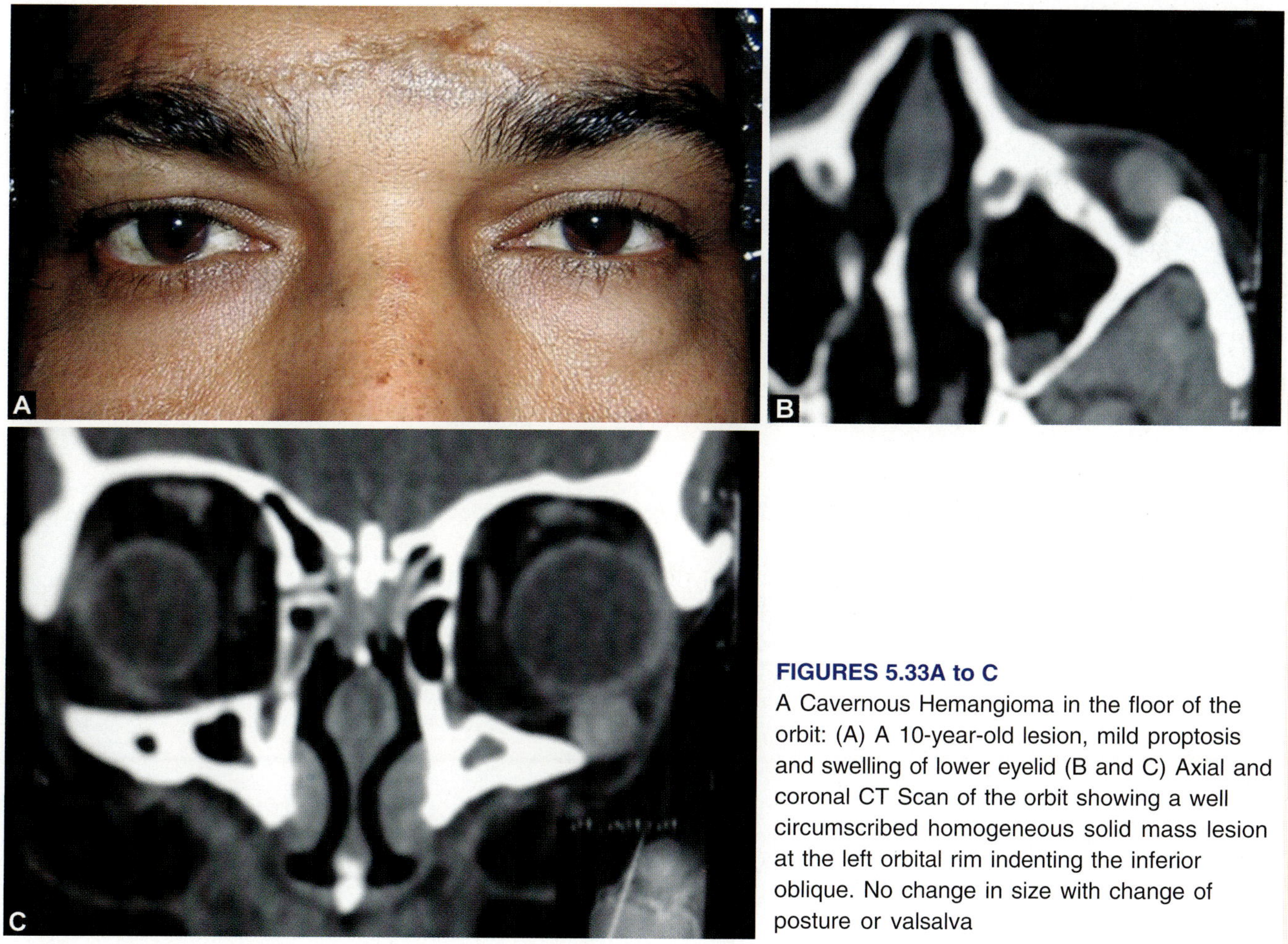

FIGURES 5.33A to C
A Cavernous Hemangioma in the floor of the orbit: (A) A 10-year-old lesion, mild proptosis and swelling of lower eyelid (B and C) Axial and coronal CT Scan of the orbit showing a well circumscribed homogeneous solid mass lesion at the left orbital rim indenting the inferior oblique. No change in size with change of posture or valsalva

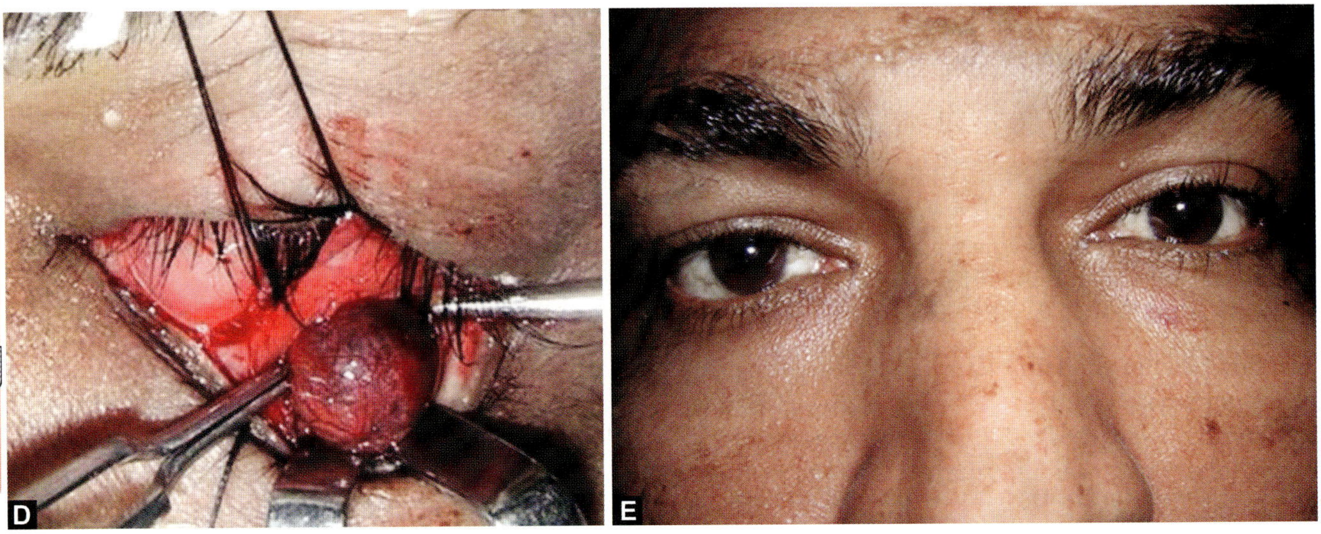

FIGURES 5.33D and E

(D) Shows the anterior inferior orbitotomy through a conjunctival incision, with a well defined red mass in postseptal area; (E) The postoperative picture. Diagnosis confirmed by histopathology

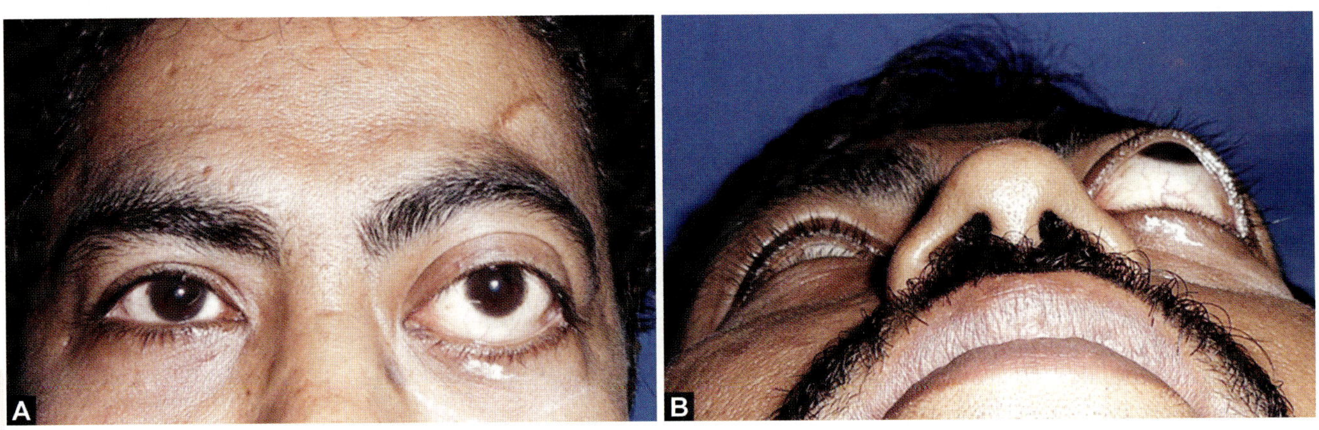

FIGURES 5.34A and B

A cavernous hemangioma with Axial Proptosis: (A and B) Shows the axial proptosis of six years duration and with gradual diminution of vision

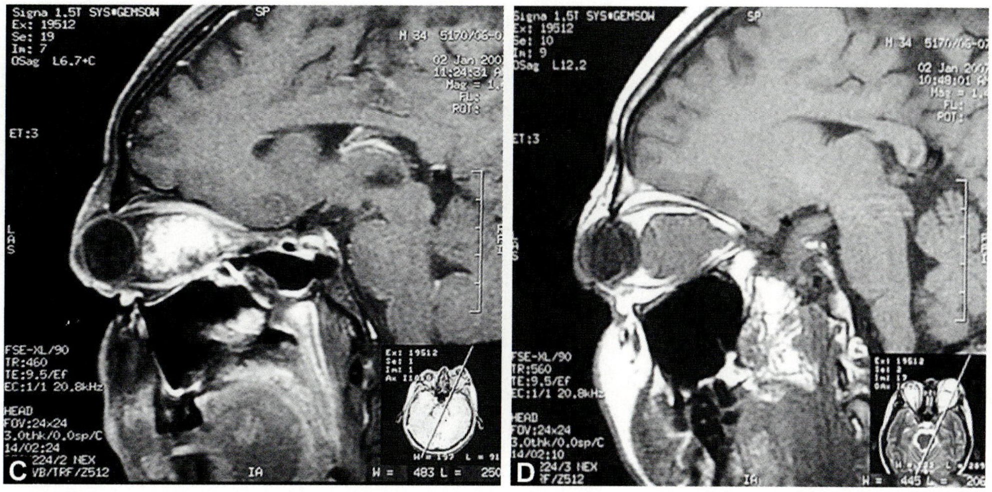

FIGURES 5.34C and D

(C and D) MRI Studies show the circumscribed solid intraconal mass inferior to optic nerve displaying an isointense signal in T1W1 and hyperintense signal in T2W1 weighted images with a homogenous central enhancement on immediate postcontrast scan. The lesion is filling the orbital cavity upto its apex

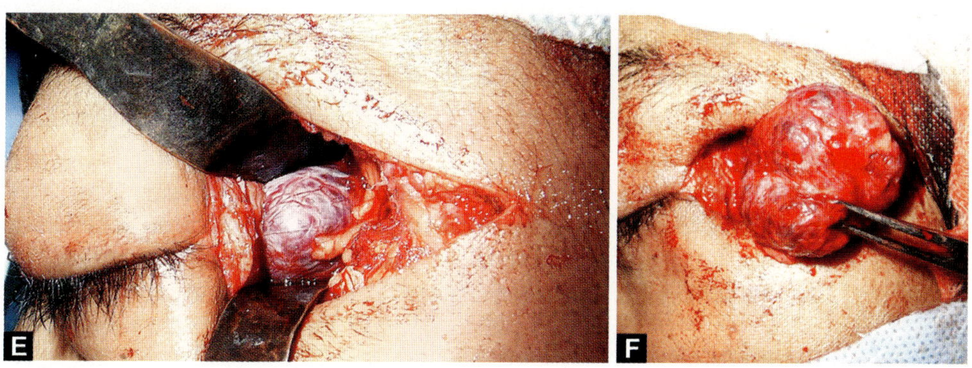

FIGURES 5.34E and F

(E and F) Lateral orbitotomy shows a large, well encapsulated red mass, intraconal, mass which was decompressed and removed. Diagnosis confirmed by histopathology

Multiple Cavernous Hemangiomas

Multiple cavernous hemangiomas are rare but can occur and must be kept in mind. The middle aged lady seen in Figures 5.35A and B, presented with a gradual onset of proptosis with no pain and no restriction of ocular movements but a diminution of vision for the past six months. Figures 5.35C to E define the extent of the lesion in a post-contrast scan. A lateral orbitotomy was done and a large well encapsulated mass was removed. As the proptosis did not completely reduce on the table, further exploration showed another mass posterior to the main mass, which was also removed. The proptosis was totally corrected but there was no significant improvement in vision, Figures 5.35F and G.

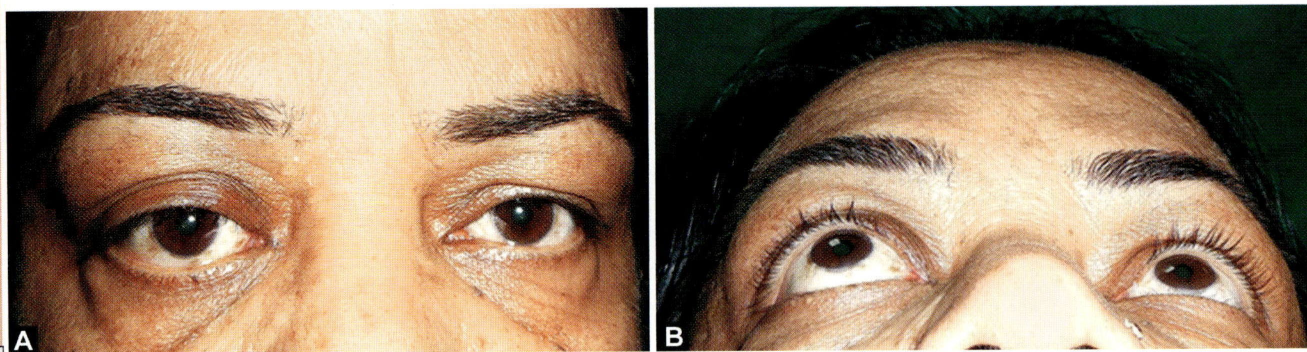

FIGURES 5.35A and B

Multiple cavernous hemangiomas: (A and B) The patient who presented with gradual onset of proptosis in right eye, with diminution of vision of six months duration

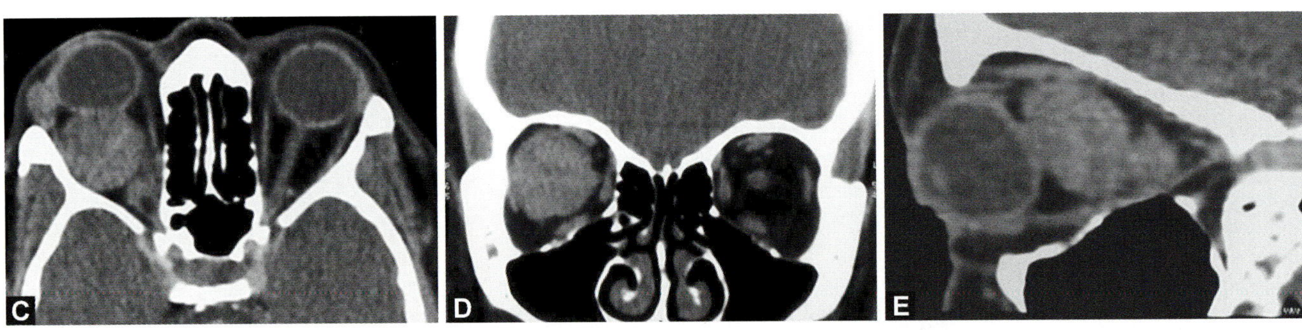

FIGURES 5.35C to E

(C to E) Shows, the axial, coronal and sagittal reconstructions in a post contrast CT study of the orbit, showing the lesions

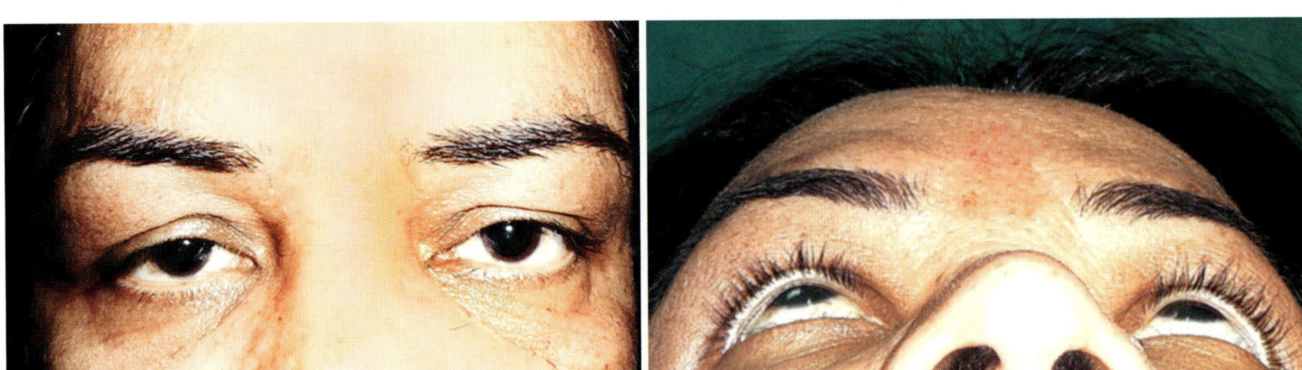

FIGURES 5.35F and G

The follow up pictures show complete disappearance of proptosis. The vision remained at the preoperative level

Removal of Cavernous Malformations — A Few Observations

Most of the cavernous venous malformations are situated intraconally. Lateral orbitotomy is the ideal choice for lesions situated in the lateral part of the orbit. In lateral orbitotomy, the lateral wall of the orbit, mainly the frontal process of zygoma is removed. The periorbita is dissected and the lateral rectus muscle is identified and retracted to enter the intraconal space.

The cavernous hemangioma is seen as a well encapsulated lobulated purplish red mass. It is easily dissected all around due to the pseudocapsule. A cryoprobe is very useful to hold the mass during dissection as the tip of the probe freezes the mass and gets stuck to it. If the mass is very large, it can be decompressed for easy removal. Usually no major bleeders are encountered. Occasionally, adhesions may be found posteriorly which have to be cauterized. Once the mass has been delivered, the reduction of proptosis is very dramatic as is obvious on comparing photographs A and B with F and G in Figure 5.35.

Medially placed lesions can be approached through transcaruncular or external medial Orbitotomy. They can also be approached with the help of a nasoendoscope through the nose via the ethmoid sinus. Multiple cavernous hemangiomas are rare but must be excluded. For lesions which are situated very posteriorly at the apex of the orbit, or very close to the optic nerve and with extension into the optic canal, the surgical approach is done via a Craniotomy (as shown in Fig. 7.7). This case was done along with a neurosurgeon by a craniofacial team.

Complications

The most disturbing complication after surgery for removal of these lesions is an adverse effect on the vision. It is rare, but can occur, if the lesion is very close to the optic nerve. It is due to direct pull on the nerve or indirectly due to an injury to the retinal vessels. Therefore, it is important to monitor the pupil throughout the surgery. As the lesion is well encapsulated and does not have any infiltrating characteristics, ocular muscle deficits are not seen.

AVMs — Arterio Venous Malformations

Congenital arteriovenous malformations of orbit are very rare. Their presence results in an almost direct flow from the arterial to the venous side resulting in a back flow in the orbital and periorbital veins. Bruits and pulsations are felt over the eyelids. Patient has severe pain and visual disturbance is noted.

Treatment is mainly by interventional radiology. Once the embolization has been done, the lesion can be surgically excised. Care must be taken to see that the nidus is removed to prevent recurrence. The patient in Figure 5.36A was 17-year-old, when she presented with a pulsatile swelling on the medial side of the right upper eyelid. She complained of pain in the area and the lesion was red and warm. A DSA study and the embolization with Cyanoacrylate glue is shown in Figures 5.36C to G. The lesion was excised a week later with an excellent result seen in Figure 5.36H.

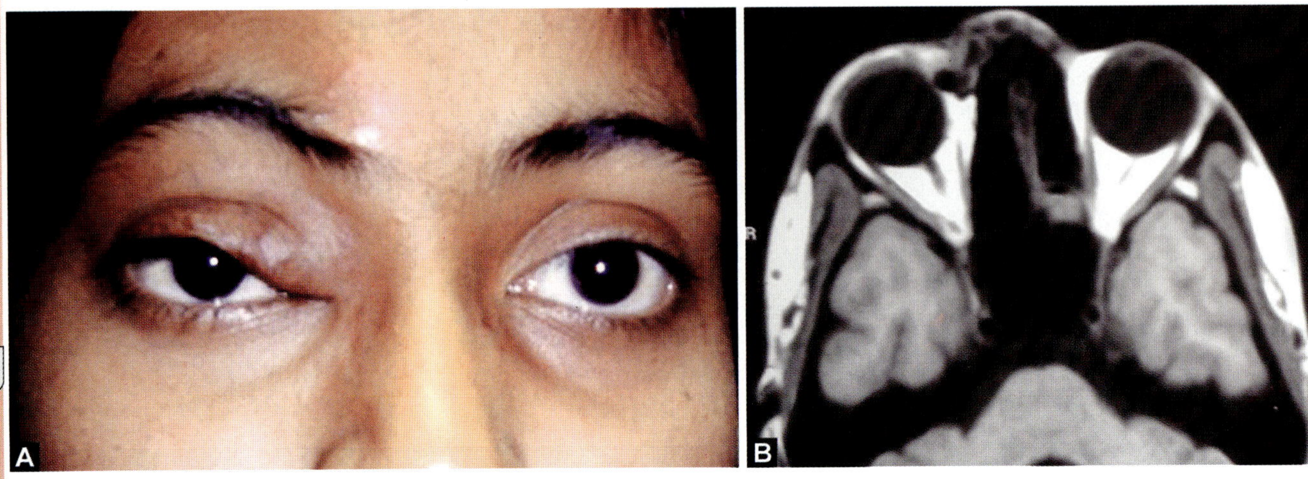

FIGURES 5.36A and B

An Arterio Venous Malformation: (A) A lesion red, warm and pulsatile in the medial side of upper eyelid; (B) An MRI image showing the lesion

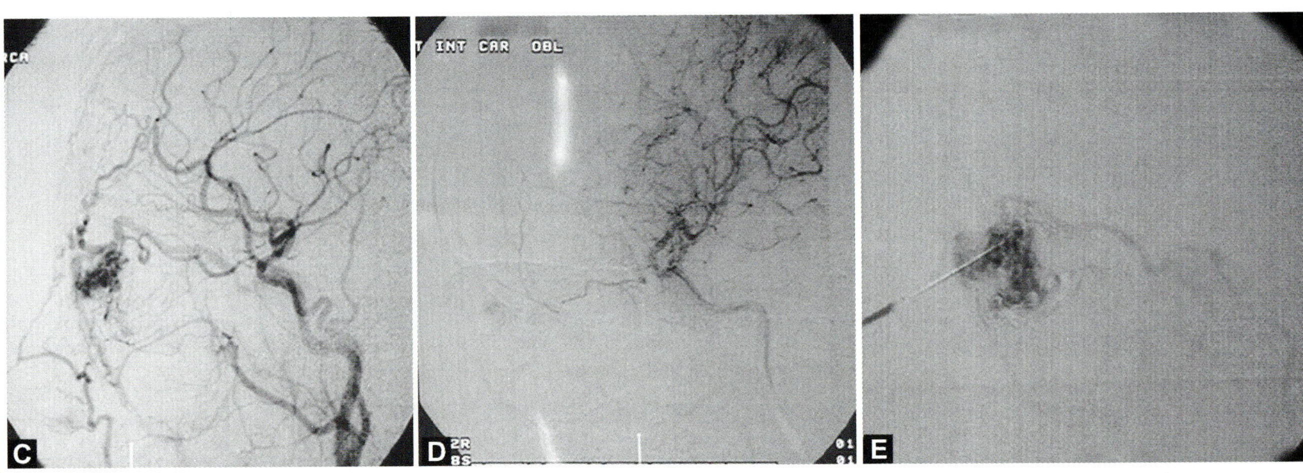

FIGURES 5.36C to E

(C) DSA of the right external carotid artery showing the nidus; (D) DSA of left internal carotid artery, lateral view showing left ophthalmic artery supply to this AVM; (E) Needle in the nidus showing contrast drained by vein

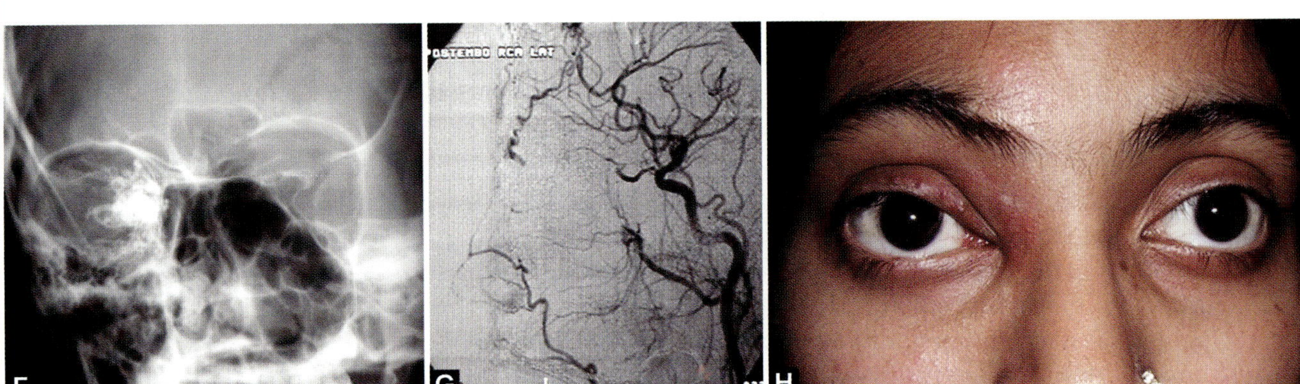

FIGURES 5.36F to H

(F) Nidus cast in cyanoacrylate glue, followed by surgery a week later; (G) A post embolization DSA. Right common carotid artery lateral view; (H) Two months postoperative follow-up

CONCLUSION

The last quarter of a century has seen a dramatic change in our approach to the understanding and classification of these lesions. Mulliken and Rootman have brought in, a lot of order to the terminological confusion and the understanding of the biological behavior of these lesions. This period has also witnessed a significant enhancement of both the diagnostic and the therapeutic armamentarium available for their management.

The advancement in imaging has enormously contributed to the differentiating of these lesions into distinct biological groups facilitating therapeutic choices. The four groups of channels with distinctive biological behavior and distinctive therapeutic responses that constitute the lesions occur singly or in varied combinations. These combinations have overlapping imaging features which makes the clinical workup very important for proper diagnosis and orderly management. It is therefore important, to be familiar with the different clinical presentations and imaging features which are characteristic of a specific lesion.

The orbit has its own special concerns:

Anatomical—The fine balance of a large number of delicate functional units in a limited space,

Functional—The fine balances that govern the vision, and

Appearance—That governs the facial aesthetics.

The treatment is conditioned by the known biological behavior of the lesion.

It should be monitored carefully when a delay in intervention is warranted.

When a therapeutic intervention is needed, it should be done early, to avoid the preventable complications especially connected with the vision and aesthetics.

As the treatment of some of the lesions is multistaged, the psychosocial aspects of the management must be kept in mind.

With research advancing to establish the cause of the vascular lesions and the development of drugs, which can control angiogenesis, the future is very promising.

The role of Plastic Surgery in the management of these lesions has been greatly facilitated and enhanced by the contributions from the departments of Imaging and Interventional Radiology. A close interaction between these two specialties is essential to their management.

REFERENCES

1. Mulliken JB, Glowacki J. Hemangiomas and vascular malformations in infants and children: A classification based on endothelial characteristics. Plast Reconstr Surg 1982;69:412-22.
2. Harris GJ. Orbital vascular malformations: A consensus statement on terminology and its clinical implications. Am J Ophthalmol 1999;127:453-5.
3. Rootman J. Vascular malformations of the orbit: Hemodynamic concepts. Orbit 2003;22:103-20.
4. Harris GJ, Sakol PJ, Bonavolonta G, De Conciliis C. An analysis of thirty cases of orbital lymphangioma: Pathophysiologic considerations and management recommendations. Ophthalmology 1990;97:1583-92.
5. Kennerdell JS, Maroon JC, Garrity JA, Abla AA. Surgical management of orbital lymphangioma with the carbon dioxide laser. Am J Ophthalmol 1986;102:308-14.
6. Tan ST, Bialosocki A. Venous malformations of the Orbit. Journal Oral Maxillofac. Surg 2004;62:1308-11.
7. Castanon M, Carrasco Margarit. Long-term follow-up of nineteen cystic lymphangiomas treated with fibrin sealant. Journal of Paediatric Surgery 1999;34.8:1276-9.

8. Boulos R. Patric: Intralesional Injection of tisseel fibrin glue for resection of lymphangiomas and other thin walled orbital cysts. Ophthalmic Plastic and Reconstructive Surgery 2005;21(3):171-6.
9. Smoker RK Wendy, Nerad Jeffrey. Vascular Lesions Of the Orbit: More than meets the eye. Radiographics 2008;28:185-204.
10. Walker RS, Nerad J. Surgical excision of periorbital capillary hemangiomas 1994;101:8, !333-40.
11. Kushner BJ. Local steroid therapy in adnexal hemangioma. Annals Ophth 1979;11:1005-9.
12. North PE, Waner H. Vascular tumors of infancy and childhood beyond capillary hemangioma. Cardiovasc Pathol 2006;15(6):303-17.
13. Karcioglu ZA, Nasr AM, Haik BG. Orbital hemangiopericytoma: Clinical and morphological features. Am J Ophthalmol 1997;124:661-72.
14. Rootman BL. Distensible venous malformations of the Orbit: Clinical and hemodynamic features and a new technique of management; Ophthalmology 1999;106.
15. Katz SE. Rootman: Combined venous lymphatic malformations of the orbit – association with non contiguous intracranial vascular anomalies. Ophthalmology 1998;105:176-84.
16. Mahesh Lakshmi, Subramanian N, Basile J. Hemangiopericytoma of the Orbit-A case report. Insight 2000;18(2) (house journal).
17. Malhotra AD, Murphy Kieran. Resection of orbital lymphangioma with the aid of intralesional liquid polymer. Am J Neuroradiology 2005;26:2630-4.
18. Zarem HA, Edgerton M. A induced involution of cavernous hemangioama following prednisolone therapy : Journal of Plastic and reconstructive surgery 1967;39:76-84.
19. Subramanian N, Selvarangan R. Intra orbital cavernous hemangiomas; JMSO 1989;263:17-8.
20. Menon S, Subramanian N. Thrombosed orbital varix—a correlation between imaging studies and histopathology 2004;13-8.
21. Stigma G, Crawford JS. Ophthalmic sequelae of infantile hemangiomas of the eyelids and orbit. J. of ophthalmology 1976;85:805.
22. Ranchod TM, Frieden I, Fredrick D. Corticosteroid treatment of periorbital haemangioma of infancy—a review of the evidence Br J Ophthalmol 2005;89:1134-8.
23. Maria I, Martinez, I, Sanchez-Carpintero, Paula E North, Martin C Mihm Jr. Infantile hemangioma. Clinical resolution with 5 percent Imiquimod Cream Arch Dermatol 2002;138:881-4.
24. Léauté-Labrèze C, et al. Propranolol for Severe Hemangiomas of Infancy. New England Journal of Medicine 2008;358(24):2649.

6

LASERS IN HEMANGIOMAS AND VASCULAR MALFORMATIONS

Shrirang G Pandit

INTRODUCTION

The term hemangioma indicates a tumor of vascular channels. In common usage this term means different things to different individuals. In fact, these are a group of lesions with varied anatomy, histology, pathology and biological behavior. They have a varied tissue structure as indicated by a plethora of terms used in their nomenclature. It is quite natural that they behave differently in regard to tissue growth, invasiveness and their biological responses.

The common denominator is the conglomeration of vascular channels. The hemoglobin in the RBCs and the water in the vessel wall, makes them a good target for laser treatment.

ADVANTAGE OF LASERS

Surgery leaves scars in its wake and non surgical solutions are gaining popularity and wide acceptance with the idea of having a scarless solution to an otherwise surgical problem. Laser energy is being harnessed to treat a large variety of lesions. In fact, hemangiomas were the first group of conditions where laser was used as a non-invasive tool.

Lasers cause photocoagulation, resulting in thrombosis of the blood vessels and involution of the lesion. Hemoglobin, oxyhemoglobin, melanin and water are some very important laser targets. They are also designated as laser target chromophores. Laser tissue interaction is the result of laser energy hitting these chromophores. This incident energy when released causes the tissue to heat up. This heat produces irreversible changes in the incident tissue, such as, coagulation of blood, charring of the vessel wall, and thrombosis of the blood vessels. When melanin is the target, it bursts the melanin into smaller molecules which are phagocytosed.

ABOUT LASERS

Theodore Maiman developed the first Ruby laser in 1960. In the years, that followed a wide spectrum of lasers were developed and a number of them became important tools in the management of vascular malformations. Laser technology too has grown by leaps and bounds, as have the opportunities to use them.

Current lasers are highly evolved electronic devices which can deliver intense specific energy to a specific target. Laser energy pulses can be delivered in nanoseconds permitting very high energy peaks. Delivery of such intense energy for very short duration to the target, results in minimal lateral tissue damage. The changes in wave lengths, Q-switching and frequency doubling, are a few ways of increasing energy intensity with nearly no lateral damage. Some lasers like CO_2 are capable of producing heat like that of the sun causing tissue to vaporize.

It is interesting to note that when the lasers were being tried out on 'hemangiomas', it was noticed that the laser treated area did not grow hair, giving birth to 'the hair removing lasers'.

Lasers and light devices, used in treating hemangiomas are:

- Neodymium YAG (Yttrium Aluminum Garnet) 1064 nm
- Intense Pulsed Light (IPL) 560 to 1200 nm
- KTP (Potassium Titanyl Phosphate) 585 nm
- Flash pump dye lasers 585 to 595 nm
- Argon laser 488 to 514.

A new method to deliver laser energy is by using a fiber. These fibers can be introduced into a blood vessel and the laser energy is delivered to the target intravascularly or in the interstitial space. The technique is freely used in the management of varicose veins. It is possible to apply the same technique in lesions, where blood vessels are accessible to fiber usage. Shortly, it may be possible to coagulate feeder vessels of the arterial malformations.

LASER PHYSICS

An insight of the basic laser physics will help to understand the science behind the methodology of laser usage, its possible benefits and more important its limitations.

Laser is an acronym that stands for 'Light Amplification by Stimulated Emission of Radiation'. Essentially, we are amplifying the light energy, which consists of photons at various levels of energy. The light as it passes through a medium, which can be glass, gas, vapor, etc. is excited by the electrical energy source like a flash lamp. These energy rich photons thus excited leave the orbit and travel in space in a coherent beam of light. They have a fixed wave length, making the light monochromatic. Laser light is a part of the electromagnetic spectrum and many wavelengths lie in the invisible light range.

Characteristics of Laser

Monochromaticity

The laser beam, which is essentially made up of photons are equally energized. Hence, the wavelength is same or lies in a very narrow band. The laser light for the same reason is monochromatic, meaning thereby that it is of one single color and not a mixture of various colors as in sunlight.

Coherence

All the photons that are emitted, vibrate in a phase agreement in space and time. Coherence relates to the quality of the waveform in its being precise. More the coherence, the greater is the potential of the laser beam to be focused accurately. The precision and accuracy are products of high degree of coherence. This quality is unique to lasers and makes them what they are precise and accurate.

Directionality

All photons travel in one direction and this unidirectional movement produces an extremely narrow beam of laser with minimal dispersion. Collimating devices in the laser delivery systems can create an intensely focused beam with a very narrow spot size, as small as 0.12 mm.

Brilliancy

The brightness or intensity relates to the level of energy. This property can be modified by, pulsing the beam or quality switching (Q-switch) to generate intense power that can be delivered in nanoseconds. This is vital as it ensures precise tissue damage and minimal collateral injury.

It is also important to understand certain terminology used in laser parlance.

LASER TERMINOLOGY

Energy: The unit of measurement is 'joules' and indicates the number of photons emitted by the laser. More the photons, higher is the energy delivered to the target. In the electromagnetic spectrum (Fig. 6.1) photons are present in varying energy states.

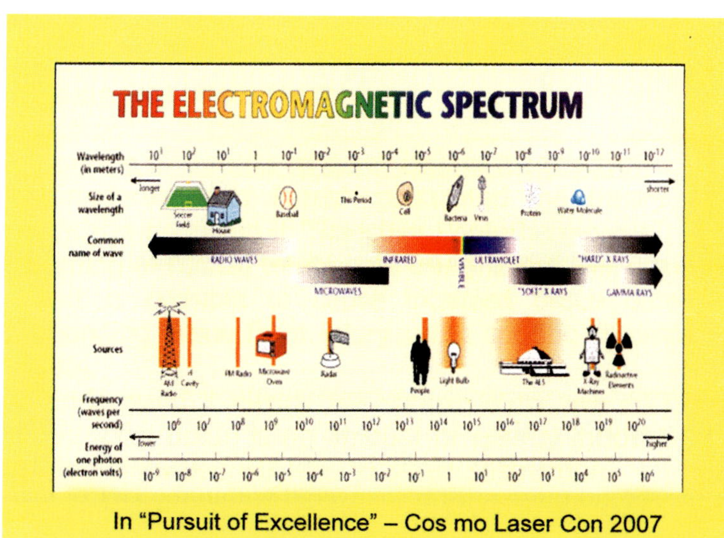

In the electromagnetic spectrum photons are present energy states.

FIGURE 6.1
The Electromagnetic Spectrum in varying energy states

Fluence: It is the measure of energy delivered per unit area expressed as joules/cm sq.

Power: It is the rate at which laser energy is delivered. It is measured in watts. One watt = 1 Joule/sec.

Irradiance: It is power per unit area measured in W/cm sq.

Wavelength Relevant to the Management of Hemangiomas

Wavelength is defined as the distance between the two subsequent peaks or troughs of a light wave and is expressed in nanometers 1×10^{-9} meters. Shorter the wavelength, higher is the frequency and a long wavelength means lower frequency. Gamma rays have shortest wavelength and the radiowaves have the longest wavelength. Wavelength is a function of energy state of the photon. Photons having a high quantum of energy will vibrate rapidly and will have a short wavelength and high frequency, while low energy state will have long wavelength and low frequency. Hence, gamma rays are most destructive while radiowaves will be the least harmful.

Flash lamp pumped dye laser or PDL has a wavelength of 585 nm and 595 nm. These wavelengths work on superficial blood vessels in the Port-wine stains (PWS) and are a method of choice for their treatment. An Intense pulse light (IPL) source with a cut off filter of 590 nm can work equally well. Frequencies of 585 and 595 nm work up to a depth of 1.2 mm. Deep seated lesions are treated with 1064 nm Nd:YAG laser which can be effective up to a depth of 8 mm.

Deep seated venous channels up to 2 mm in diameter can be targeted by rapid synchronized pulses. The medium sized channel and the slow flow rate will permit vessel coagulation effectively. Small caliber varicose veins can be thus treated.

Sequence of Events in Laser Tissue Interaction

Earliest known light tissue reaction is photosynthesis. It was Anderson and Parrish *(1983)* who postulated the theory of laser tissue interaction, which they called "selective photothermolysis." It was the true beginning of clinical treatment using lasers, because we came to understand, that it was possible to cause localized tissue damage and spare surrounding tissue from injury using specific chromophores as laser targets.

To understand this clearly, two concepts are relevant:

- Threshold fluence of a tissue is the amount of energy incident on the tissue, which if equalled or exceeded, will lead to tissue destruction, and
- Thermal Relaxation Time (TRT) is the time required by an object to cool by 50 percent of the initial temperature reached.

For tissue damage to occur, the laser wavelength needs to be selectively absorbed by the chromophore in the target tissue and not by the surrounding tissue. Once the temperature is raised, the second pulse needs to reach the target before it cools too much. Hence the second pulse must be delivered within the TRT of that target to be effective.

Variables to be Controlled for Effective Treatment

The laser surgeon has to effectively manipulate three modalities:

a. *The wavelength:* As discussed above, it leads to the choice of the source, pulse duration and energy level.

b. *The pulse duration:* It is the duration of time for which the laser emission is on. This leads to the determination of the total energy that will reach the tissue. Repeated laser pulses can be delivered at specific intervals to prevent tissue from recovering from the damage and at the same time protecting surrounding tissue. It is possible to deliver these pulses in nanosecond and millisecond domains and effectively control a highly selective damage.
c. *The energy level:* When the energized photon comes into contact with the target chromophore, it transmits its energy to the target. This energy can produce thermal, mechanical or chemical changes in and around the chromophore. The thermal changes are the most important, when we are dealing with vascular lesions.

Skin Type and Delivery of the Energy

The Fitzpatrick classification of skin typing, which is a good indicator of skin melanin content, will decide on the efficacy of a particular laser beam. Excess skin melanin will make deep delivery of laser energy difficult as melanin, a more superficial competing chromophore, will absorb and take away large amounts of energy.

The Logic of Laser Usage in Hemangiomas

For treating hemangiomas, we need lasers that have affinity to hemoglobin and oxyhemoglobin. The laser beam will deposit its energy into hemoglobin, produce intense heat and coagulate the blood. This is a direct transfer of energy. This heat, if transferred to the vessel wall, will coagulate the blood vessel. This is an indirect transfer of heat. Direct effect will be seen if the chromophore is water and the laser energy gets released in the vessel wall itself.

Factors Affecting the Efficacy of Laser Treatments

These are:

- Amount of hemoglobin or oxyhemoglobin in the area
- Size of the blood vessel
- Velocity of blood flow
- Volume of blood flow
- Depth of the blood vessel from skin surface
- Laser wavelength
- Adequate energy transfer over enough length of time.

Cooling used during the procedure and pressure of treatment head, are technique related issues. Too much cooling can reduce effective coagulation. Too much pressure on the blood vessel can empty the vessel and move the laser target away and make the treatment ineffective.

If the blood flow is fast, there would not be enough time for the heat to be effective. Hence, the laser will not work effectively in high flow lesions. If the flow is large, the heat will dissipate and again the laser will not be effective.

If the lesion is located in the depth, the energy will be lost in transit and a short wave length may not reach the target tissue.

If higher energies are used to compensate losses in transmission, it is possible that the target chromophores like melanin situated in the superficial layers may take up excess heat and get burnt.

Venous lakes or large sinuses will dilute the heat energy and make the treatment ineffective.

Too much energy can burst the blood vessels causing hemorrhage and purpura.

It must be abundantly clear that the lasers have a limited role to play and are useful for very specific and carefully chosen indications. Capillary hemangioma of infancy, Port-wine stain, involuting hemangioma, superficial cavernous hemangioma, spider nevi, small venous lakes, superficial varicose veins less than 2 mm in diameter, Telangiectasias, visible facial veins are principal indications for laser treatments.

Transvenous Ablation as for Varicose Veins

Recently fibers have been developed that can be inserted through the draining vein into venous varicosities. The fiber is advanced under 2D echo control up to the sephano-femoral junction and then gradually withdrawn by an automated process. During withdrawal, bursts of energy are delivered at 1 mm interval to coagulate the vein. Perforators and intermediate varicosities can be dealt with, in a similar manner. This is a minimally invasive procedure performed under 2D ultrasound control and is done under local or regional anesthesia. Different frequency of Nd:YAG laser is used to target the hemoglobin or the water in the vessel wall.

The venous destruction is very clearly demonstrated by Doppler.

A venous malformation with structural similarities can be dealt with, in a similar manner.

Carbon Dioxide Laser and Radiofrequency

CO_2 Laser and RF (radiofrequency) machines are excellent surgical adjuvants for treatment of some lesions.

Radiofrequency in cutting and coagulating mode can ablate superficial lymphangiomas and capillary malformations. The treatment is swift, relatively painless and can be repeated frequently to control recurrence if any.

Surgical handpiece on a CO_2 laser is a great tool for surgical excision of lesions. It is possible to use this evaporative energy to cut and coagulate blood vessels at the same time. It is possible to dissect involuting lesions easily. The laser incision spot is 0.2 mm in size and works as a hot knife. The sleek and ergonomic handpiece permits full flexibility to the surgeon. This being a non contact energy delivery it is possible to work in the depth easily.

A powerful smoke evacuator is essential to take away the tissue plume that kicks up when laser vaporizes the tissue. Ultrapulsing produces minimal or no charring and wound healing proceeds smoothly, albeit a bit slow at times.

CLINICAL APPLICATIONS OF LASERS IN VASCULAR MALFORMATIONS

From amidst the whole spectrum of hemangiomas and vascular malformations, the use of Lasers is optimally indicated for capillary malformations, commonly labeled as Port-wine stains (PWS). These are common on the face as a part of the Sturge-Weber Syndrome. Usually present at birth they grow relentlessly into a dark thickened nodular lesion, making the treatment more difficult. Hence early treatment is recommended. The most suitable Lasers for managing these lesions are the Nd:YAG Laser or the intense pulse light (IPL). In children with thin skin, and no significant hyperkeratinization, IPL would be the better choice.

The child shown in Figure 6.2A was born with the vascular malformation on the face which had grown slowly. She was 4 years old when 1st seen (Fig. 6.2A) and was treated with 3 sessions of Nd:YAG laser with significant involution and benefit Figures 6.2B to D shows the patient a year later. Figure 6.2E shows the patient another 2 years later with mild recurrence with ecstatic vessels which are generally more difficult to treat with lasers.

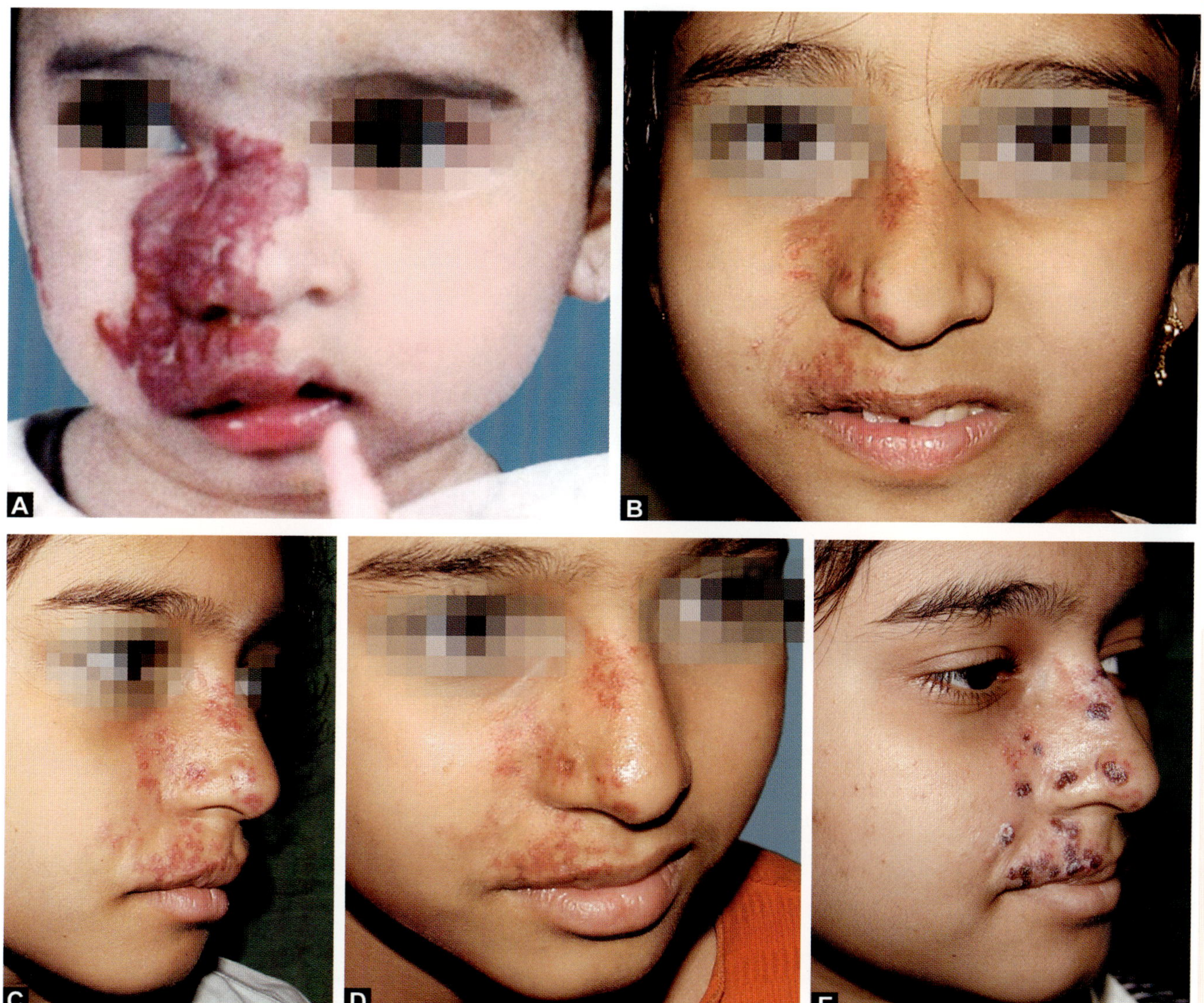

FIGURES 6.2A to E

(A) A port-wine stain (PWS) on the nose and adjacent cheek; (B) Three sessions Nd:YAG; (C) Good involution assisted by Nd:YAG laser; (D) one year later; (E) Two years later some recurrence with ecstatic vessels

The patient (Figs 6.3A and B) is a case of bilateral V3 Sturge-Weber syndrome (PWS) treated with two sessions of IPL. The IPL has the advantage of having a very large spot size. This helps in producing a very uniform effect, with an even color. The texture too is satisfactory, with an absence of any honeycomb appearance.

As mentioned earlier, the character of capillary malformation changes with growth. There is thickening of skin, increased keratinization and nodularity. All of these affect the response of the skin to laser.

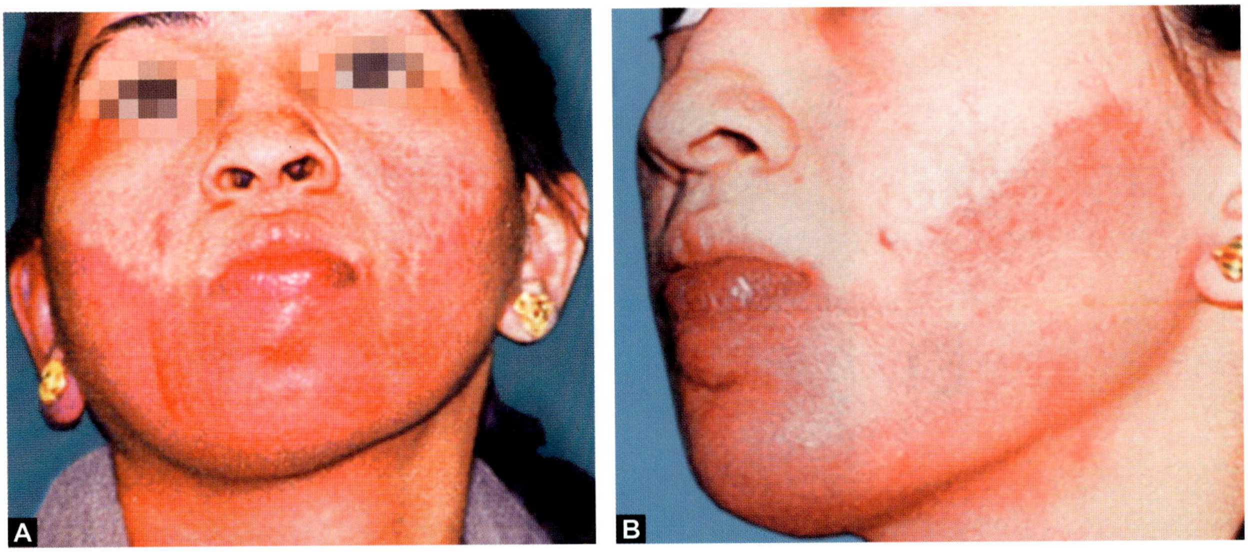

FIGURES 6.3A and B

(A) Bilateral V3 Sturge-Weber syndrome — PWS; (B) After 1st sitting of IPL

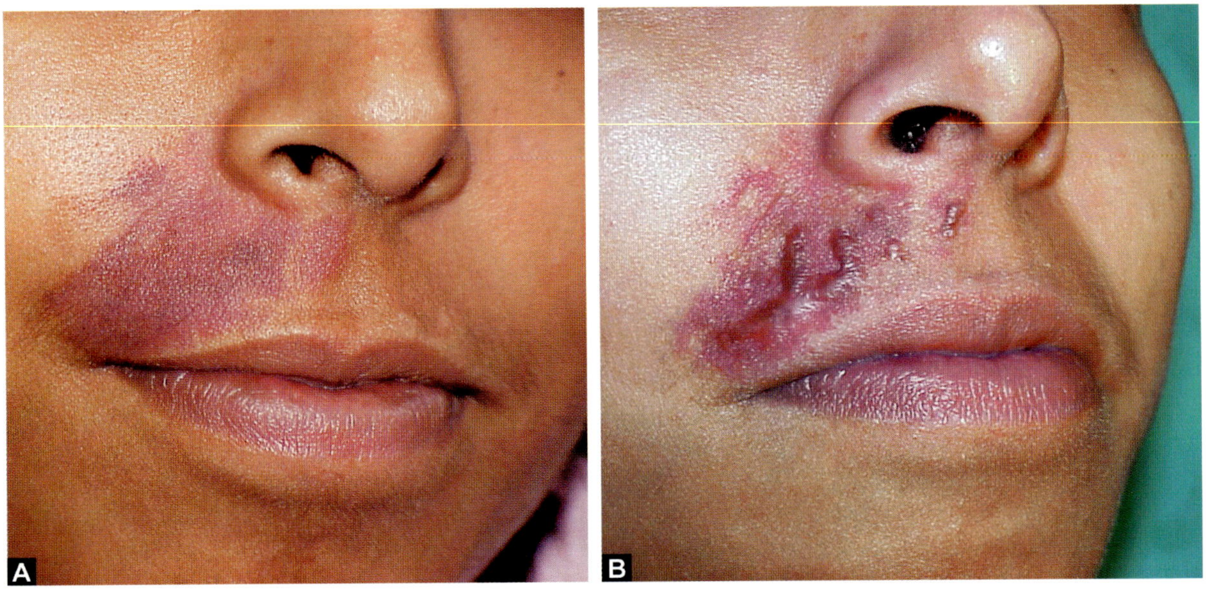

FIGURES 6.4A and B

The hyperkeratinized capillary malformation in an adult: (A) Before intervention; (B) Post-treatment scarring following a single session with a Nd:YAG laser;

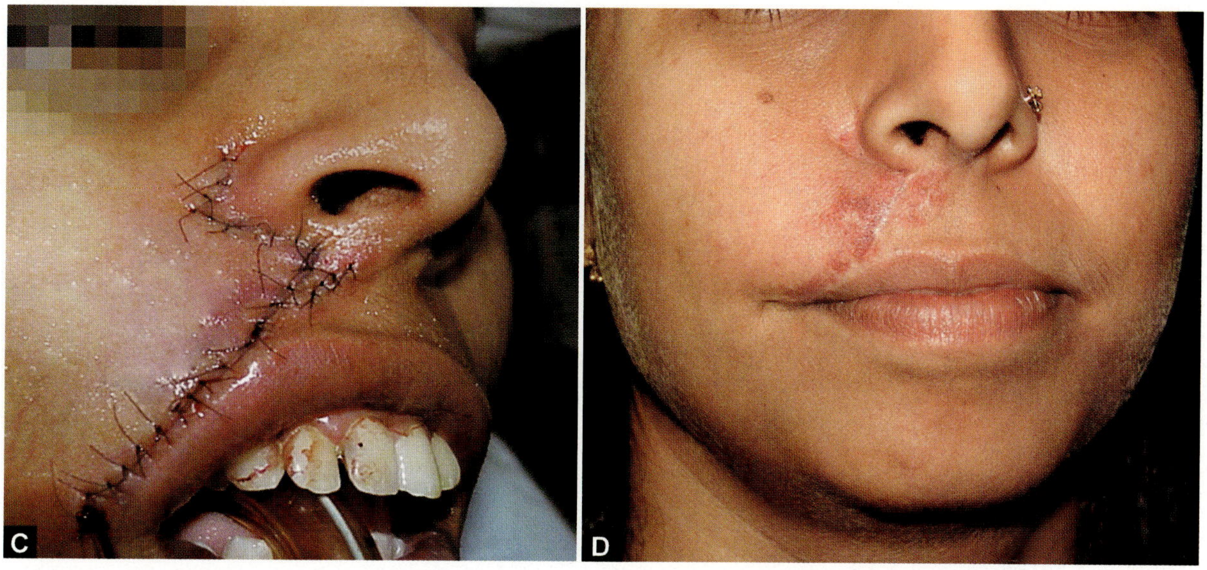

FIGURES 6.4C and D
(C) Surgical management; (D) Ten years later after treatment.
Note: Recurrent ecstatic vessels below nose

Figure 6.4A shows a PWS in an adult who has some of these changes. Following treatment with one session of Nd:YAG laser he developed heavy scarring (Fig. 6.4B). An effective surgical intervention, (Fig. 6.4C) gave a satisfactory result. Figure 6.4D shows a tiny recurrence after 10 years. These are probably ecstatic vessels which usually are extremely difficult to treat with lasers.

A long standing capillary malformation (Sturge-Weber syndrome) with many areas of hyperpigmentation, hyperkeratinization and nodularity, involving both the eyelids and the adjacent face is illustrated in Figures 6.5A and B. The patient was treated with two sessions of Nd:YAG laser, with changes as shown in Figures 6.5C and D. Note the heavy deep scarring in the area of deep nodular lesions. The circles in Figure 6.5D represent the 'spot size' of the laser beam. The eyelids have been left alone.

She had multiple Nd:YAG laser sessions and the same laser treated skin was used as thin flaps which were raised for the purpose of serial excisions and reconstruction. This demonstrates that laser irradiated skin retains its vascularity well enough to be able to raise thin skin flaps from the same area.

Following this, the patient had three sessions of IPL treatment and the replacement of the eyelid skin with a full thickness skin graft. The honeycomb areas (Fig. 6.4D) are very resistant to future laser ablation. The areas unaffected by Laser were treated with three sessions of IPL with the final result as shown in Figures 6.5E and F.

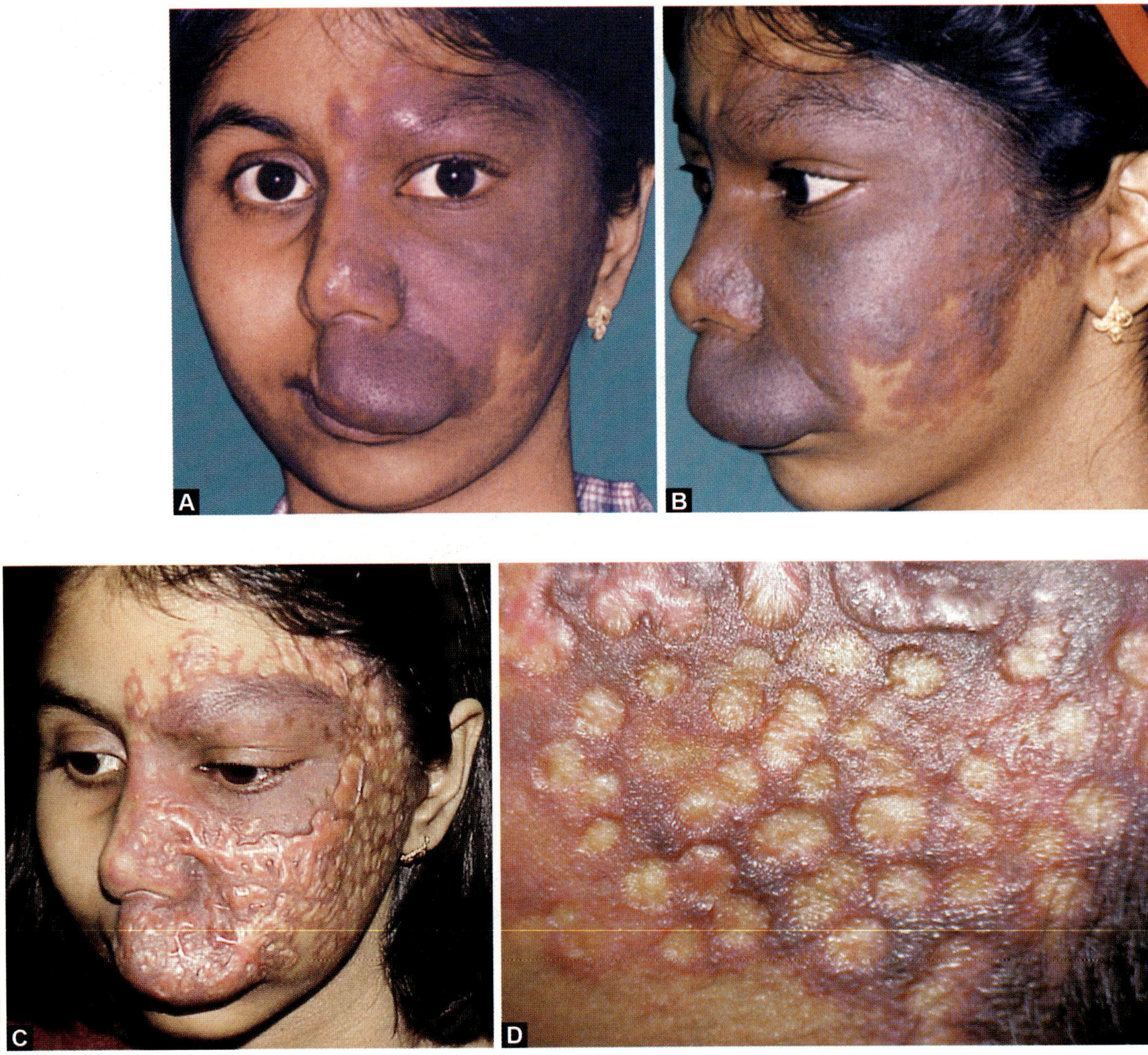

FIGURES 6.5A to D

PWS with marked hyperkeratinization and nodularity: (A and B) Front and Profile; (C) After two sessions of Nd:YAG Laser shows d. Deep scarring in the areas of marked nodularity; (D) The circles represent the spot size of the laser beam

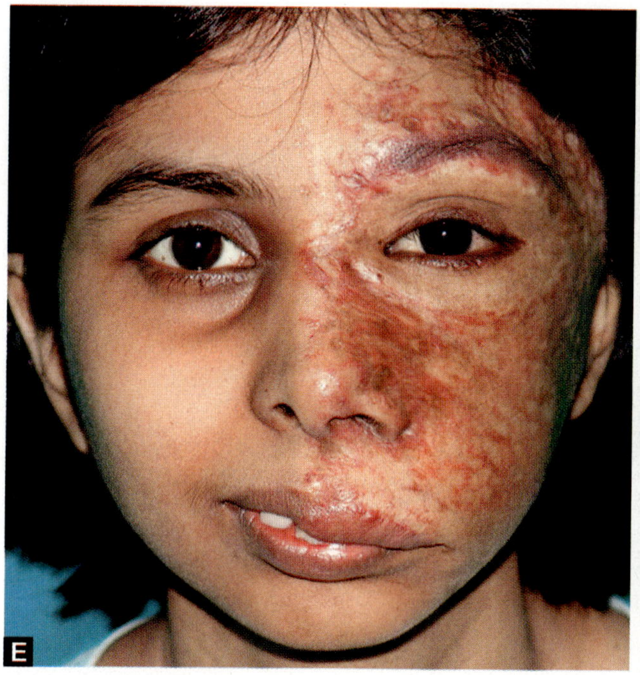

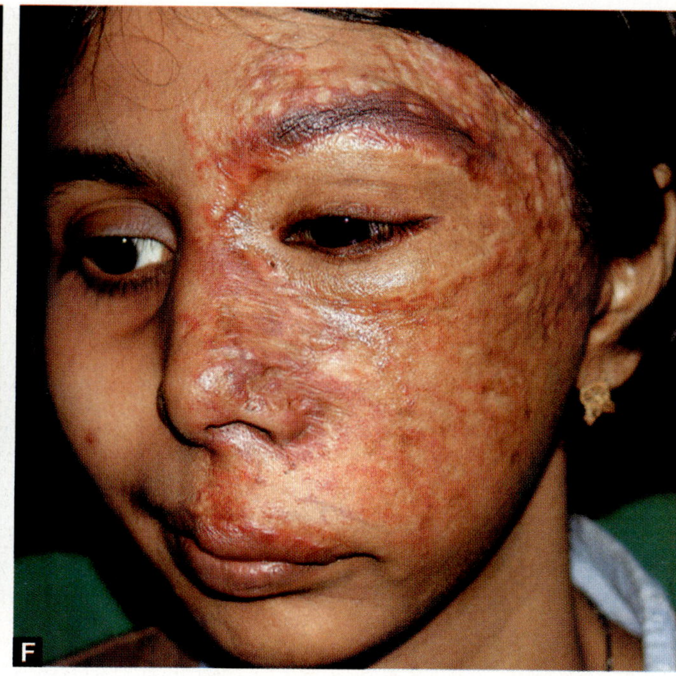

FIGURES 6.5E and F
(E and F) The final result after a full thickness skin graft for both the eyelids and 3 sessions of IPL

The patient shown in Figure 6.6 shows a capillary hemangioma (Sturge-Weber Syndrome V2) with hyperkeratinization, fibrosis and nodularity. He needed multiple surgical interventions, involving excisions using CO_2 laser. Serial excisions were carried out for covering the cheek. The flaps could be raised repeatedly from areas

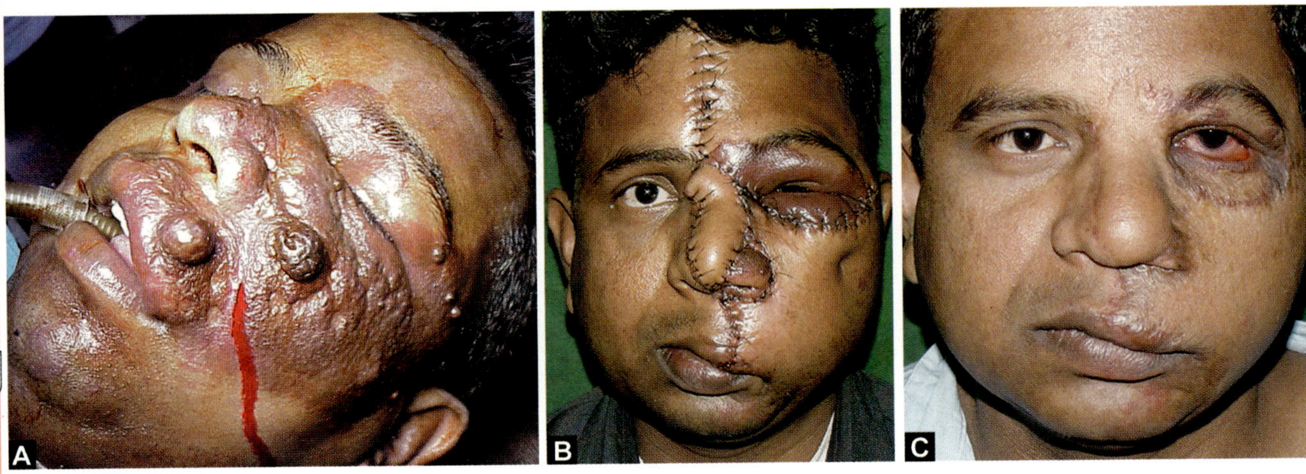

FIGURES 6.6A to C

(A) A long standing capillary malformation (Sturge-Weber syndrome). IPL and Laser Nd:YAG used on three occasions; (B) The last stage of serial excisions and the setting in of the median forehead flap. CO_2 laser was used to incise and dissect; (C) Postoperative result

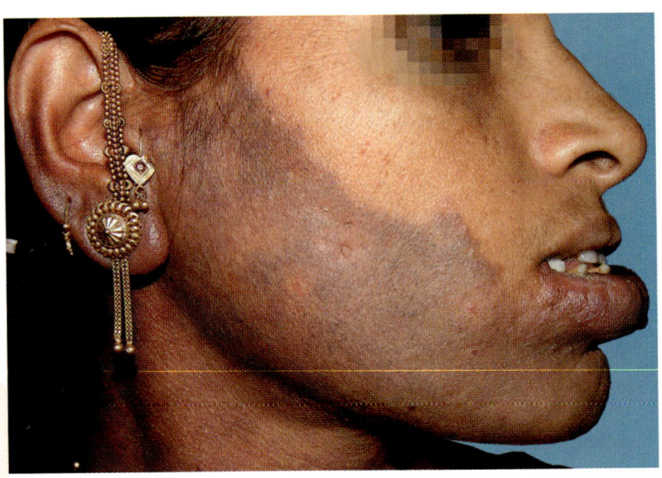

FIGURE 6.7

Endpoint of Nd:YAG session showing graying of lesion and circular impression of the laser spot

skin retains its vascularity well enough to be able to raise thin skin flaps repeatedly from the same area. Figure 6.6A shows the lesion at the start of the surgical intervention. Figure 6.6B shows the last phase of the serial excision and the setting in of a median forehead flap to resurface the nose. The Figure 6.6C shows the final result.

Decision on when to stop laser treatment is important. Figure 6.7 shows a long standing PWS under treatment with Nd:YAG laser showing graying of the lesion and circular impressions of the laser spot which indicate the end point of laser therapy.

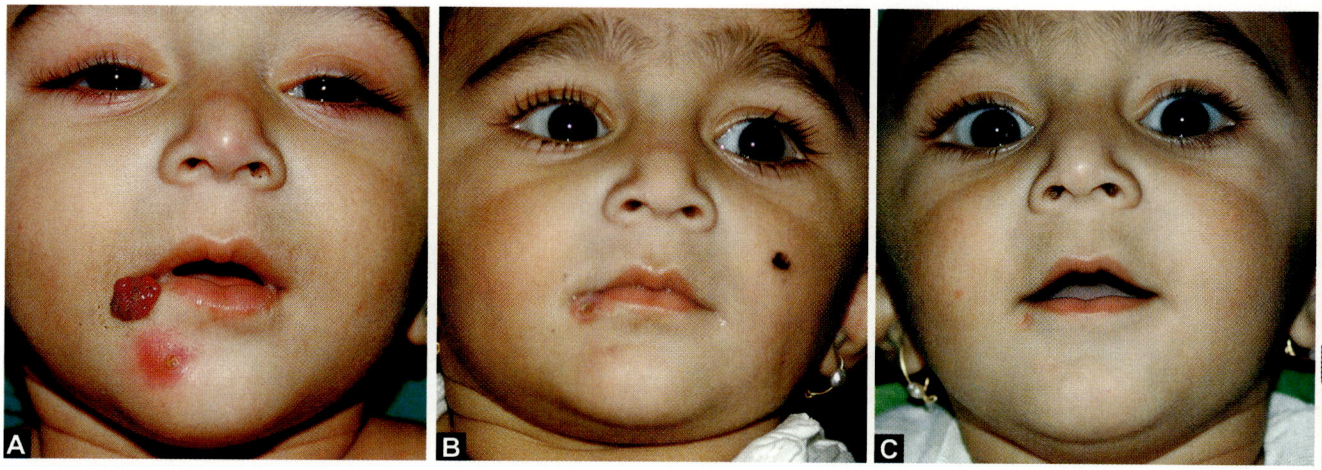

FIGURES 6.8A to C
(A) The lesion capillary hemangiomas of infancy; (B) Soon after ablation; (C)The final result

Lasers in Capillary Hemangiomas of Infancy

The capillary hemangioma of infancy are normally self curing, but occasionally an ablation becomes a necessity and lasers come in handy. The patient shown in Figure 6.8 A shows a CHI with a proclivity for repeated hemorrhages. A laser ablation came in handy for a clean ablation (Figs 6.8B and C).

Lasers for Precision Hemostasis

Because of its precision in energy release, Laser and RF energy can be used to precisely arrest hemorrhage as shown in Figures 6.9A and B. A child had a severe bleed from a tiny conjunctival varix, on the conjunctiva of the left upper eyelid. Patient was treated with bipolar radiofrequency device. A single treatment resulted in total relief (Fig. 6.9C). In a procedure like this, a total corneal protection is absolutely important. The protection device is illustrated in Figure 6.9D.

Lymphangioma Treated with RF

RF superpulse is very useful for treating lymphatic malformations as illustrated in Figures 6.10A and B.

What to Expect When Treating Hemangiomas with Lasers?

The laser energy will show immediate effect by changing the lesion to a ash gray color. This signifies vessel coagulation and obliteration of capillaries. It is clinical endpoint of treatment.

Small blood vessels will turn gray and stop filling and emptying. They will become cord like and over next few weeks disintegrate and gradually disappear.

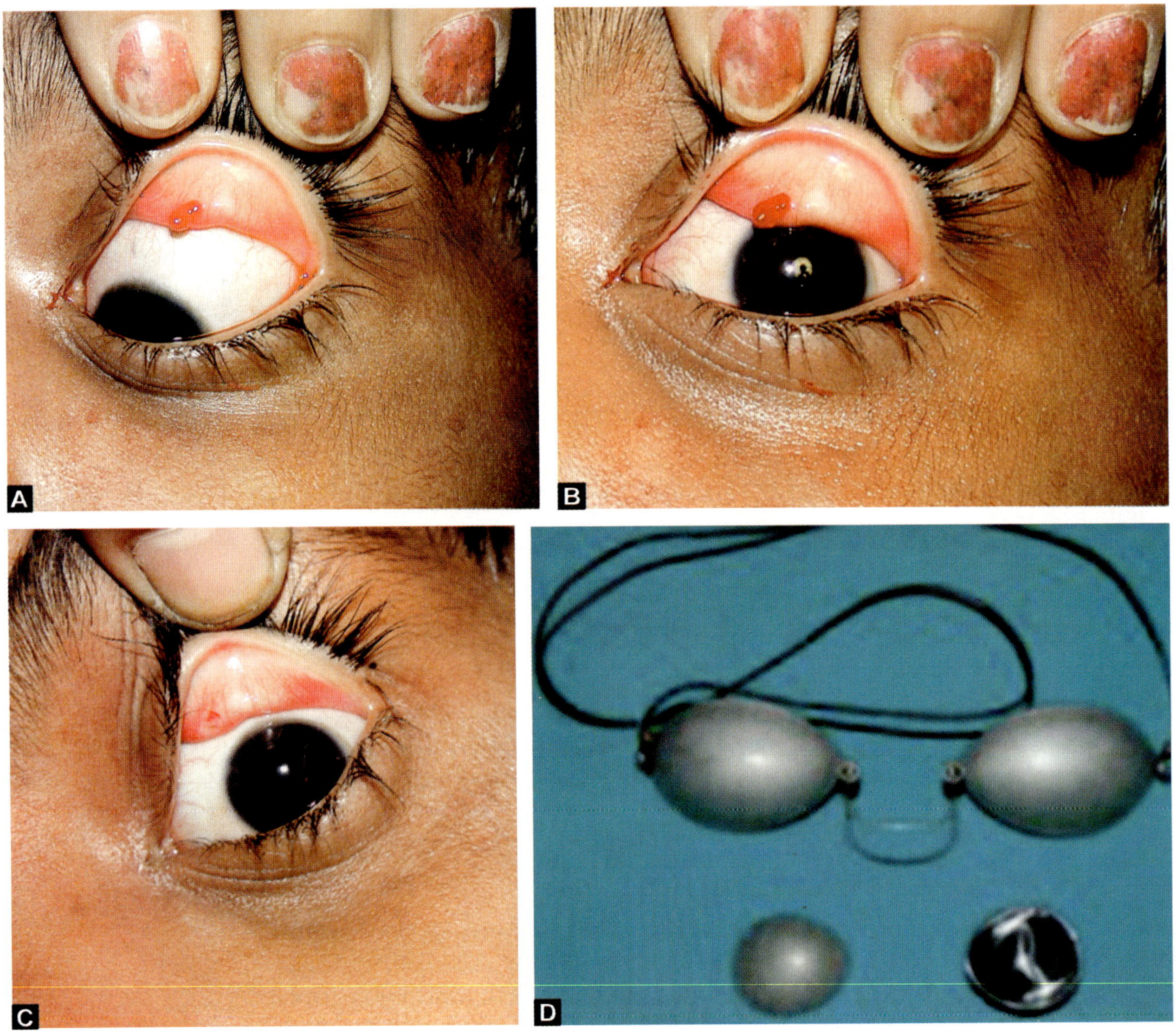

FIGURES 6.9A to D

(A) The vascular malformation; (B) Appearance at the end of the procedure; (C) The final result; (D) The metallic eye-shield

The pink spongy look will go away and flattening will be visible. This takes some time, as in the immediate post-treatment phase the part swells up and may show blisters and some weeping. A steroid antibiotic application is very soothing and rapidly reduces inflammation.

It is not uncommon to find significant scarring in spongy areas of the lesion. This is due to the coagulation of a large volume of blood which produces a lot of heat and damages the superficial tissues producing scarring.

Commonly, there will be a flattening and lightening of the lesion. The rate of vascular proliferation is reduced and the lesion tends to involute rapidly. The skin

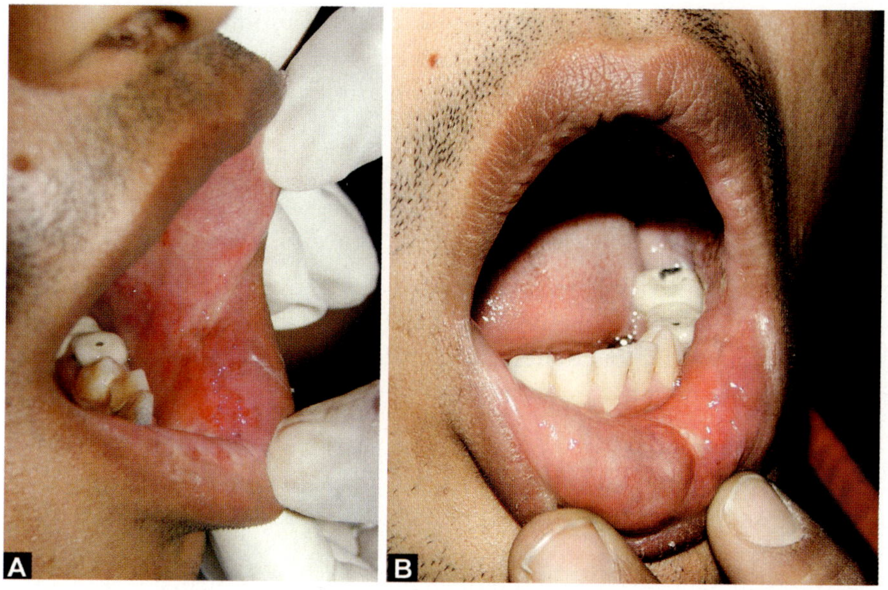

FIGURES 6.10A and B
A surface lymphangioma of lip before RF; and after RF ablation

changes are rewarding, as the lesion assumes skin color and has a decent texture. However, it is a bit glossy and lacks the dermal support and may look wrinkled at times. This skin can be used as flap, as the blood supply is intact and withstands the surgery.

Aftercare

The laser treatments are generally office procedures. They may be performed under topical Prilocaine anesthesia or nerve blocks. Often no anesthesia is required.

It is common to prescribe an oral analgesic like paracetamol or diclofenac for a day or two. Topical application of antibiotic and steroid combination is routinely used.

Postinflammatory hyperpigmentation (PIH) is a serious worry and is best avoided by diligent care. Patient is asked to observe total sun protection. Mechanical barriers like caps, scarves and sunscreen cream of 30 SPF and above, are prescribed.

Lesions are reviewed as often as needed. In rapidly proliferating lesions, repeat sessions can be done as early as 15 days apart.

Laser Safety

No writing on study of lasers can be complete without understanding and implementing the issue of safety of lasers. Lasers are extremely potent and powerful devices and therefore can be dangerous too. The laser beam is generally invisible to the naked eye and hence is not seen. It can inflict severe injury to the eye, cornea and retina.

It is vital to understand that the patient, the laser surgeon, the assistants and the accompanying people are at risk from laser irradiation injury.

There must be warning signs on the entry to the Laser room, on the covered windows and access points, about of risks from laser exposure. Everyone at risk, should wear properly designated and certified eyewear at all times when the laser in on.

When treating lesions on the face, metallic eye shields on cornea or extraocular shields must be worn at all times by the patient through out the procedure.

Recurrences

It will be good to remember here that recurrences do occur and are common. They may be seen as late as after 10 years and are believed to be due to the development of new blood vessels in that area. Unfortunately, they retain their telangiectatic nature. Secondary treatments are not always successful.

Complications

Laser induced purpura is a known entity due to vessel rupture in the management these vascular lesions with lasers.

Burns and the resultant scarring are the other known complications.

Treatment Advances

Rapid progress is being made in improving laser applications. Cryogen sprays, contact cooling, cold air spray, internally cooling sapphire tips reduce pain, protect the epidermis and permit delivery of higher quantum of energy to the target. Sometimes, this cold can cause vasoconstriction and take away the target chromophore making the treatment ineffective.

SUMMARY

The advent of lasers in surgery has brought a new perspective and a potent tool to the management of hemangiomas and vascular malformations, particularly the later. Being a nonsurgical option, less invasive, with minimal scarring and less morbidity, the therapy is readily accepted and the compliance is better. It can be done at any age and can be periodically repeated.

Undoubtedly, it needs strict protocols, therapeutic discipline and methodology to avoid disasters.

Lasers are invaluable in the management of small channel low flow systems. To this, if one adds the power of the harnessed radiofrequencies, the whole spectrum of the small channel lesions has been brought under fair control.

Lasers with a wavelength of 1064 mm or IPL are ideal to effectively control. Capillary malformation, if used before the age of 7 or 8, before keratinization sets in, will not merely eradicate a blemish but also prevent hideous and difficult to treat deformities.

The use of radiofrequency has emerged as the mainstay of managing lymphangiomas.

The Lasers and RF together, have significantly contributed to the management of Lymphangiomas and Capillary malformations which are otherwise difficult to treat. They are also useful in the management of port-wine stains, superficial lymphatic and venous malformations, varicosities, spider Nevi, and Telangiectasias.

Applying the Management oriented classification, it can be said that small channel slow flow lesions will respond best to laser treatments. Here too, the small channels carrying blood, capillaries and venules would respond better. Since they are often intermingled with lymphatics, these too would be destroyed. Their superficial location, small vessel size, presence of hemoglobin the target chromophore, and slow velocity of blood flow will lead to a safe and effective obliteration of the channels.

Small channel high flow lesions (capillary hemangiomas of infancy) can be dealt by using high energy, large laser spot sizes and using compression to partially empty the blood vessel and reduce flow velocity.

Large channel high flow and large channel slow flow lesions will render laser ineffective due to rapid cooling and heat dispersion in the vessels.

Radiofrequency and CO_2 laser are excellent surgical tools to excise the lesions with minimal blood loss.

Lasers have a very important role in management of vascular lesions. The learning curve is rather steep. At times, it is difficult to keep up with technological advances as newer and newer devices hit the market with amazing regularity. The downside aspect is the costs involved in buying and maintaining the laser machines. This however, does not undermine their utility in handling this perplexing problem.

BIBLIOGRAPHY

1. Anderson RR, Parish JA. A selective photothermolysis, precise microsurgery by selective absorption of pulsed radiation. Science 1983;220:524-7.
2. Cosman B. Clinical experience in the laser therapy of port-wine stains. Lasers Surg. Med 1980;1:133.
3. Galileo.phys.virginia.edu/..../introduction.htm
4. Landthaler M, Hohenleutner U. The Nd Yag laser in cutaneous surgery. In: Lasers in cutaneous and aesthetic surgery. Philadelphia: Lippincott Raven; 1997:pp.124-49.

7

VENOUS MALFORMATIONS (VMs)

A LARGE CHANNEL LOW FLOW LESION

KS Goleria

Venous malformations (VMs) are fairly common, usually in the pure form, but not uncommonly associated with capillary venous malformations (CVM) or with lymphatics (LVM). In their pure form, VMs are a conglomeration of venous channels of varying sizes. In the larger channels, thrombi are frequently seen, some with dystrophic calcification identified in radiological studies as phleboliths and considered as diagnostic of VMs (see Figs 7.2E and F).

MANIFESTATION

All VMs are probably present at birth. Their presentation is varied, depending on size, location and depth. When located on the surface, their presence is easily seen as identifiable varicosities—thin walled, soft, compressible and purplish vascular structure, frequently seen in a conglomeration. These veins are thin walled with decreased smooth muscle cells, often arranged in clumps rather than concentrically. When located at a depth, they may be noted at a later age. Whatever be the presentation, they are characterized by a swelling, soft, bluish, easily compressible, nonpulsatile, and growing slowly. Intralesional clotting is known to occur particularly in dependent parts and its expression may vary from simple fibrin deposition to the pathognomonic phleboliths.

Being thin walled, low pressure and low flow channels, the venous malformations are easily compressible. They are essentially low pressure systems fed by veins and drained by veins. Illustrated is a small venous malformation, (Figs 7.1A and B) which is fed by a single afferent vein and drained by a single efferent vein. (I have seen only one more such a VM located in the subclavicular area with both the afferent and the efferent vessels lying near each other, the lesion literally suspended by this pedicle).

BIOLOGICAL BEHAVIOR — FEATURES AND GROWTH

Mostly multiple, interconnected malformations are primary lesions which gradually enlarge, possibly adding new connections. They grow slowly, expand slowly and possibly undergo both the processes. The effect is to expand the space occupied by

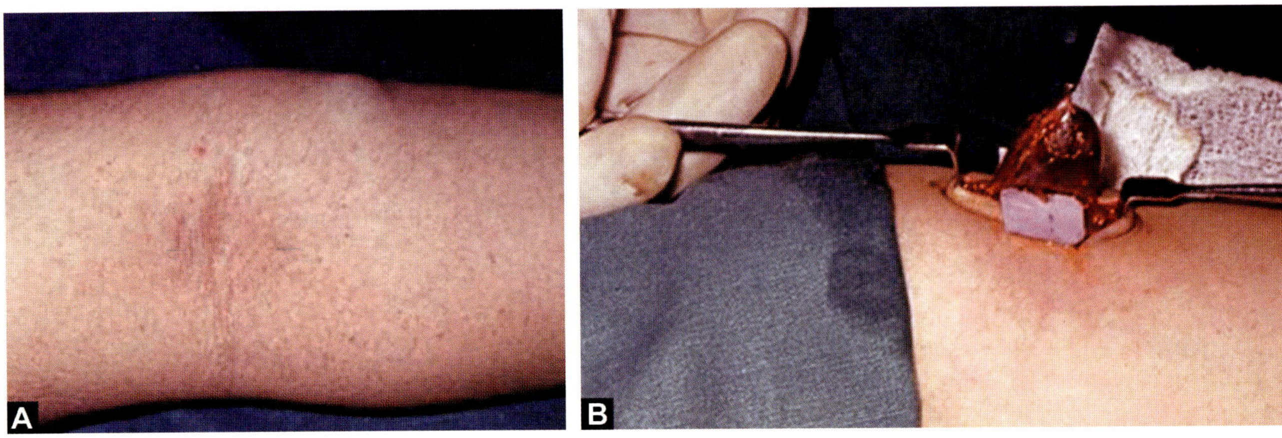

FIGURES 7.1A and B
A small VM with a single afferent and a single efferent vessel

them without violating its borders and preserving excision planes. They all have afferent tributaries and efferent drainers. During their excision, as far as possible, the input must be ligated before the output.

Head and neck lesions often expand with a Valsalva test. Posture too, may affect the judgment of extent — a characteristic that some venous malformations share with macrocystic lymphatic malformations (cystic hygromas). These lesions in the head and neck may be hardly noticeable in the vertical posture but become prominent on lying down.

Figure 7.2 illustrates a venous malformation of the neck hardly noticeable in the vertical posture and prominent when recumbent (Figs 7.2A and B). Axial sections of the CT scan (Figs 7.2C to E) show the close relationship of the carotid sheath with the structures of the neck. The coronal reconstruction (Fig. 7.2F) demonstrates, the size and the extent of lesion, tissue displacement as typified by the displacement of the external jugular vein, numerous phleboliths and the close contact of the malformation with the terminal portion of the internal jugular vein. The tiny space between them, not only marked the most dangerous part of the operative exercise but also indicated its possibility.

The supraclaircular transverse part of the incision helped identification and preservation of the Thoracic duct looping across the terminal portion of the malformation as also the draining vein. The tiny space between the internal jugular vein and the draining vein, enabled a surgical separation without damage to the internal jugular vein.

The postoperative status (Fig. 7.2G) clearly shows the significant atrophy of the soft tissue, associated with these malformations.

DIAGNOSTIC ERRORS AND INADEQUATE EXPOSURES CAN BE DISASTEROUS

Initial treatment of the patient shown in Figure 7.3, was carried out elsewhere. As per the history given, she appears to be a victim of diagnostic confusion. A lesion in her left parotid region was first noted at the age of 3 months. She was operated at the age

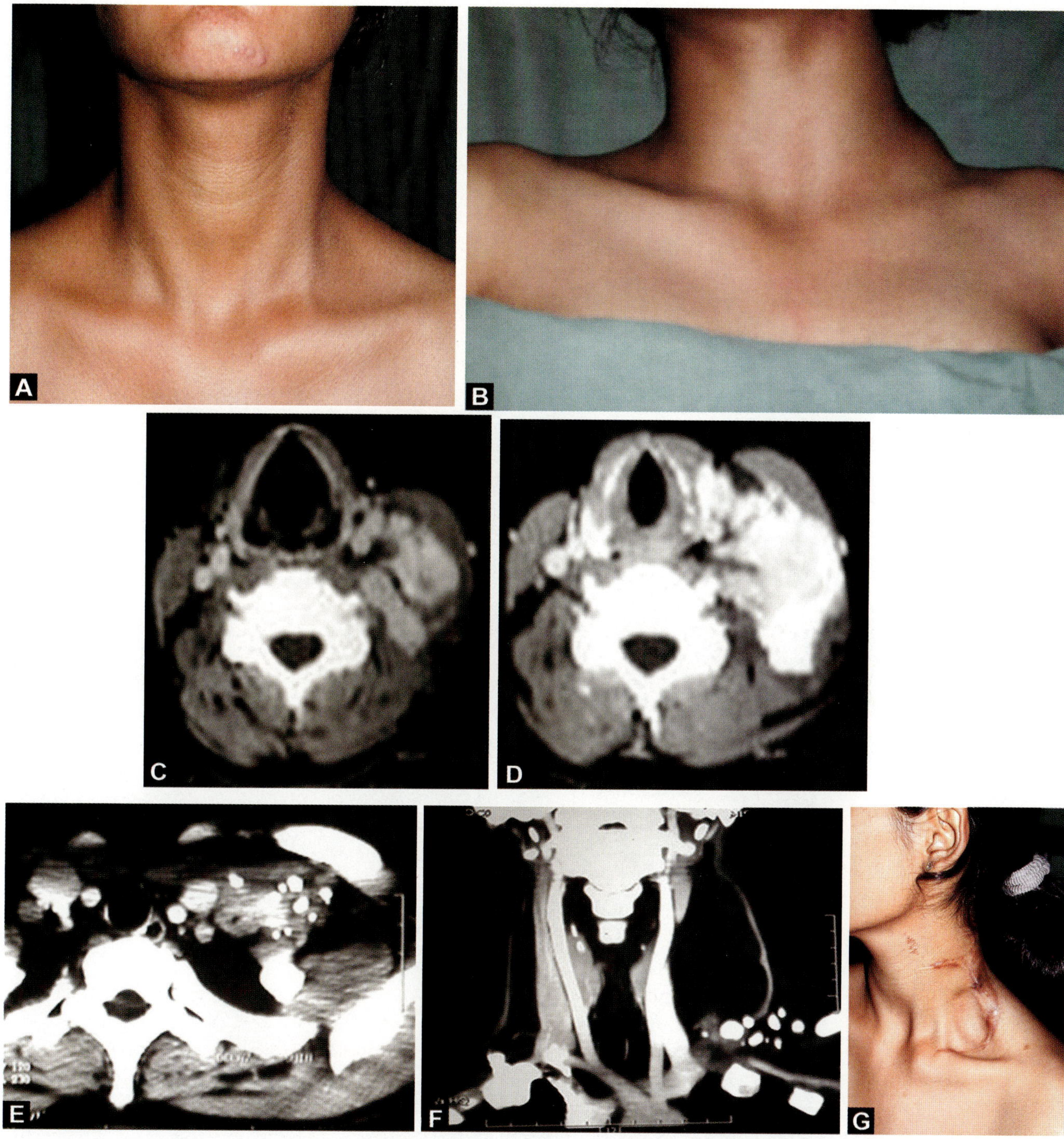

FIGURES 7.2A to G
A Venous Malformation of the Neck: (A and B) The lesion hardly noticeable in vertical position but prominent in the recumbent position; (C) A CT study to show the extent of the lesion and its relationship with the carotid sheath; (D) At the level of the lower border of the mandible; (E) At mid neck; (F) The coronal reconstruction, at the level of the clavicle. Note the close contact between the internal jugular vein and the lower end of the venous malformation and the tiny space between them; (G) The postoperative status showing the soft tissue atrophy associated with the VM

of 1½ years with the diagnosis of a lymphangioma by a pediatric surgeon, on the basis of a senior opinion, clinical translucency and a plain CT scan. The operation was abandoned due to hemorrhage. Subsequently, the child appears to have been administered a couple of hot saline or boiling water injections. When first seen by us at the age of 19 years, she showed heavy iatrogenic scarring (Figs 7.3A and B) but an unaffected facial nerve. A CT scan confirmed a VM. Iatrogenic scarring is a known drawback of the use of all sclerotic agents.

Our incision closely followed the scar borders and at the upper end, turned back to continue as a parotid incision. Through this adequate exposure, the facial nerve could be identified and protected and the venous malformation is ablated (Figs 7.3C and D). A follow-up 12 years later (Figs 7.3E and F) showed a good appearance and no recurrence.

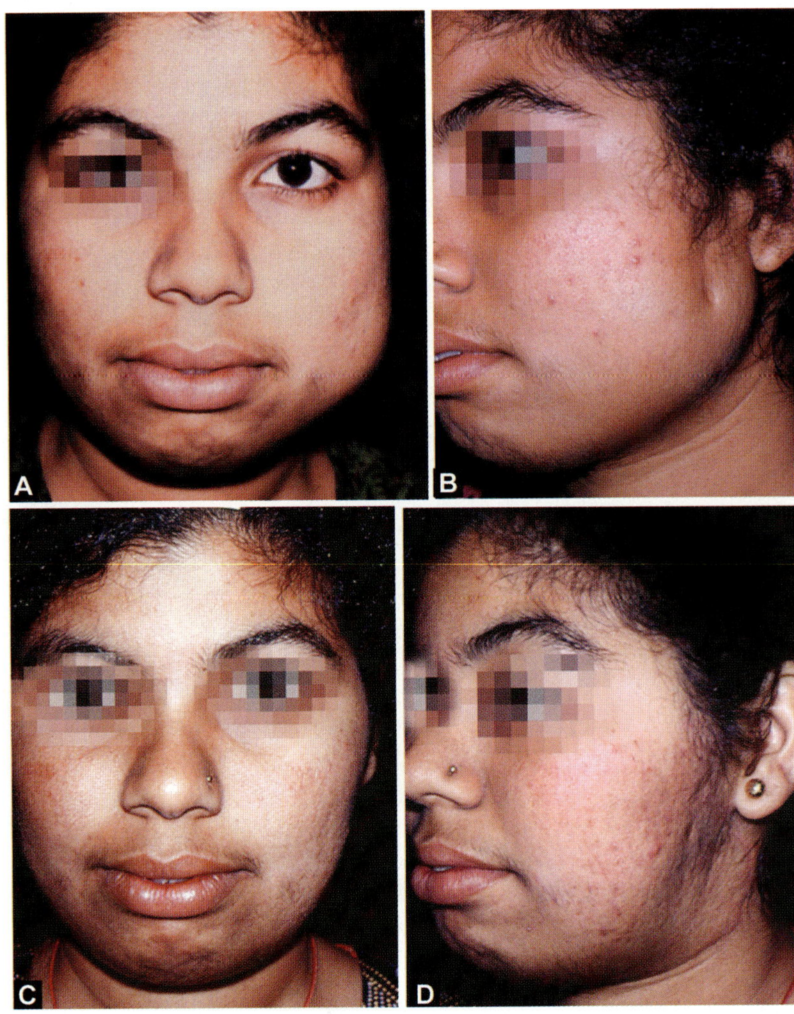

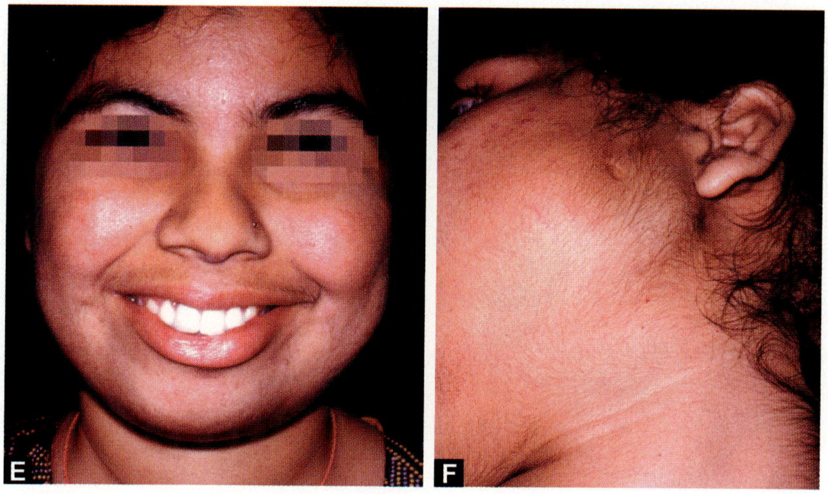

FIGURES 7.3A to F
(A and B) Preoperative appearance; (C and D) Early postoperative appearance; (E and F) Follow-up after 12 years

SOME OTHER FEATURES RELATED TO VMs

Excessive growth of the lesion, following partial excision is reported in literature. I have not seen this happen. Possibly, the cause is the ligation of efferent vessels without obliterating the afferent vessels. Hence, a centripetal dissection to the extent possible is always advisable.

Phlebothrombosis with associated pain and swelling, is common in venous malformations of the extremities, but not commonly seen in head and neck lesions.

Location in muscles: VMs are known to be located in the muscles of mastication. They are comparatively more common in the masseter muscle (Fig. 7.3) and very rare in the temporalis muscle.

Transgression: Transgressions of muscles is attributed to these lesions. This transgression involves not only the muscles but, also the adjacent tissues. It does not appear to be due to growth, but merely an expression of a preexisting malformation. However, it does pose problems in their management. Figs 7.4A to E illustrate such transgressions. The lesion here goes across the temporalis muscle and permeates the subtemporal, sub-mandibular and cervical regions. An adequate access was provided by a parotid incision extending upward into the temporal region. The lifting up of the zygomatic arch, gave an access to the subtemporal region.

The proximity of the malformation, to the internal jugular vein (Figs 7.4C and D), prompted the decision to dissect in the submandibular region from the periphery towards the vein. This was a useful decision because the malformation opened directly into the internal jugular vein. The opening was closed and the continuity of the internal jugular vein was maintained (Figs 7.4E and F).

Familial inheritance has been reported as an autosomal dominant with its association mapped to chromosome 9q. There is evidence of genetic basis in Turner's syndrome (lesions in intestine and feet), familial cutaneous mucosal VMs, and cerebral cavernous VMs. The concerned gene is KRITI 1.

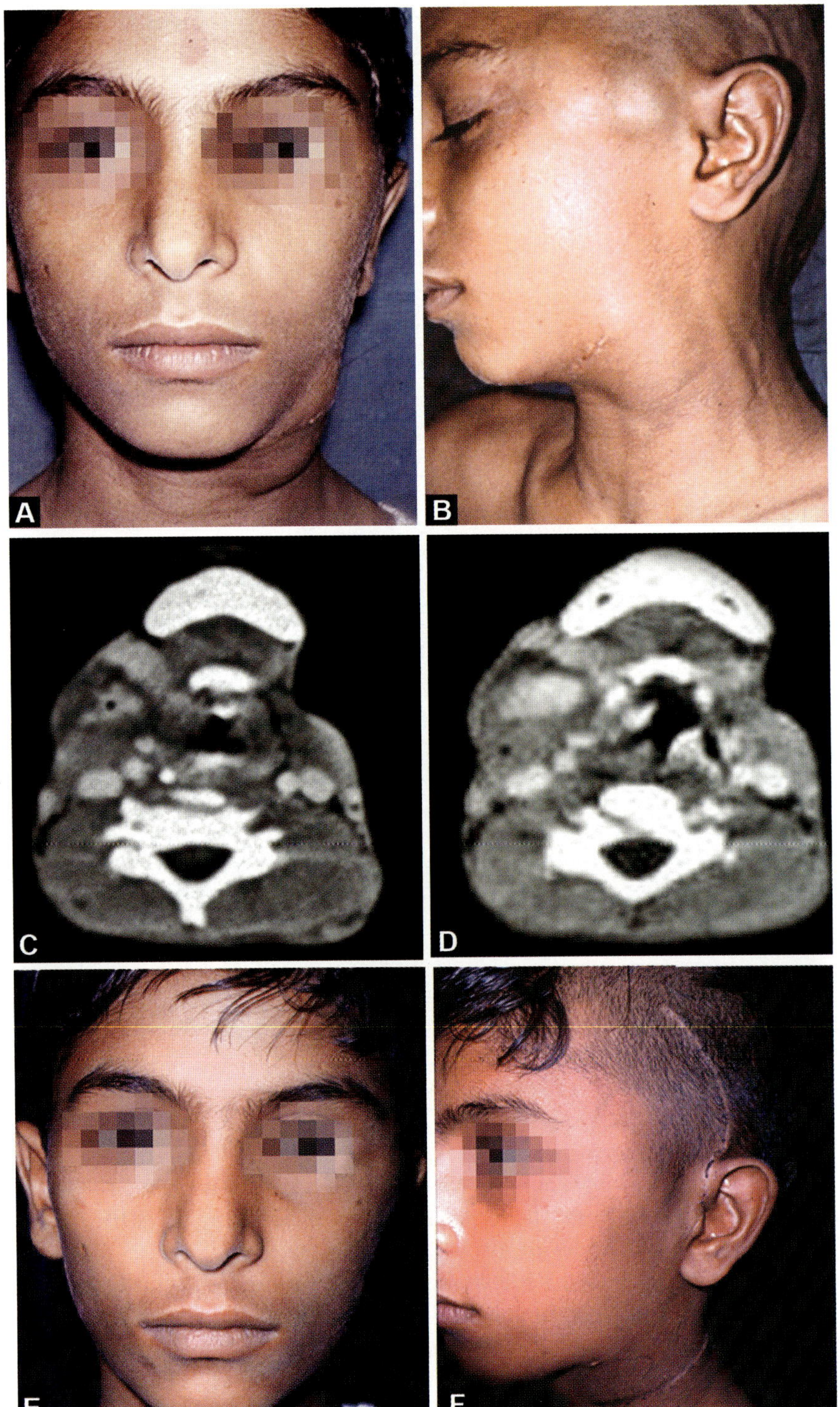

FIGURES 7.4A to F

Venous malformation — left side of the face: (A) Note prominence of left side of the face and upper neck; (B) In addition note the prominence of the veins; (C and D) Axial CT studies to show proximity of the VM to the internal jugular vein; (E and F) Show the postopretive result, the extent of the incision, the restoration of the facial symmetry and absence of the injury to the facial nerve

A couple of syndromes are associated with these lesions:

a. Blue Rubber Bleb Nevus Syndrome—Multiple VMs with occasionally problematic GI bleeding.
b. Maffuci syndrome—Multiple VMs associated with enchondromas, begins at adolescence, Skeletal lesions may degenerate into malignancies.

MANAGEMENT

Investigations

The presence of phleboliths, even in a plain radiograph is diagnostic of a venous malformation. Being a purely venous structure, a color doppler study is diagnostic and adequate to confirm the clinical suspicion.

A CT study and/or an MRI are useful to define the extent and the important relationships and thereby help in planning the surgical intervention.

To achieve precision and avoid disasters, sclerotherapy too, if used, should also be preferably controlled by an appropriate and available imaging guidance.

Preoperative evaluation of the coagulation profile is important.

Coagulopathies, if present, should be corrected preoperatively. The patient is monitored for them, postoperatively.

Skeletal deformities or asymmetry can be well documented by appropriate radiological images or 3D reconstructions.

THERAPEUTIC MEASURES

Sclerotherapy: Ablation using a variety of local sclerosants like boiling water, alcohol, quinine, sodium morruhate and others have been advocated. All these blind procedures, are characterized by a poor control on the extent of eradication and the safeguarding of normal tissue. Sclerotherapy can produce secondary deformities, due to heavy scarring and renders subsequent surgical ablation more difficult.

There is also a risk of severe hemorrhage when blindly dealing with large channel lesions.

It should preferably be done under imaging guidance. Ultrasonography is the most commonly used imaging modality. Doing a direct venography under fluoroscopic control, to identify the extent and morphology of the lesion and the location of the efferent veins is useful.

In head and neck lesions, there being no scope for using a tourniquet to produce circulatory stasis, sclerosants can be useful only in small lesions where the spread of the sclerosant can be effectively controlled by local pressure, till the sclerosant is fixed.

When injecting sclerosants, it is important to block the efferent vein by external pressure—a difficult task in the head and neck.

I prefer to use sclerosants only for residual pockets. However, there are lesions or their residual parts which may not be easily accessible to the surgeon or the excision may be a very dangerous exercise. These could be considered for well-controlled sclerotherapy, which should be done under anesthesia and under fluoroscopic control by an interventional radiologist. A direct venogram defines the limits of the lesion and identifies the draining veins which must be temporarily blocked or closed off before injecting the sclerosants.

Haphazard attempts at sclerotherapy can be counterproductive and make subsequent management by any modality more difficult.

My preferred sclerosant, for my limited use has been sodium tetradecyl sulphate injection — 30 mg per cc. It can be used for both venous and lymphatic malformations.

It is less painful and less toxic than ethanol and the use is relatively safe in the venous channels.

Ethanol is currently the most commonly used sclerosant in various parts of the world, with a fairly high percentage of patients needing repeated sessions. Ethanol has been maximally used because of its potential for total destruction of the tissue with which it comes in contact, obliterating the channels and ensuring a good result. However, ethanol can have systemic effects and the permitted dosage that can be injected in a single session of treatment is 1 mg/kg of body weight. In addition, it can damage any other structure with which it may come in contact, including nerves, vessels and muscles. Therefore, particularly in head and neck, the use of sclerosants should be practiced with extreme caution, only by experienced teams and under effective controls. We have no personal experience of using ethanol in the management of vascular malformations.

Embolization

Attempt at embolization of VMs can be dangerous as also the embolization of an arterial inflow to a venous anomaly. (Demuth et al. 1984).

Preoperative Direct Embolization — NBCA Glue

Preoperative direct percutaneous obliteration of the VM cavity with *N*-butyl 2-cyanoacrylate NBCA glue, holds promise of facilitating easier and bloodless dissection of a venous malformation (Cil et al, 2008). The authors share their experience of thirteen patients treated over a period of about three years. The patients were referred from the plastic surgery department. Angiography ruled out an arterial element in the malformation before embolization. They had used NBCA diluted with iodized oil at a ratio of 1:6 (18%) injected percutaneously through a 21 gauge needle. A few patients required more than one session. The Surgical intervention was undertaken about 10 to 15 days later, giving the surgical team a clean field.

Embolization with NCB Glue is a potent tool to facilitate blood less excision. However, in VMs it should be used with extreme caution, ensuring that afferent vessels are effectively blocked to prevent systemic embolization.

Surgery

Surgery for VMs is curative. If anatomical limits of the lesion are accessible, even with some difficulty, surgery is my first choice. The use of sclerosants is reserved for residual lesions. In the nascent lesions, the dissection planes are clean and bloodless surgery is possible. However, blood should always be kept ready, for it may suddenly be needed particularly when dealing with a part of the lesion with a difficult access.

Planning — Surgical Intervention deserves to be carefully planned, contrast imaging gives a fair idea of directions, tributaries and extent. A study of these considerably aids planning.

As far as possible, the input must be ligated before the output. It is easy and obvious in the situation in Figure 7.1 to differentiate the input and the output, but more difficult in larger lesions.

Differentiating the 'Feeders' and the 'Drainers'

When there are a number of 'feeders', to differentiate between the 'feeders' and the 'drainers', is morphologically not so obvious. Locations and directions are important. Peripherally, radially located 'feeders' are likely to be true feeders. The 'drainers' are more centripetally located, sometimes bunched and directed towards the main draining veins. Ligating them primarily is likely to cause ballooning of the malformation, increase the blood loss significantly and make the dissection extremely difficult. Differentiating the 'feeders' and 'drainers' can be considerably facilitated by color Doppler and other imaging techniques. Surface and deep lesions pose different problems.

Surface lesions, when extensive, are extremely difficult to treat without accepting some deformity. This residual deformity is associated with the technique used for skin cover and the deformity already created by the lesion itself. However, comparatively localized surface lesions, even full thickness, if conveniently located, can give good results following ablation and reconstruction. A considerable circumference of the right side of the mouth in the patient shown in Figures 7.5A and B, was pervaded by a venous malformation. A conservative but total excision and reconstruction using an Abbe'-Estlander flap, and a minor touch-up thereafter was rewarding (Figs 7.5C to E).

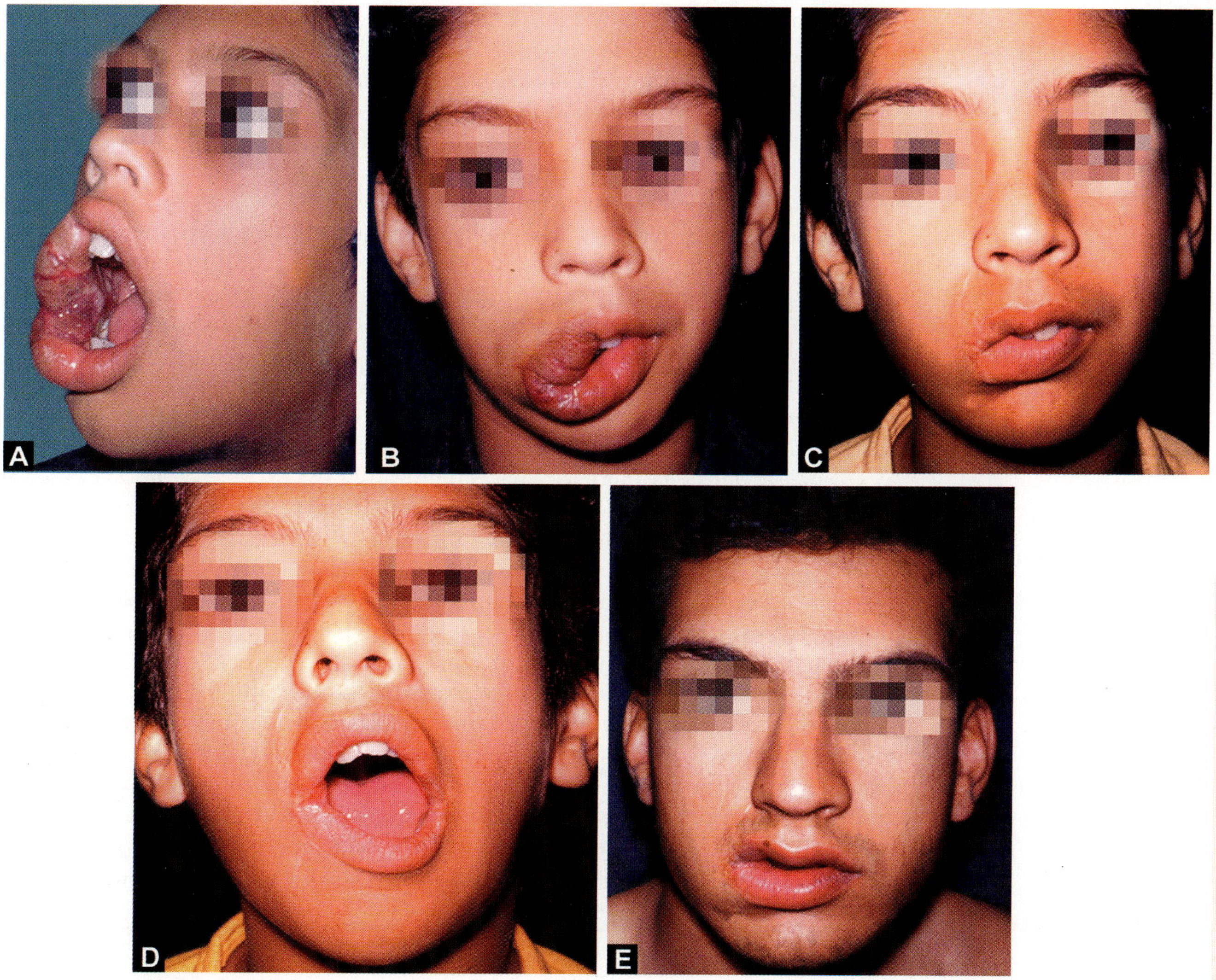

FIGURES 7.5A to E

Vascular malformation — Superficial and extensive: (A and B) A full thickness lesion involving the margins of the right side of the mouth including the angle. (C to E) After excision and reconstruction of the angle using Abbe-Estlander Flap. (C) soon postoperative; (D) 5 months later; (E) 7 years later

Deeper lesions. The modalities generally used are sclerosants, surgery and their combinations. I prefer surgery whenever possible and restrict the use of sclerosants only for the residual lesions. Their primary and extensive use causes fibrosis and disturbs the surgical planes and the surgical field. Even in these lesions, total excision is the treatment of choice. For the sake of safety or in presence of inaccessibility, one may be constrained to leave behind small pockets, some of which can be obliterated by sclerosants.

Partial excision has been recommended for a persistently painful area in a venous malformation and for contouring a deforming malformation. I feel, that such interventions are rarely justified, because the residual lesion continues to grow.

For the ablation of the deep lesions, selecting the approach is important.

The Choice of Approach

In these benign meandering lesions of the head and neck, the choice of approach is overwhelmingly important to avoid damage to important structures. In general, the incisions and the route to be adopted, have to be carefully planned. The incision should be aesthetically placed and the route, should not transgress or endanger any vital structure, even at the cost of leaving a small residual lesion.

The location decides the approach and the extent of surgical intervention as demonstrated by the cases shown in Figures 7.4 and 7.6.

The patient shown in Figure 7.4 demonstrated an extensive yet discrete approach to large VM of the left side of the face and the importance of the centripetal approach. Here, in the sub-mandibular area, the malformation drained directly into the internal jugular vein. The centripetal approach helped both, the identification and localization of their communication and its management.

The patient in Figures 7.6A and B had a large venous malformation situated on his left cheek. It extended up, to the zygomatic arch and posteriorly going deep to the carotid sheath and then medially to the posterolateral wall of the pharynx and the adjacent palate (Figs 7.6C and D). This configuration led to the assumption that the facial nerve except its buccinator branch, lay superficial to the malformation. It was decided to explore and ablate the lesion, through the left buccal incision below the level of the parotid duct and if necessary, leave the lateral pharyngeal extension for subsequent sclerotherapy. He did extremely well as seen about 8 years later (Figs 7.6E and F).

Figure 7.7 shows a young mother, of a three year old child with a proptosis caused by a VM sitting on the optic nerve and extending to the optic canal (Figs 7.7A to C). To assure adequate access not only to the orbit but also to the optic canal (Fig. 7.7D) the transcranial approach was preferred. The approach followed was a bicoronal incision, the transcranial route and the exposure of the orbital contents through the orbital roof (Fig. 7.7E). The periorbita was opened between the frontal and trochlear nerves, giving us a bloodless route to the hemangioma and the optic nerve. The VM was exposed, the exposure completed by deroofing the optic canal and the whole of the malformation removed in a clean field and under direct vision.

Atraumatic Technique and Choice of Instruments

The use of the atraumatic technique is relevant to all vascular malformations but is particularly important to large channel malformations. Here a careful choice in the

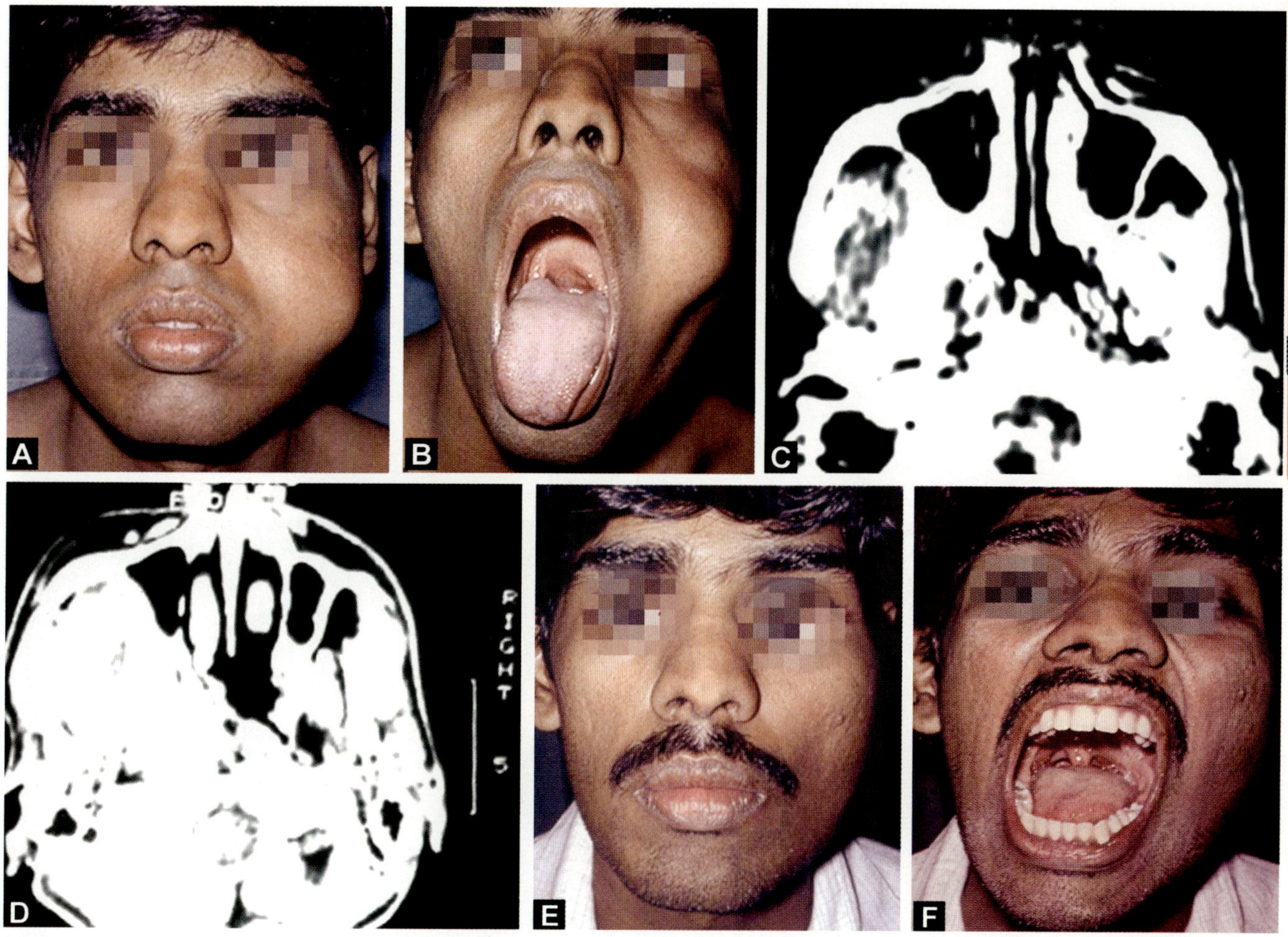

FIGURES 7.6A to F

A large venous malformation situated in the left cheek: (A and B) The preoperative status; (C and D) CT images showing the extent from the cheek to the posterior lateral pharyngeal wall and the proximity to the carotid sheath; (E and F) The postoperative status confirming no damage to the facial nerve

selection of instruments and technique makes a lot of difference to the execution of the surgical task and prevention of blood loss.

Near the venous malformation, the use of toothed forceps and conventional hemostats should be avoided. I only use atroforceps and atroclamps.

To dissect in the plane between the vessels and the normal tissues, my choice is blunt pointed, sharp, and narrow scissors.

I find the use of neurosurgical lint patties useful to aid protection, retraction and compression of the vascular tissue.

Whenever possible, the feeders should be underrun and ligated. Hemostats should be used, only if the whole circumference of a vessel can be identified and the vessels can be divided between two clamps and ligated.

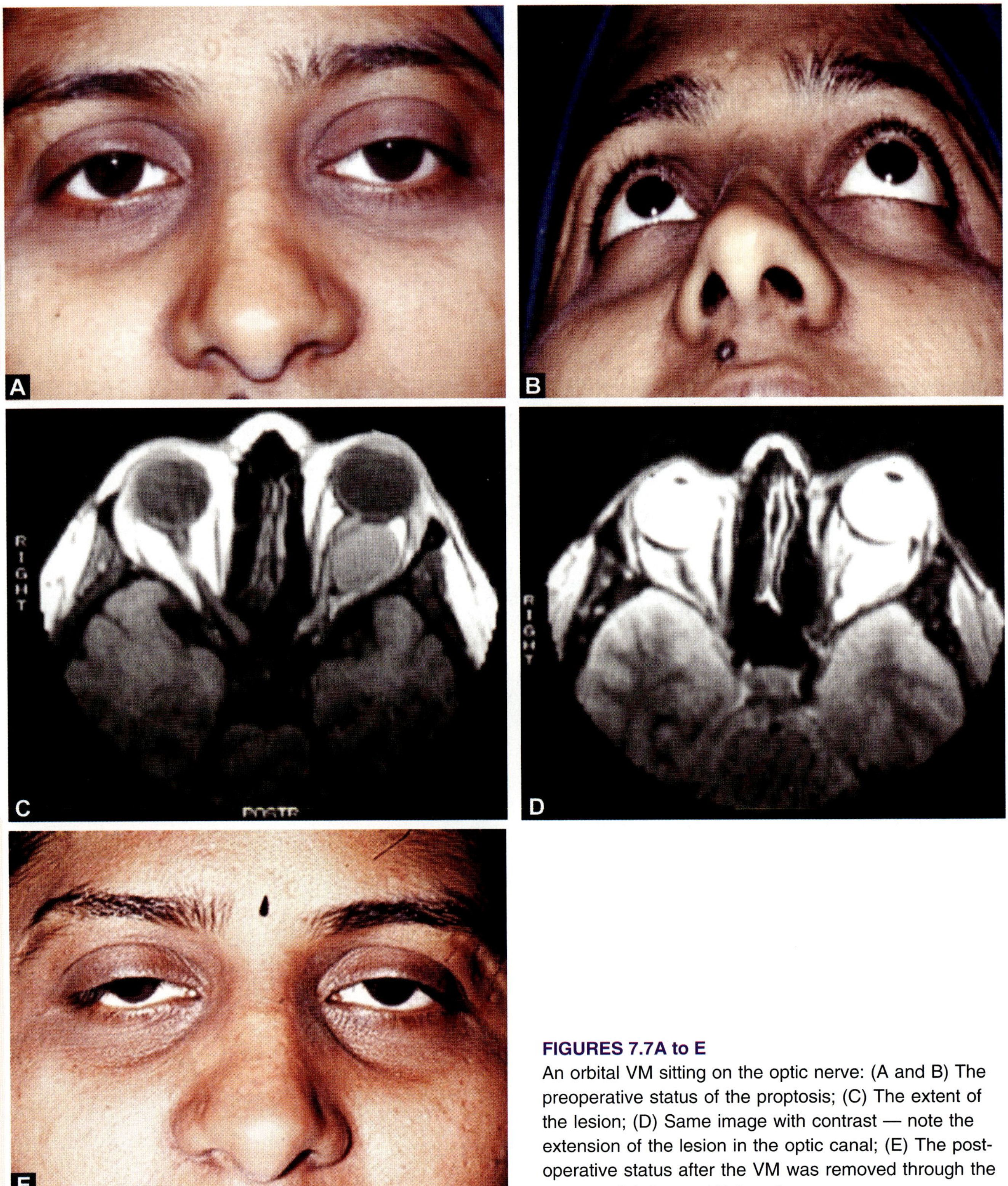

FIGURES 7.7A to E

An orbital VM sitting on the optic nerve: (A and B) The preoperative status of the proptosis; (C) The extent of the lesion; (D) Same image with contrast — note the extension of the lesion in the optic canal; (E) The post-operative status after the VM was removed through the transcranial, transorbital route

It has to be remembered that the wall of VMs are usually very thin and severe bleeding can start by trying to catch the walls of the malformation blindly.

Often, gentle pressure over a neurosurgical pattie can effectively control the bleeding, while the surgeon proceeds to find enough room for a proper ligation.

Free use of local coagulants, gelfoam and patience is extremely useful.

The separation of the VM from the internal jugular vein Figure 7.2 is an illustration of the caution and patience required in these dissections.

Bipolar cautery is very useful. Radiofrequency coagulative instruments, both unipolar and bipolar are superior when dealing with vascular malformations.

SUMMARY

Venous malformations are vascular lesions causing a bulge, which is usually compressible. When large, local atrophy, especially of the fibrofatty tissue is common. If reasonably localized, it is best removed surgically using a centripetal and atraumatic approach. Adequate and a carefully planned exposure is a necessity.

In operating all Vascular Malformations particularly the venous malformation, as far as possible, the input must be ligated before the output and the dissection should be in a centripetal fashion wherever possible. Ultrasound and contrast imaging give a fair idea of directions and tributaries.

Carefully done surgical ablation can be fairly bloodless. However, blood should always be kept ready.

Early intervention is recommended, because with the passage of time, enlargement and possibly the development of new channels and connections, would make the task more difficult. If totally removed, recurrence is unlikely. Small residual lesions can grow slowly. They are suitable for sclerotherapy or may be excision by another approach.

Asymptomatic deep seated lesions can be left alone.

Surgery for Venous Malformations has been very rewarding and preferred over haphazard and often imprecise sclerotherapy.

BIBLIOGRAPHY

1. Cil BE, Vargel I, Geyik S, Peynircioglu B, Cavusoglu T. Venous vascular malformations of the craniofacial region: Pre-operative embolisation with direct percutaneous puncture and N-butyl cyanoacrylate. British Journal of Radiology 2008;81:935-9.
2. Demuth RJ, Miller SH, Keller F. Complications of embolization treatment for problem cavernous hemangiomas. Ann. Plast. Surg 1984;13:135.
3. Gomes AS. Embolization therapy of congenital arteriovenous malformations: Use of alternate approaches. Radiology 1994;190:191-8 [Abstract/Free Full Text].
4. Han MH, Seong SO, Kim HD, Chang KH, Han MC. Craniofacial arteriovenous malformation: Preoperative embolization with direct puncture and injection of n-butyl cyanoacrylate. Radiology 1999;211:661-6 [Abstract/Free Full Text].
5. Jackson IT, Carreno R, Potparic Z, Hussain K. Hemangiomas, vascular malformations and lymphovenous malformations: Classification and methods of treatment. Plast Reconstr Surg 1993;91:1216-30 [Medline].
6. Küppers GLE, Eichhorn E, Hoeve LJ, Verwoerd CDA. A venous malformation of the neck: Otorhinolaryngol nova 1998;8:73-75 (DOI: 10.1159/000027815), a single case report

8

VASCULAR MALFORMATIONS OF THE BRAIN

Anil Karapurkar

PIAL ATERIOVENOUS MALFORMATIONS (AVM) AND ATERIOVENOUS FISTULA (AVF)

Pial AVM consists of a bunch of blood vessels where the intervening capillaries have not formed. Within the bunch of blood vessels called AVM nidus, there may be intranidal arterial aneurysms or intranidal A-V fistulae with direct communication between artery and vein. There may be a single arterial feeder and single draining vein, multiple feeders and single vein or multiple feeders and multiple veins. The veins are arterialized and carry red blood and show reflux into multiple tributaries.

Associated venous anomaly with absence of deep venous system, anomaly of the venous dural sinuses, stenosis of the draining veins or aneurysms (varices) along draining veins are common. AVM may be compact like a tumor or show a diffuse spread over a large part of the hemisphere. Most brain AVMs are congenital but acquired AVMs have been documented. Usually they are single but multiple lesions are not rare.

Pial arteriovenous fistula (AVF) is formed by direct communication between a large artery and a draining vein. There may be a single hole fistula fed by a single artery and drained by a single large arterialized vein or a multiple hole fistula with multiple feeders but single vein. Because the vein is arterialized, venous aneurysms and stenosis along the course of the vein are common. Usually pial AVFs are single but multiple are not unknown. AVMs and AVFs are most common in the middle cerebral artery distribution. They may be cryptic, small or large and even giant sized involving the whole hemisphere.

There are no true epidemiological studies. Incidence of AVM, according to different studies varies between 0.94 to 15 per 100,000 population. (Stapf 2000, Warlow 2001, Berman 2000, Jessurun 1993). Though AVMs are congenital, but have rarely been found in families and no genetic predisposition has been identified (Kamiryo 2000, Aberfeld and Rao 1981, Yokohama 1991). AVMs are usually single, but multiple AVMs may be found in hereditary hemorrhagic telangiectasia (HHT), Rendu-Osler-Weber disease and Wyburn Mason disease. Multiple AVMs have also been described in CAMs and PHACE by Lasjauinas and Bhattacharyya.

Clinical Presentation

Hemorrhage, epilepsy, progressive neurological deficit and headache are the common presentations. In recent years, CT or MRI scans done for various indications may show incidental AVMs. Hemorrhage is the most common and devastating presentation. Various studies have been done to estimate the risk of bleeding. It is estimated to be about 2 to 4 percent per year of life. It is commonly believed that small AVMs present with devastating hemorrhage and large AVMs present with epilepsy. Hemorrhage is more common if there is an associated juxta or intranidal aneurysm, single draining vein, stenosis or aneurysm along the draining vein, or associated venous anomaly. Hemorrhage may be small as a warning leak with mild headache or may be devastating, leading to rapid coma and death. The commonest age of presentation is in the second and third decade. Intracerebral hemorrhage is the most common presentation. Rarely, there may be pure intraventricular hemorrhage (IVH) or subarachnoid hemorrhage (SAH).

Epilepsy may be focal or generalized. It is due to gliosis of the brain adjacent to the AVM or irritation of the cortex by the AVM nidus. It is more common in large AVMs. The type of epilepsy varies according to location. Temporal lesions may present with complex partial seizures, those around motor or sensory cortex with Jacksonisan epilepsy, occipital lesions with visual symptoms and frontal lesions with generalized epilepsy.

Progressive neurological deficit is often seen in large deep AVMs. It is either due to pressure on the internal capsule by the mass of the AVM or due to ischemia of the adjacent brain due to steal into the high flow AVM nidus.

Headache is usually seen when there is dural supply to a pial AVM. It can be intractable.

Investigations

Plain X-rays may show nodular calcification of the adjacent ischemic brain or a calcification of an old healed hematoma.

Plain CT scan may show the calcification. Large AVM may be seen as a hyperdense shadow. A small AVM is not seen.

Contrast CT Scan usually shows the AVM nidus. Large feeding arteries and draining veins may be seen. Associated hematoma, IVH or intracerebral hemorrhage (ICH) are well seen. Mass effect and compression and shift of brain and ventricles can be appreciated.

CT Angiography shows the nidus, feeding arteries and draining veins. There may be one or more feeding arteries. Large AVMs may be fed by all three arteries, i.e. anterior, middle and posterior cerebral artery. Feeding veins superficial and deep may be well seen. Associated aneurysms are usually seen but some may be missed. No idea can be had of the rate of flow across the AVM.

MRI shows the nidus well. Feeding arteries and veins may be well seen. Associated aneurysms may be documented. Mass effect is well seen.

MRA shows the architecture of the AVM well, but usually is not very useful in planning treatment.

DSA is the gold standard. For a therapeutic decision, DSA is mandatory. It shows all the feeding arteries, draining veins, associated arterial and venous aneurysms, venous anomalies like stenosis or absence of veins. Remote aneurysm on the circle of Willis may be identified. Rate of flow across the AVM is well seen.

When analyzing the AVM one looks at the site of the nidus, size of the nidus, feeding arteries, draining veins, associated arterial or venous aneurysm, rate of flow across the nidus, associated venous anomaly and superficial or deep venous drainage.

Natural History of Brain AVM

The precise natural history of brain AVMs is not known. There are many studies on the natural history. Hillmans study on population based analysis from Sweden throws some light on the natural history. The incidence of hemorrhage is about 2 to 4 percent per year of life. If an AVM has already bled the natural history changes and it is about 6 to 10 percent per year of life. By age 40 years, 50 percent of patients harboring AVM will have bled at least once and about 40 percent will have succumbed or have developed major neurological deficit. Spontaneous thrombosis of an AVM is rare.

Treatment

There are following possibilities:

a. No treatment
b. Surgical excision
c. Embolization
d. Radiosurgery (SRS)

No Treatment

Treatment of AVMs should be a team effort. The team should consist of neurosurgeon, interventional neuroradiologist, neurologist and radiotherapist. Every case should be discussed and pros and cons of different modalities analyzed.

Should all AVMs be treated? There is no consensus on which AVMs should be treated. The risk of treatment should be less than that of the natural history of the disease. If one undertakes treatment, one must obliterate the AVM completely. Partial treatment is more dangerous and hemorrhage is more common and disastrous. Targeted treatment of "weak spots" is also controversial. Weak spots are associated aneurysms arterial or venous, associated AVF, stenosis of draining veins and absence of a deep venous system.

Medium and large incidental AVMs need not to be treated. Large AVM presenting with epilepsy need not to be treated except for weak spots. Small accessible non-eloquent AVMs associated with hematoma must be treated by surgical excision or embolization. AVMs associated with hemorrhage must be treated.

Surgical Excision

Spetzler Martin classification is widely used to determine the risk of treatment (Table 8.1).

TABLE 8.1
Pial AVM classification — Spetzler Martin score

Parameters	*Score*
Size	
<3 cm	1
3 to 6 cm	2
>6 cm	3
Venous drainage	
Superficial	0
Deep	1
Eloquence	
Noneloquent	0
Eloquent	1
Least risk for surgery (minimum)	1
Highest risk for surgery (maximum)	5

The three parameters considered are:

A. Size of nidus — less than 3 cm — point 1, 3 to 6 cm — points 2 and more than 6 cm — points 3.
B. Non-eloquent point 0, eloquent brain point 1.
C. Superficial venous drainage — point 0 and deep venous drainage — point 1. They are graded from Grade 1 to 5. The ideal AVM for surgical excision is small (less than 3 cm), lying in noneloquent brain like frontal or temporal pole of nondominant hemisphere and having only superficial veins draining the AVM. The risk for Grade 5 AVM is very high and is best left alone.

Surgical excision of AVM is always performed through a large craniotomy. If there is clot a small cortical or sulcal incision is made to enter it. The clot, is evacuated by gentle irrigation and suction. There is always a gliotic plane around the AVM nidus. This gliotic plane is gradually dissected clipping or coagulating feeding arteries until the nidus is hanging free. The draining vein is finally clipped or coagulated and the nidus lifted in one piece. If there are multiple draining veins, one of these can be divided early in the course of the surgery and used as a handle for gentle traction.

Total excision should be confirmed by intraoperative DSA. If there is a small residue, it is excised immediately. There is high-risk of hemorrhage from the residual AVM. Break through bleeding has been described after excision of large high flow AVMs. This is assumed to be due to a gush of blood into the hitherto relatively ischemic brain. Hence, for high flow large AVMs, embolization followed by excision reduces the risk of high mortality and morbidity and is the better option.

Many surgeons do not agree with the concept of breakthrough bleeding. They believe this is due to hemorrhage from tiny fragile arterial feeders which retract into the brain and are missed despite a diligent search.

The operative morbidity and mortality should be less than that of natural history. In most series, it varies between 5 and 15 percent.

Embolization

It can be curative especially for small and medium size AVMs. It can be adjunct to surgery or Radiosurgery. For preoperative embolization, it is ideal to occlude supply from the deep perforators as cortical arteries are accessible and can be easily tackled. Embolization for SRS should be sectorial, to allow planning. For large or inaccessible AVMs, targeted embolization for obliteration of "weak spots" such as aneurysm or an intranidal AVF is attempted. Management team makes a definitive plan before commencing treatment. The aim of embolization is to deposit liquid embolic material, histoacryl or Onyx into the nidus. If the feeding artery is occluded and the nidus is left behind it recruits feeders from adjacent arteries which make subsequent treatment with embolization or surgery very difficult. If particles such as gel foam, polyvinyl alcohol (PVA), avitene or silk thread are used, the nidus escapes and the feeders get occluded. This form of embolization may give immediate fantastic result but the AVM nidus very soon recruits blood from adjacent arteries and is now a multiheaded monster. If the nidus is obliterated, the AVM does not recur. In principle, one does embolization from distal to proximal or posterior to anterior. Small and medium AVMs may be obliterated in a single session. Large AVMs may need several sessions, four to six weeks apart.

Complete cerebral angiography with bilateral internal and external corotid and bilateral vertebral artery angiography is done. All feeders, draining veins, associated aneurysms and AVMs are analyzed. The artery providing direct access to the AVM is identified and catheterized. The microcatheter is placed as close to the nidus as possible, or within it, with the help of a supple microwire. Histoacryl or N-Butyl-2 cyanoacrylate, a liquid embolic agent (glue) is a rapid setting polymer which hardens as soon, as it comes in contact with blood, saline or contrast. The polymerizing time is modified by adding Lipiodol which also makes it radiopaque and visible on fluoroscopy. For high flow AVMs, 50 to 66 percent glue is injected. For low flow AVMs, 20 percent glue is injected slowly under fluoroscopy.

The rate of cure from glue alone is about 30 percent (Figs 8.1 and 8.2). Today the liquid embolic agent of choice is ONYX (Ethyl Vinyl Alcohol Copolymer, DMSO or Di-methyl-sulphoxide and tantalum powder) (Fig. 8.3). The injection is made slowly over several minutes. The rate of cure has gone up from 30 percent with glue alone to 60 percent with Onyx alone. The main risks are erratic embolization and hemorrhage. After the learning curve has been ascended, the risk of complication is about 8 to 10 percent (Figs 8.3A to H).

Radiosurgery (SRS)

In radiosurgery a single large dose of radiation is delivered to the AVM nidus in a single sitting. SRS is performed by gammaknife, X-knife, Cyberknife and proton beam. Gammaknife SRS is done by 201 sources of Cobalt 60 placed in a helmet. In X-knife and Cyberknife X-rays are used. The tube containing the source of X-rays rotates around the head which is at the isocenter. Planning is done by fusing images of MRI, CT scan and DSA, so as to minimize injury to normal brain and deliver a large dose to the nidus. The average dose is 25G to the isocenter. After SRS, there is gradual thrombosis of the AVM nidus and on an average the AVM disappears after 2 years (Figs 8.4A to H). CT scan or MRI is done at 6, 12, 18 and 24 months. DSA is done after

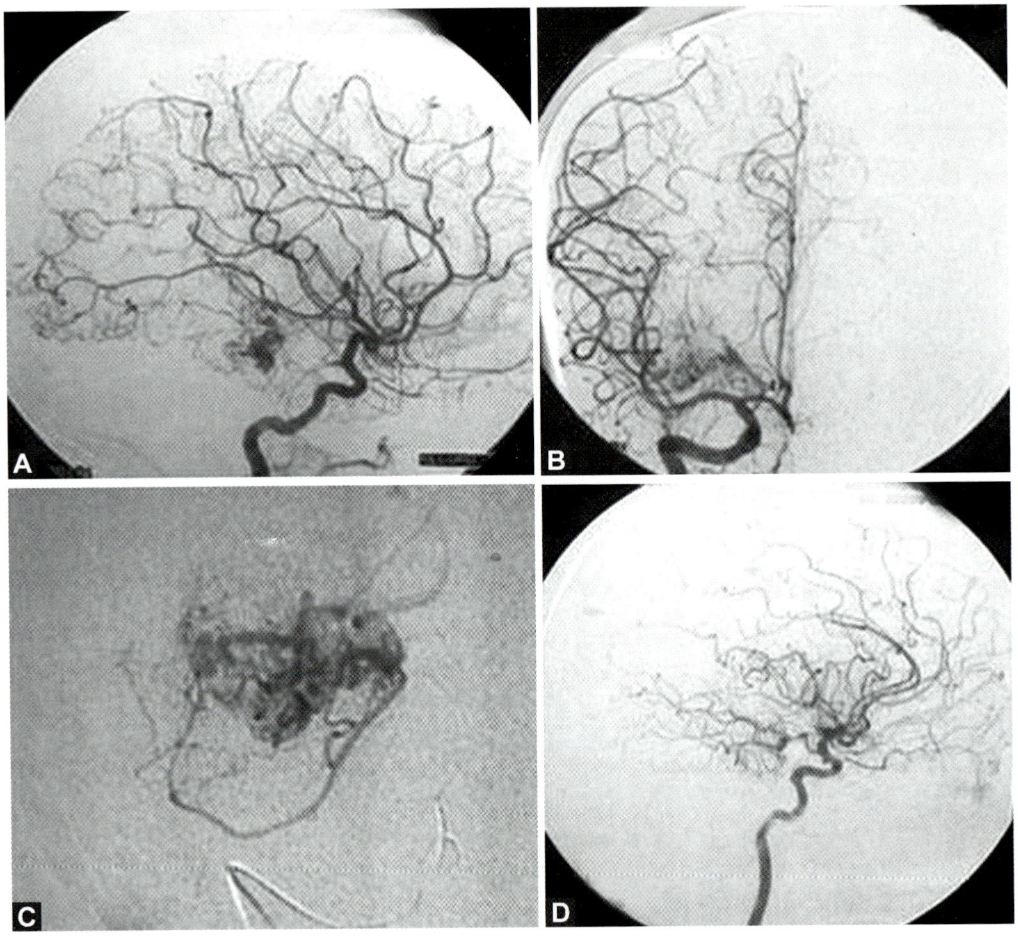

FIGURES 8.1A to D
Titrated with N-Butyl and cyanoacrylate glue: Small deep temporal AVM; (A and B) Pre-embolic ICA angiography showing small deep temporal AVM; (C) Superselective angiography showing AVM nidus, and draining vein; (D) Post glue embolization lateral angiography showing obliteration of the nidus

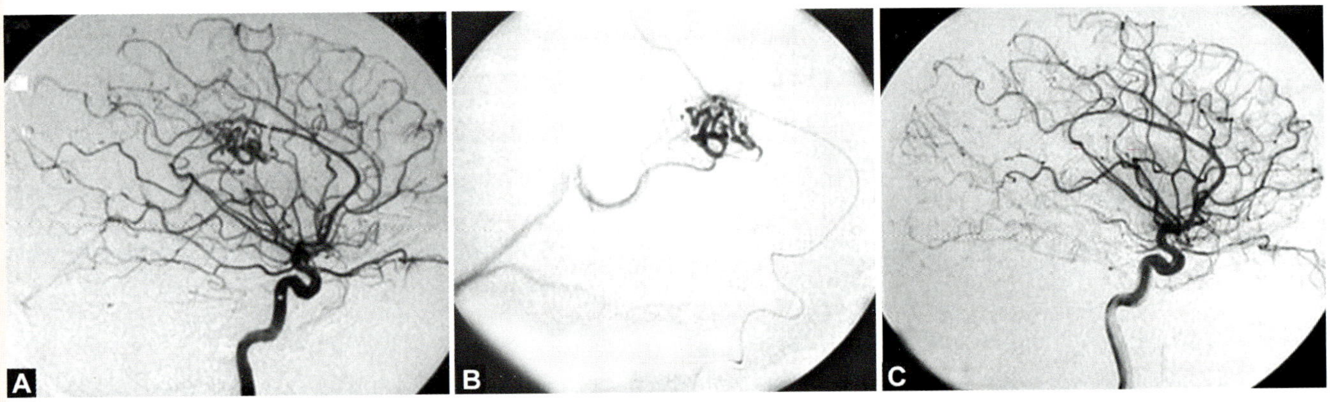

FIGURES 8.2A to C
Callosal AVM with intraventricular hemorrhage: (A) ICA lateral angiography to show AVM nidus in corpus collosum before embolization; (B) Superselective lateral view showing AVM nidus; (C) Follow-up after 1 year showing persistent obliteration of AVM nidus

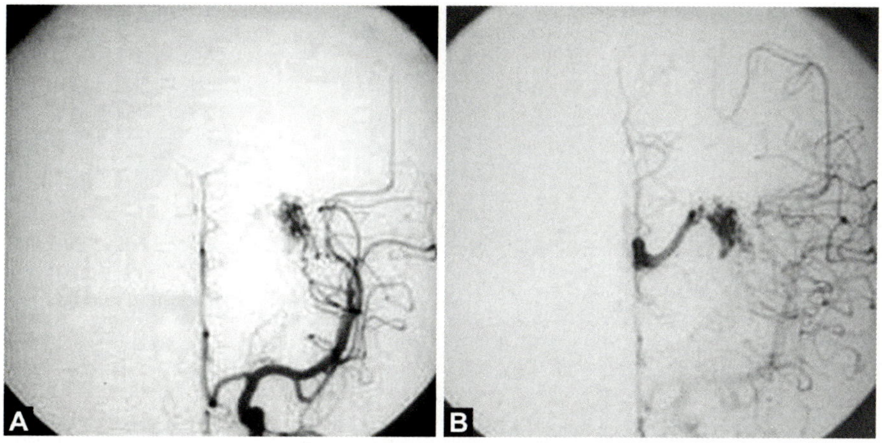

FIGURES 8.3A and B
Left ICA Pre-AP showing small deep paratrigonal AVM

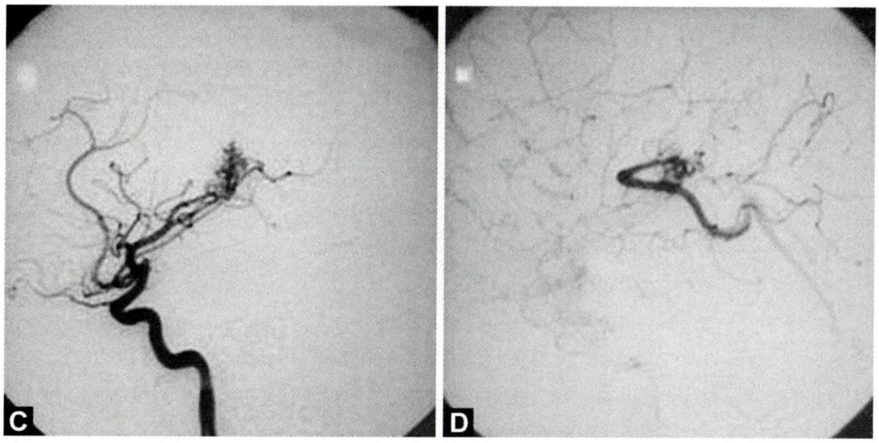

FIGURES 8.3C and D
Left Pre-embolization lateral view showing AVM draining into deep vein

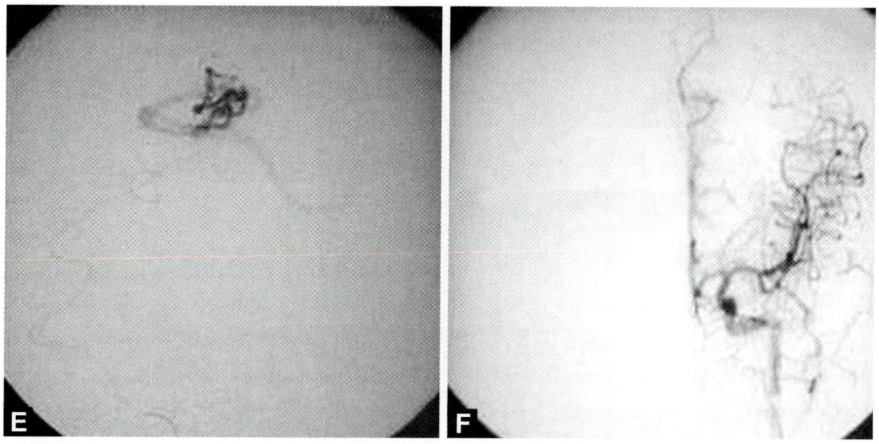

FIGURE 8.3 E
Superselective injection shows compact AVM nidus

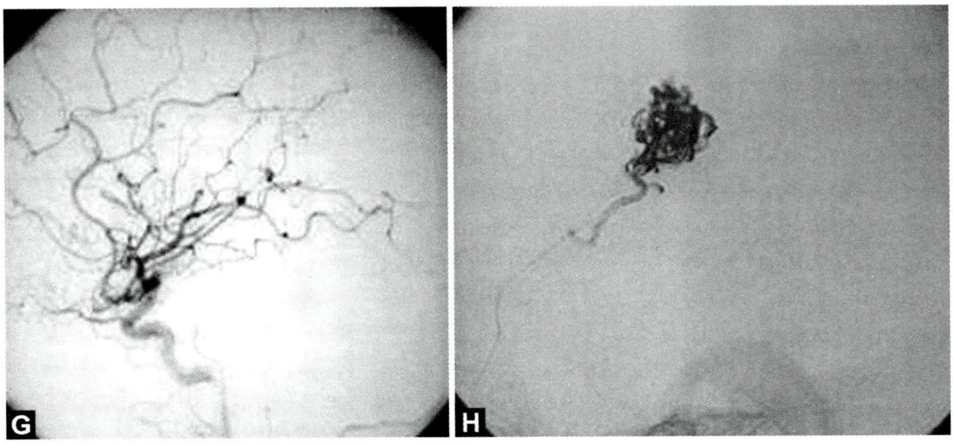

FIGURES 8.3 F to H
Obliterations with ONYX: (F and G) Lateral ICA postembolization AP and Lat view showing obliteration of nidus; (H) Plain X-ray lateral view showing ONYX cast

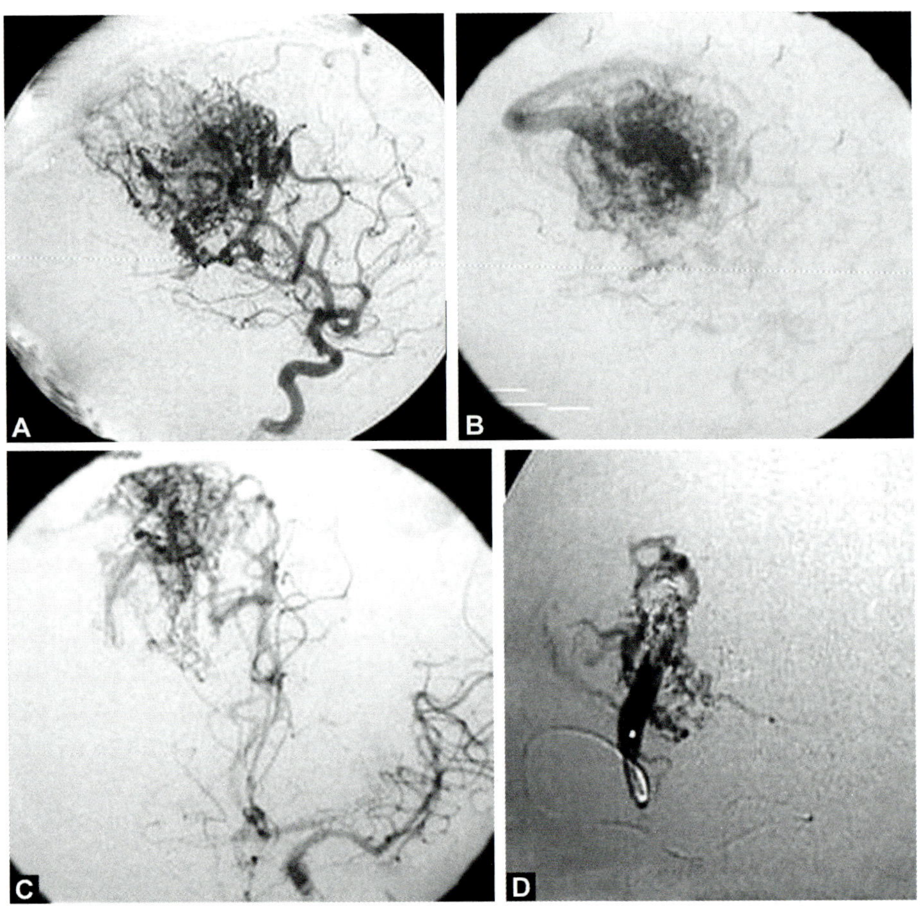

FIGURES 8.4A to D
Large Right Parietal AVM: Glue embolization followed by SRS: (A and B) Lateral view of right ICA; (C) Towne view of Left ICA angiography to show MCA and ACA supply to large right parietal AVM; (D) Superselective angiography showing AVM nidus

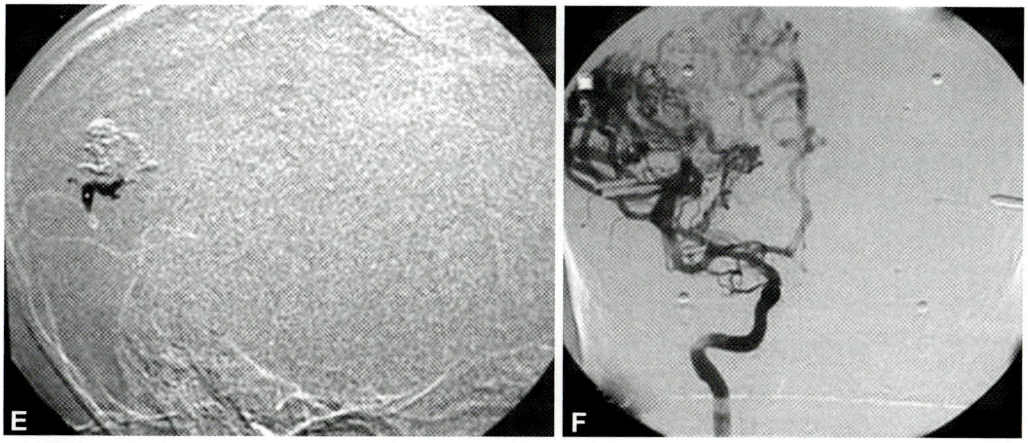

FIGURES 8.4E and F

(E) Glue injection into AVM nidus; (F) ICA angiography after glue and before SRS showing residual nidus

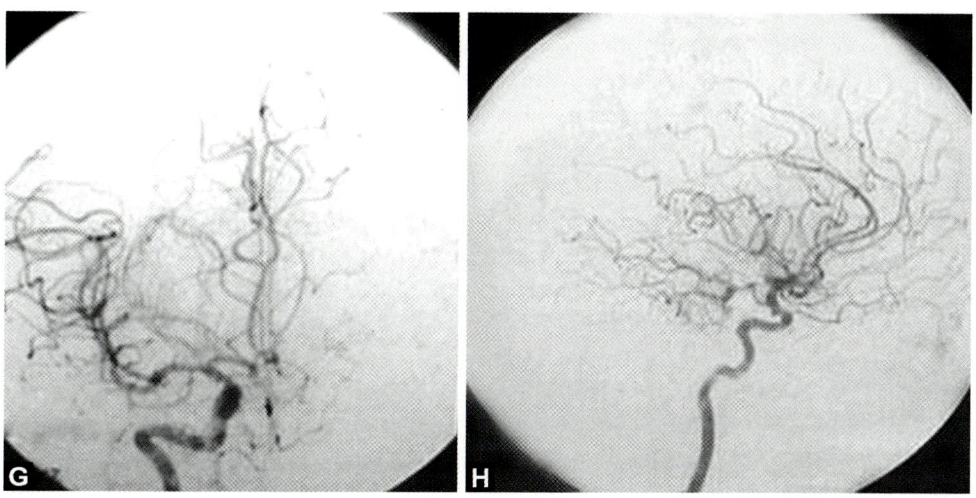

FIGURES 8.4G and H

Large Right Parietal AVM: Glue embolization followed By SRS: (G and H) 30 months after SRS. No trace of AVM

24 months. If there is residual AVM, a second course of SRS may be administered after 3 years.

DURAL ARTERIOVENOUS MALFORMATIONS (DAVMs)

DAVMs are abnormal vascular connections between arteries and veins in the wall of dural venous sinuses. DAVMs are rare lesions supplied by meningeal arteries. A high flow, or even low flow, DAVM is very hungry and annexes blood supply from every artery carrying blood towards the head.

The venous outflow is into a dural venous sinus, which may be open or occluded, or into a cortical vein. There may be a tangle of vessels in the dura or multiple small and large direct AV shunts. The DAVM is frequently associated with occlusion of dural venous sinuses, stenosis of draining veins or aneurysms along draining veins. Most DAVMs are acquired. Rarely, they are congenital. They may develop in pre-existing small dural arteriovenous shunts or from angiogenesis, when an occluded venous sinus recanalizes. They may occur anywhere in the head or spine. They are most common in the junction of transverse and sigmoid sinuses. They are also found in the wall of the transverse sinus, cavernous sinus, superior sagittal sinus and tentorium, draining into the vein of Galen, the dura of Foramen magnum and the spine. The exact etiology is unknown but they often occur after thrombosis of the sinus. The author has several cases of thrombosis followed a few months or years later by formation of a DAVM. They may follow infection in the mastoids or inner ear, trauma, surgery of the cranium or mastoid. Sudden decrease in estrogen levels after menopause has been implicated in the thrombosis of cavernous sinus in women.

Congenital DAVM may follow intrauterine thrombosis of a venous sinus or developmental anomalies of the venous system. The author has treated a 2-year-old girl who had a large high flow dural AVF of the transverse-sigmoid junction.

Clinical Presentation

It depends on the location and venous drainage of the DAVM. Low flow DAVM of the cavernous sinus presents with increasing redness of the eye, which is severe in the morning on waking up and wanes as the day waxes. Later, there may be persistent conjunctival injection followed by axial proptosis. DAVM of the transverse sinus commonly presents as bruit synchronous with pulse. If there is reflux into cortical veins, there is intracerebral or cerebellar hemorrhage. SAH is a rare presentation. The most foxing is the presentation with raised intracranial pressure (ICP). In high flow DAVM with direct AVF, the draining veins are arterialized and there is reflux into opposite transverse or sigmoid sinus, superior sagittal sinus (SSS) and into cortical veins either directly or through superior sagittal sinus (SSS). As a result, there is obstruction to normal venous outflow of the brain. This leads to progressive back pressure and progressive loss of cerebral functions. There may be loss of cognitive functions which is followed by progressive dementia with or without focal neurological deficit.

This may progress to coma and death. Headache and diminished vision progressing to blindness due to papilledema going into secondary optic atrophy is common in long standing high flow DAVM. Often, the headache disappears with the onset of blindness.

Investigations

Plain and contrast CT Scan may be normal. Occluded venous sinus may be diagnosed by delta sign. On CT Angiography, the large network of arteries and veins may be seen. Many times, the CTA may not show the lesion. MRI or MRA also may not show the lesion. Sometimes the mesh of vessels, draining veins and occluded sinuses are seen. Thrombosis of TS and SSS may be visualized. However, MR venogram shows the thrombosis unequivocally. DSA is the gold standard. Bilateral ECA, bilateral ICA, bilateral VA, angios are mandatory. All arteries supplying the DAVM are identified.

The arterial supply is usually from all meningeal branches of ECA of the same side, often of the opposite side, meningeal branches from ipsilateral, contralateral or both VAs, one or both ICAs, one or both ophthalmic arteries, pial arteries such as PCA or SCA. The precise location of the AVF is identified. Arteries providing direct access to AVF are defined. The venous outflow is visualized. Is the dural sinus occluded or open? Is it incarcerated with no direct outflow into sinus but only into cortical vein? Is there reflux into adjacent venous sinuses? Is there reflux into cortical or deep veins? Are there anomalies of the draining veins such as stenosis or venous aneurysms? What is the competition between the outflow of the DAVM and the normal brain? If the normal brain drains into the outflow of the DAVM, the sinus cannot be occluded.

Treatment

Low flow DAVM may thrombose spontaneously and usually no treatment is needed. Thrombosis may be promoted by intermittent digital compression of the carotid artery in the neck. Thrombosis following angiography has been documented. This is especially seen in the low flow cavernous sinus and sigmoid sinus DAVM in old female patients.

High flow DAVMs with cortical venous reflux must be treated urgently, as the draining vein may rupture leading to cerebral hemorrhage.

High flow DAVM associated with high ICP and must be treated urgently. High flow lesions with open sinuses and antegrade venous outflow need not be treated, if the patient can tolerate the bruit. Treatment is either surgical or endovascular, with the latter, if feasible, being the treatment of choice.

Endovascular treatment: The route depends on the location and may be arterial, venous or by direct puncture. Cavernous sinus lesions are treated by the venous route. Access is obtained either through the inferior petrosal sinus or the ophthalmic vein.

An occluded inferior petrosal sinus (IPS) may be recanalized by careful technique. Once the cavernous sinus has been accessed, it is packed with platinum coils, until the DAVM is obliterated. Rarely, if there is good access via a meningeal branch, embolization is done with Onyx. Glue Histoacryl can also be used (Figs 8.5A to J).

For DAVM of TS, SSS, vein of Galen and petrosal sinus, the preferred route today is arterial. The meningeal branch providing direct access to the feeder is identified. It is catheterized with Marathon or similar Onyx-compatible catheter with the help of a microwire. The tip is placed as close to the site of DAVM as possible. Onyx 34 is injected slowly if the flow is very rapid. Onyx 18 is injected after the flow is slowed. Onyx injection is made over one to two hours until DAVM is completely obliterated. Onyx usually first fills the network on the dura, then the vein or sinus and from the latter it flows backwards into all the feeding arteries (Figs 8.7A to H). If onyx cannot be used Histoacryl (glue) is injected through the feeding artery. The polymerizing time of Histoacryl is modified by adding Lipiodol to make different concentration. In a high-flow dural AVM 70 percent glue is injected in less high-flow AVM 50 percent is injected and in low-flow AVM 20 percent is injected. It is difficult to obliterate the dural AVM using glue and the cure rate is about 35 percent.

DAVM, is injected slowly. The aim is to traverse the tangle in the dura and occlude the foot of the draining vein. If the draining vein is not occluded the, DAVM recurs. Complete obliteration is confirmed by doing complete angios. of both ECAs, ICAs and VAs. If there is no arterial access the venous route is taken. The guiding catheter travels from the femoral vein through the inferior vena cava, superior vena cava, jugular vein, sigmoid sinus to TS. Sometimes, access is obtained through the jugular vein by direct

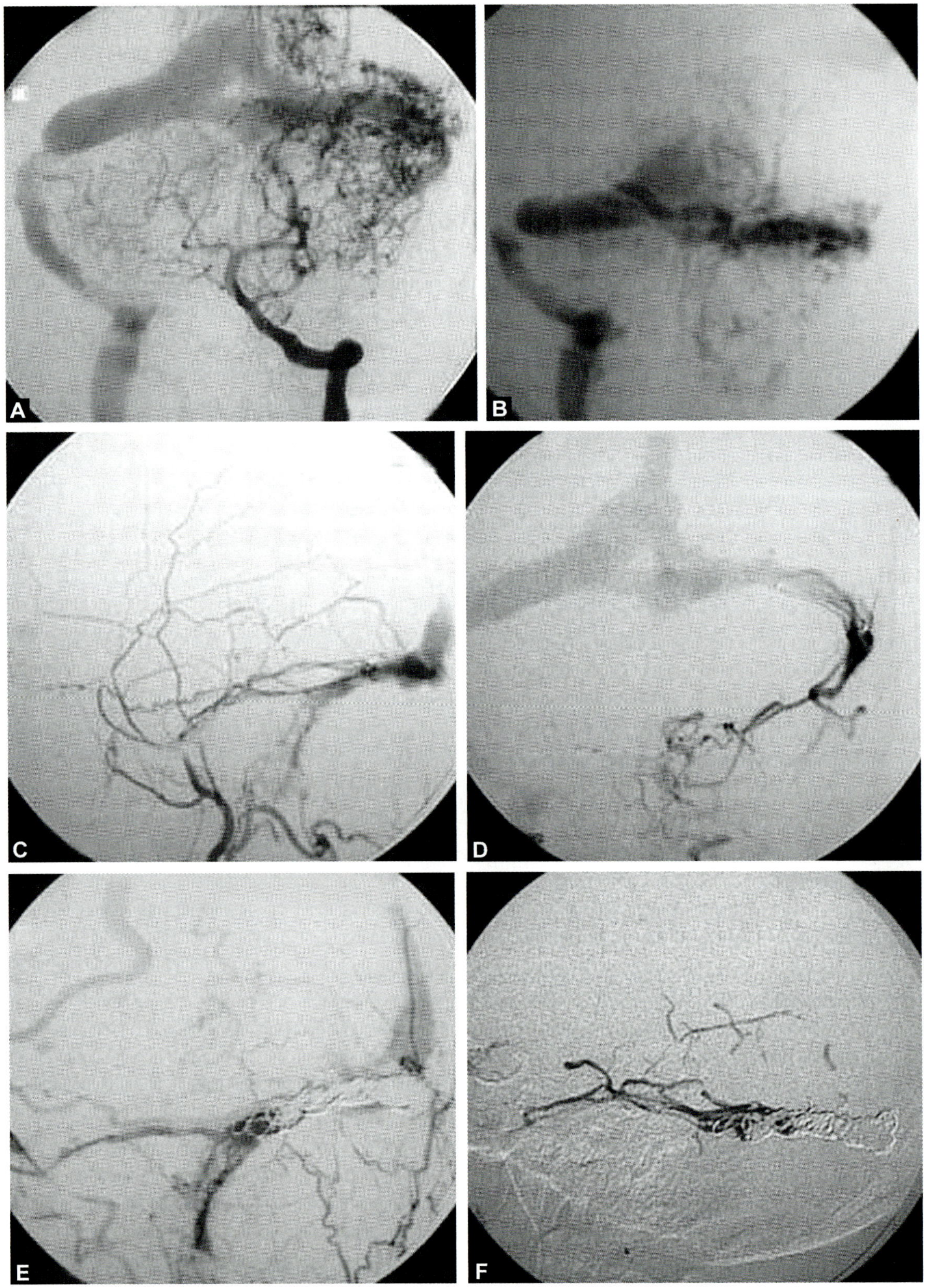
A
B
C
D
E
F

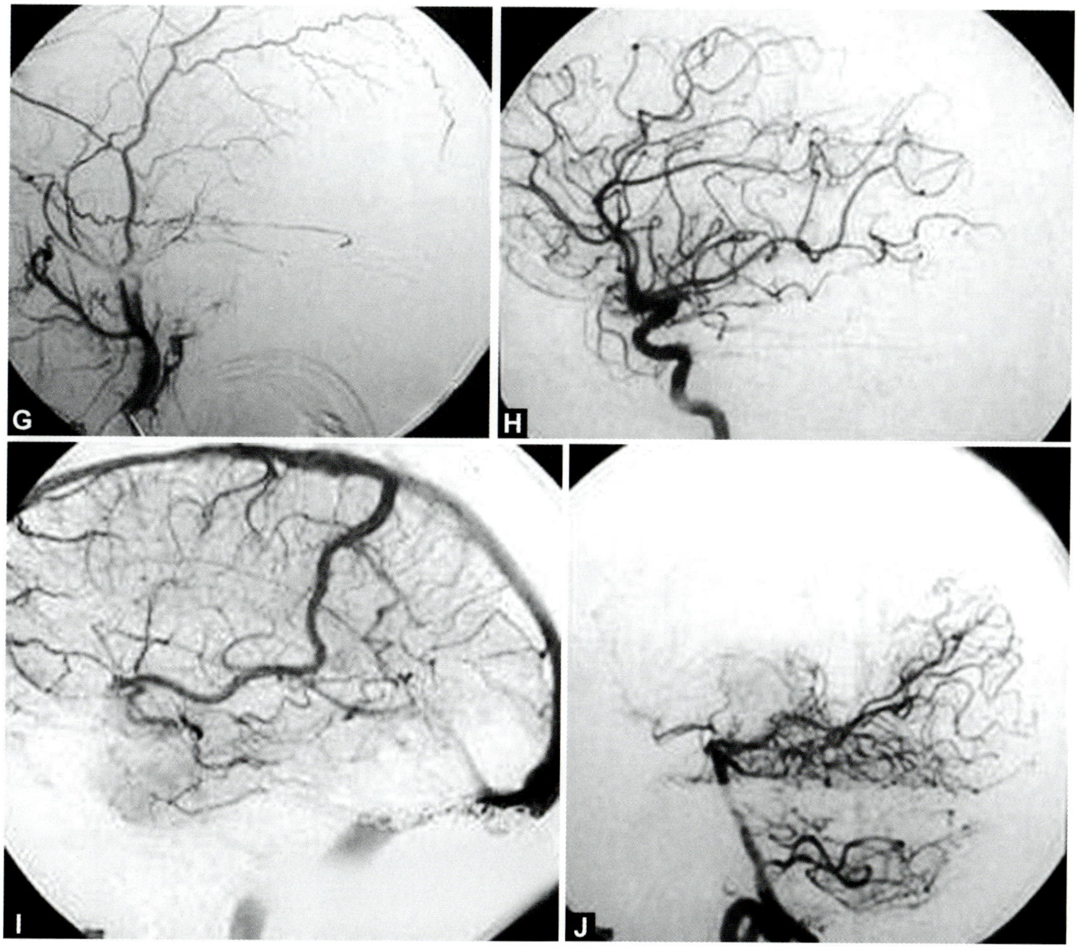

FIGURES 8.5A to J
Left Transverse sigmoid junction DAVF with occlusion of left sigmoid sinus and stenosis of right Transverse Sigmoid junction: (A and B) Left VA Towne's; (C and D) Left ECA Lat and AP; (E) Post left TS SS junction coiling, left ECA angiography shows opacification of shunts; Glue inj. decided for residual shunt; (F) Glue injection; Final Post; (G) Left ECA; (H and I) Left ICA Lateral; (J) Left VA Lateral

puncture in the neck. The microcatheter is then placed in the sinus to be occluded with the help of a microguide wire. The sinus is occluded opposite the AVF by tight packing with platinum coils sometimes supplemented by the injection of glue or Onyx (Figs 8.6A to T).

If the sinus is incarcerated and there is no arterial or venous access, a burr hole or small craniectomy is made over the occluded dural venous sinus. Intraoperative angiography is mandatory. The dura is punctured with an angiocatheter and a microcatheter is introduced into the sinus. It is then occluded with coils or glue or both.

Surgery is usually done only if endovascular treatment is not possible. If there is cortical venous outflow, it is always into a single vein with reflux into other tributaries. It is important to identify this draining vein before the tributaries. Coagulation or

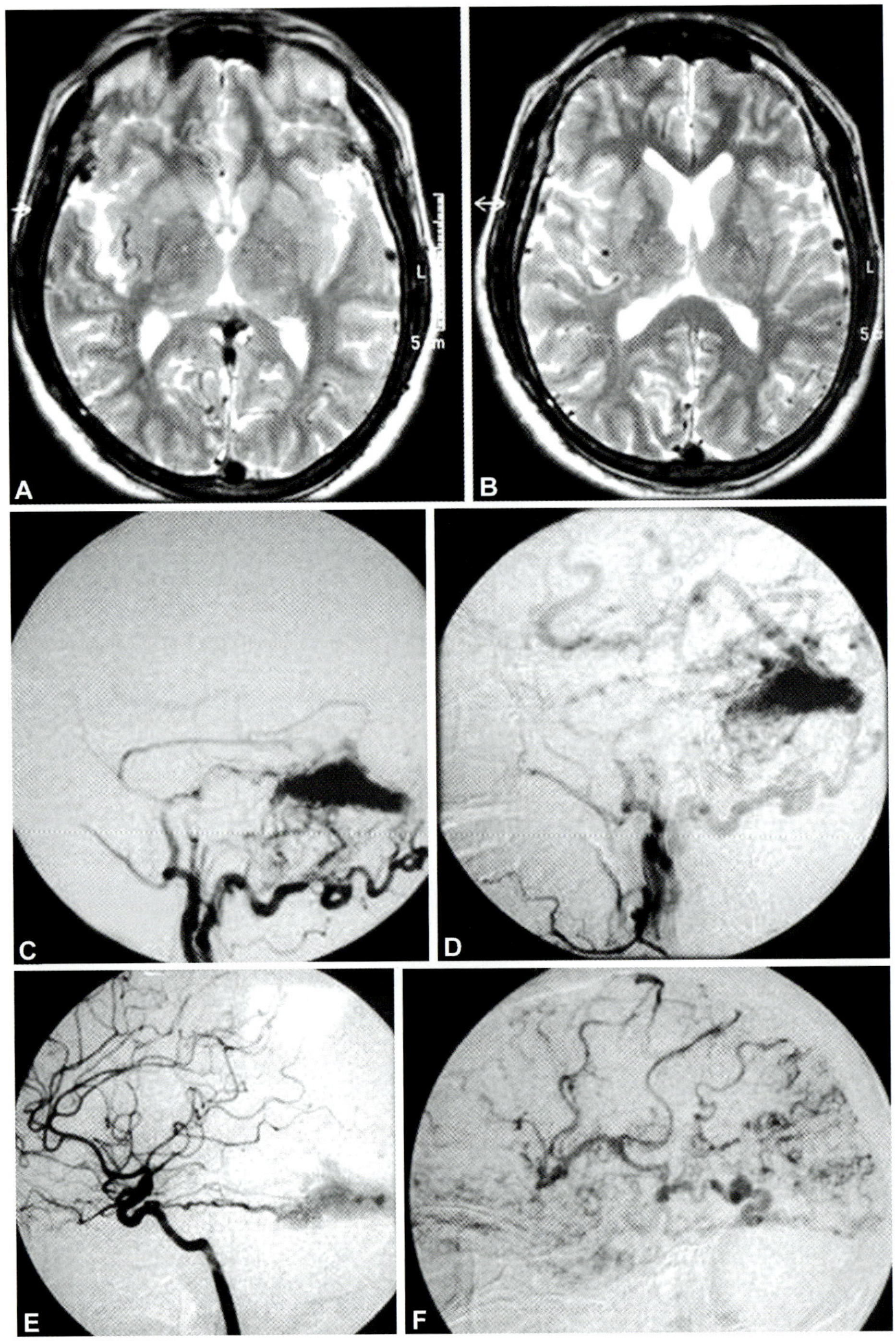

FIGURES 8.6A to F
ONYX embolization of dural AVM in a thirty-five year old gentleman who presented with signs of raised intracranial tension: (A and B) MRI showing multiple flow voids in both sylvian fissures; (C to F) Right ECA and ICA angiogram show sequestrated right transverse sigmoid junction fed by dural arcade of posterior fossa and severe venous congestion

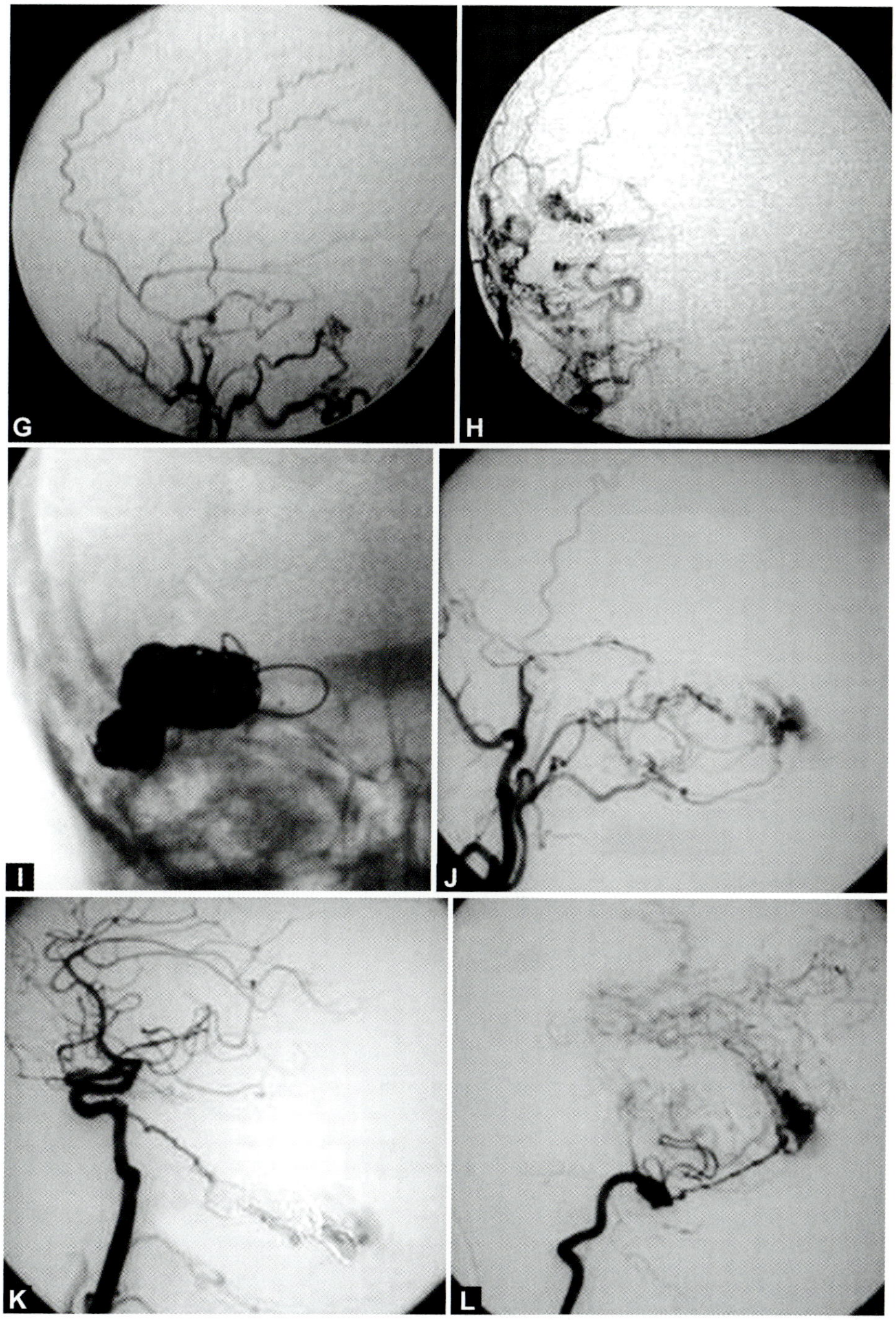

FIGURES 8.6G to L

ONYX embolization of dural AVM in a thirty-five year old gentleman who presented with signs of raised intracranial tension: (G and H) After coiling of right transverse and sigmoid sinus junction, right ECA angiogram shows minimal opacification of residual dural AVM; (I to L) Plain X-ray, ECA, ICA, VA angiogram showing recurrent AVM two years later

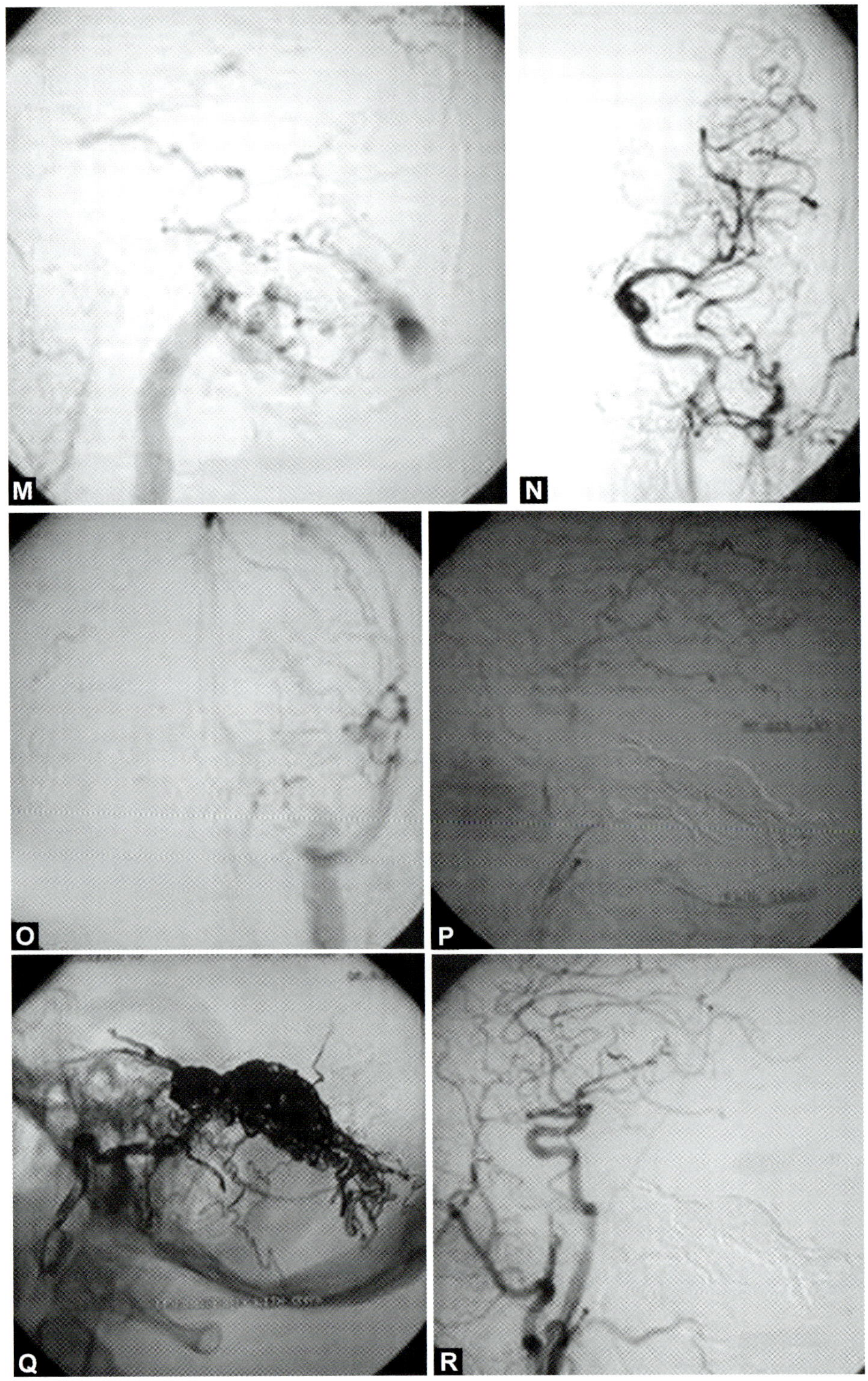

FIGURES 8.6M to R

ONYX embolization of dural AVM in a thirty-five-year-old gentleman who presented with signs of raised intracranial tension: (M to P) Angios showing reflux into cortical veins and occluded transverse sinus and open sigmoid sinus; (Q) Plain X-ray showing ONYX cast in the dural AVM, feeding arteries and draining veins; (R) Angio showing obliteration of AVM

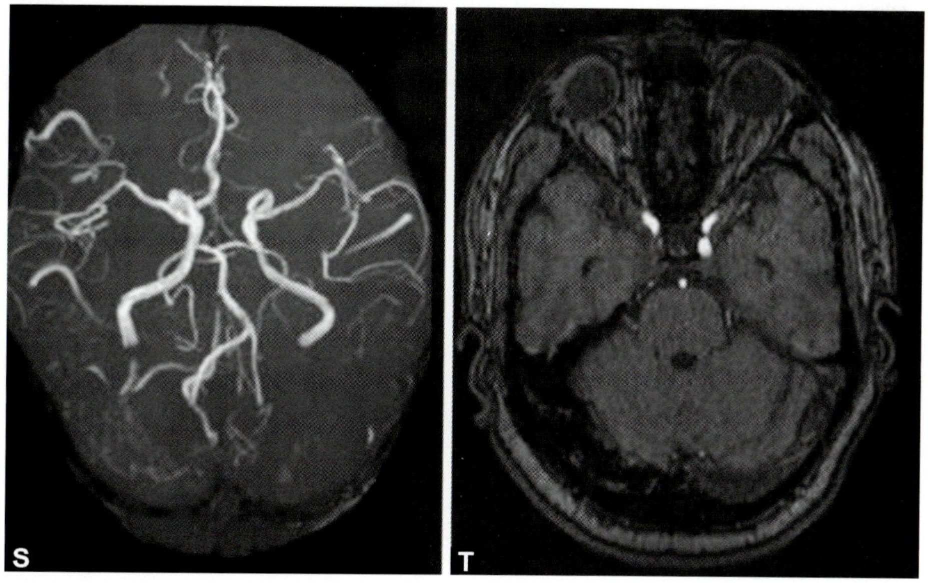

FIGURES 8.6S and T

ONYX embolization of dural AVM in a thirty-five year old gentleman who presented with signs of raised intracranial tension: (S and T) MRI two years after embolization showing no residual or recurrent dural AVM

clipping and dividing this vein results in complete cure. There is no need to excise the network on the dura.

If the DAVM must be treated and there is no cortical venous outflow and no arterial access, surgical treatment is carried out. This is a formidable procedure as there is profuse hemorrhage throughout the operation. The scalp, the bone, the dura and the brain bleed profusely. The affected dura along with the occluded sinus is excised. This major operation is usually required for DAVM of the tentorium, torcula, olfactory groove and petrosal sinus.

Radiosurgery has been recommended in the treatment of inaccessible DAVM. Reconstruction of the dural venous sinus using a self-expanding stent has also been done.

Results

Today with excellent endovascular techniques, the outcome in sick patients is excellent. Most comatose patients and those with profound neurological deficit do very well and often make a complete recovery. However, treatment must be planned individually for every case.

DEVELOPMENTAL VENOUS ANOMALIES (DVAs)

DVAs are the most common vascular malformations. These consist of radiating medullary veins in the form of caput medusae which drain into a collecting vein which may be cortical, deep or dural. DVAs drain normal brain. The pressure in the veins is not raised. In one third of cases these are associated with a cavernoma. A *de novo* appearance can occur. They may also be associated with a sinus pericranii or with anomalies of neuronal migration.

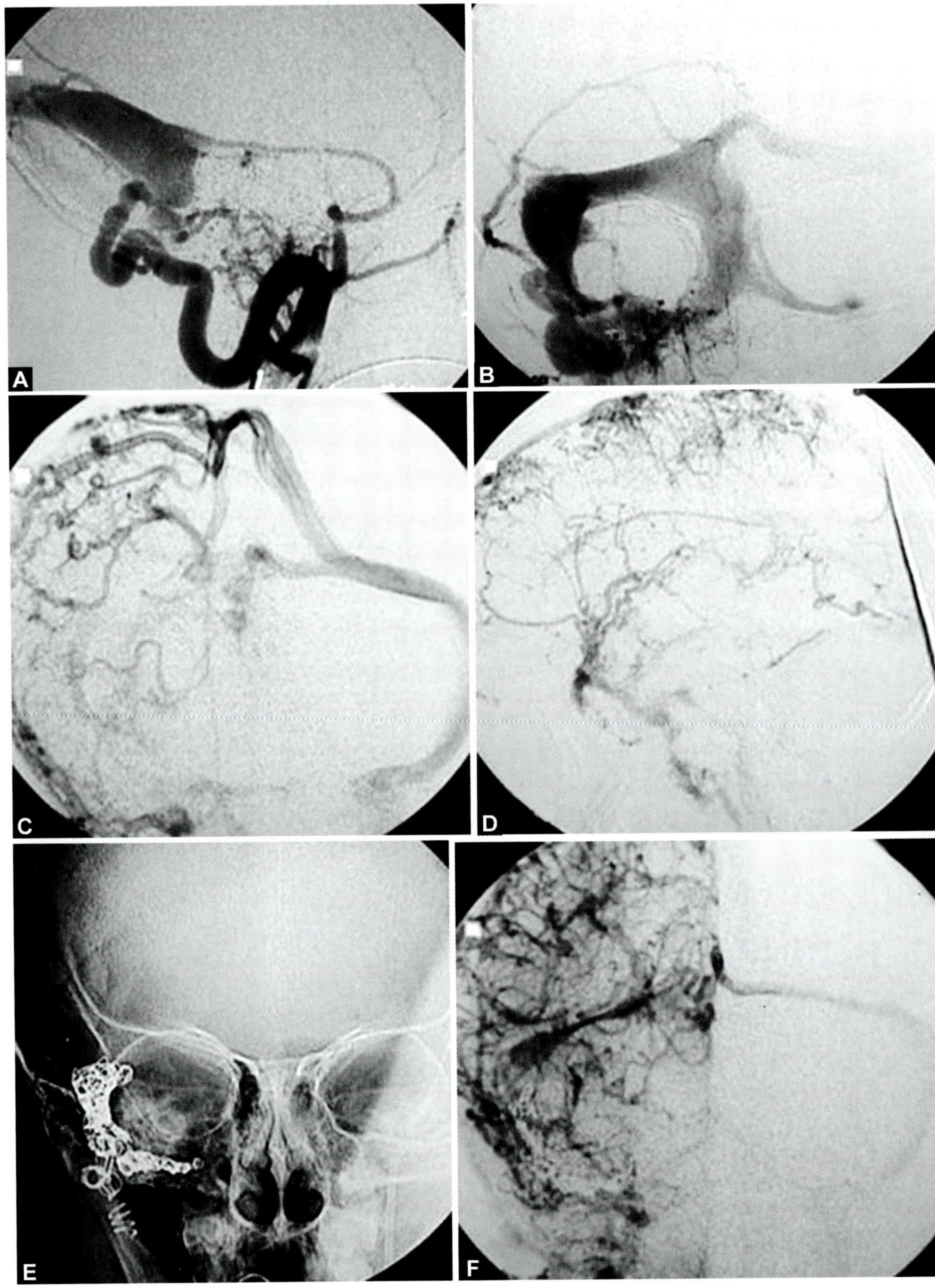
A
B
C
D
E
F

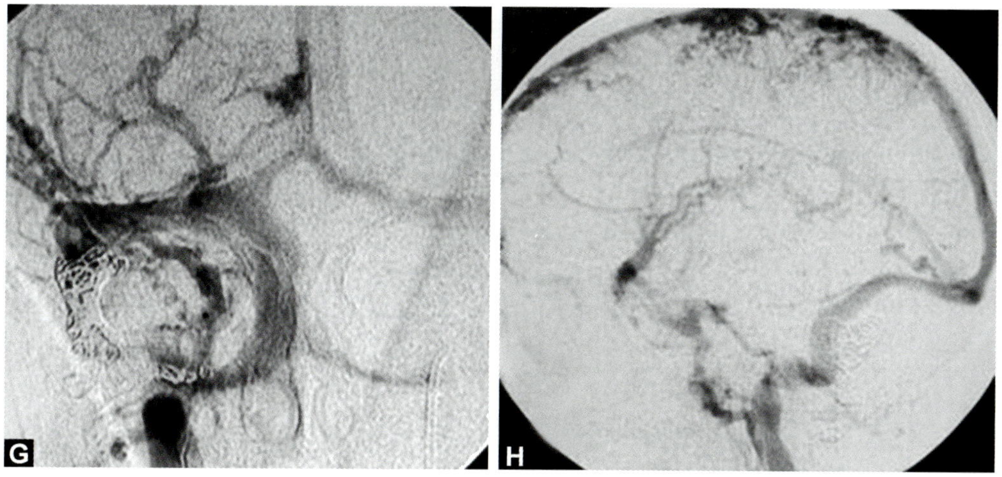

FIGURES 8.7A to H
Four year girl presented with tinnitus on left side: (A to D) Rt. ECA angiogram shows Dura AVF of right Transverse Sigmoid junction fed by hypertrophied mastoid branch of occipital artery with severe stenosis of right Jugular bulb and persistence of bilateral medial occipital sinus. Signs of supratentorial venous congestion are evident; (E) Occlusion of right SS achieved with free coils; (F to H) Postcoiling right CCA angiogram shows no opacification of shunt and adequate venous adaptation in the form of cavernous rerouting

They are usually asymptomatic but may cause mild symptoms like giddiness, vague headache, or convulsions. Headache, focal or generalized epilepsy, intracerebral hemorrhage, are usually not due to the venous malformations but have been attributed to the associated cavernoma. Trigeminal neuralgia has been reported when the malformation or a collecting vein lies close to the trigeminal nerve.

Investigations: CT scan may show the caput medusae or collecting vein or both. Associated cavernoma may be seen. MRI shows the caput medusae, can show the draining vein and the associated cavernoma. Associated abnormalities like heterotopia may be seen. DSA is done if an AVM is suspected. DSA will show the venous angioma and the draining vein well.

Management: By themselves, they are almost never the cause of symptoms and no surgical or endovascular treatment is required. In fact, the developmental venous anomalies should not be excised, as they may follow an abnormal course and yet drain normal brain. Rarely a venous angioma may undergo spontaneous thrombosis and produce neurological deficit. Microvascular decompression has been done to relieve trigeminal neuralgia.

CAVERNOMA

Cavernomas consist of endothelium lined sinusoidal blood cavities without muscular or adventitial walls and without incision of cerebral tissue. Most cavernomas are congenital, non-familial or hereditary. Some may be acquired following radiotherapy, or without any reason. They may be single or multiple. They may occur anywhere in the brain. They are often associated with venous angioma.

Clinical presentation may be: (A) Hemorrhage with or without neurological deficit; (B) Epilepsy; (C) Cavernous sinus syndrome; (D) Headache; (E) Hemispheric cavernomas present with epilepsy or hemorrhage. Epilepsy may be focal or generalized. Hemorrhage from a cavernoma is usually not large, does not cause a mass effect and is not life threatening, except when occurring in the brainstem. Annual bleeding rate is about 0.25 to 0.7 percent per year. Recurrent hemorrhage and profound neurological deficit are common in the brain stem cavernomas. Some cavernomas may enlarge by osmosis of fluid from adjacent brain and some may show calcification.

Investigations: On the CT scan, a cavernoma can be easily missed. Calcification associated with old hemorrhage may be seen. On the MRI, cavernomas have a typical "pop-corn" appearance. They are not seen on DSA, as flow across them is slow. Associated venous malformation may be seen on DSA and MRI.

Management: Cavernomas presenting with epilepsy are treated with anticonvulsants. Surgical excision is indicated for cavernomas presenting with recurrent hemorrhage in non-eloquent areas of the brain. Most cavernomas do not need to be excised, however repeated hemorrhages may necessitate surgical excision.

Intracerebral cavernomas should be excised, if they have become large and have repeated hemorrhages. Excision should be done under intraoperative image guidance as most of them are located deeply in the brain. Cavernomas in the brain stem are far more dangerous, as repeated hemorrhages cause profound neurological deficit and may result in death. Cavernomas in the brainstem, especially those close to the surface form an indication for surgical excision. SRS has been reported to reduce the incidence of hemorrhage and has been recommended for cavernomas which cannot be excised.

CAPILLARY TELANGIECTASIA

These are composed of thin-walled vascular channels with normal brain parenchyma interspersed within the capillaries. It is not clear whether the capillaries have normal walls. Growth and bleeding have not been observed however hemosiderin indicating old hemorrhage may be seen in surrounding tissue. They are most common in the pons.

They are sporadic and nonhereditary. They may occur with cavernomas or DVA. Hereditary hemorrhagic telangiectasia (Rendu Osler Weber disease) is not associated with cerebral telangiectasia but with other vascular malformations. Usually, these are asymptomatic. They may cause vague headache, giddiness or tinnitus.

Investigation: They are easily diagnosed on MRI as a homogeneous, irregular contoured lesion in the brain stem particularly in the pons. Two-thirds show a draining vein only. DSA is normal. They do not merit any treatment.

CEREBROFACIAL ARTERIOVENOUS METAMERIC SYNDROME (CAMS)

Cranial AVMs are sometimes associated with maxillofacial arteriovenous malformations. Historically, these lesions are categorized as Wyburn-Mason or Bonnet-Dechaume- Blanc or Sturge-Weber syndromes.

Pierre Lasjaunias et al (2006) suggested segmental patterns of involvement in what is likely to be a disease of the neural crest and/or adjacent cephalic mesoderm. A newly proposed rational classification reflects the putative, underlying disorder and calls for a new label: Cerebrofacial arteriovenous metameric syndrome (CAMS) (Bhattacharya et al. 2001) (Fig. 8.8). CAMS is associated with various lesions along the metamere extending from skin to neural tissue involving ectoderm, mesoderm and endoderm. These lesions are not seen at the same time. These may appear over years as the child grows. Successive lesions may be seen over years. They may be dormant and become evident later and may be misinterpreted as new lesions, the so called "pseudo de novo lesions" as described by Lasjaunias.

i. *CAMS 1:* A midline prosencephalic (olfactory) group with involvement of hypothalamus (hypophysis) and nose.
ii. *CAMS 2:* A lateral prosencephalic (optic) group with involvement of optic nerve, retina, parietal, temporal occipital lobes, thalamus, and maxilla.
iii. *CAMS 3:* A rhombencephalic (optic) group, with involvement of cerebellum, pons, petrous bone, and mandible.

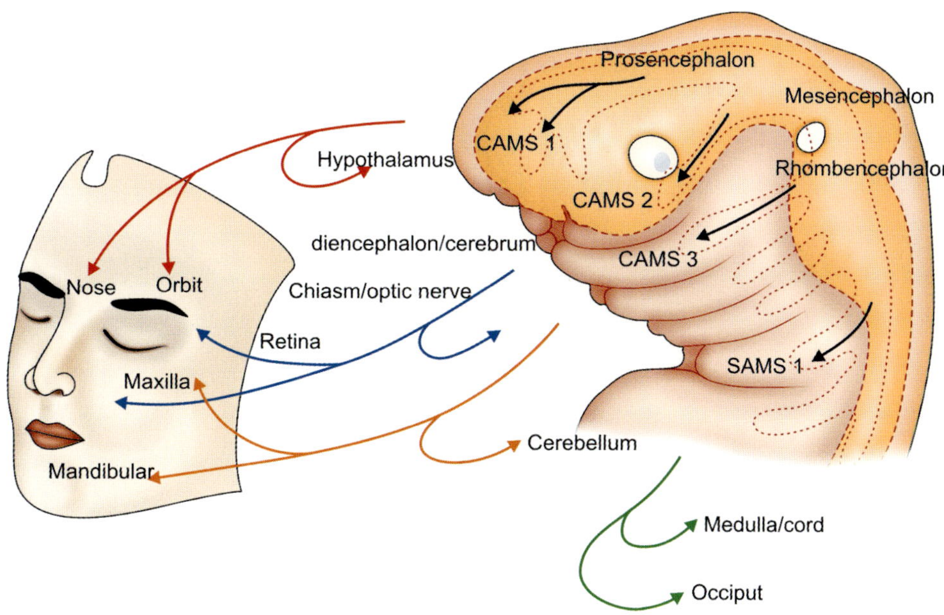

FIGURE 8.8
Cerebrofacial arteriovenous metameric syndrome (CAMS) (*With permission from Bhattacharya JJ)*

Bone Hemangiomas

Intraosseous cavernous hemangiomas of the bone are uncommon tumors, accounting for 0.7 to 1 percent of all bone neoplasms. Intraosseous hemangiomas (Valentini) are classified as benign tumors of vascular nature. Some authors describe them as hamartomas. They originate and expand inside bone structures. They are usually congenital, rarely of post-traumatic origin.

In the Maxillofacial Surgery departments of the Universities of Rome "La Sapienza" and "Tor Vergata," from 1990 to 2004, 11 cases of intraosseous hemangioma have been diagnosed. In 6 cases, the neoplasm was localized in the zygomatic region; in 3 cases, at the mandible level; in 1 patient, in the maxillary site; and in 1 patient, in the frontal bone. Literature review and the case of a male patient affected by left orbitozygomatic hemangioma are described. The preferred treatment is complete tumor removal with normal bony margins.

Sometimes, the classic radiographic appearances are not evident. Consequently, the diagnosis is most often made during surgical resection (Naama 2006). Satoh reported on hemangioma of the forehead which included skull tumors.

Vascular tumors of the maxillofacial bones in adults account for less than 1 percent of all osseous neoplasms (Dorfman 1971). In the jaw, they behave like slowly growing benign tumors and usually occur in females (female : male = 2:1) in the second decade of life (two-thirds of the patients reported by Batsakis 1979).

Bony hemangioma are usually of the capillary type and are highly vascularized, although some may not be visualized during angiographic studies (cavernous or fibrous type). If the lesion is large, enlarging and causing cosmetic deformity, these should be treated by radical excision (Figs 8.9A to G).

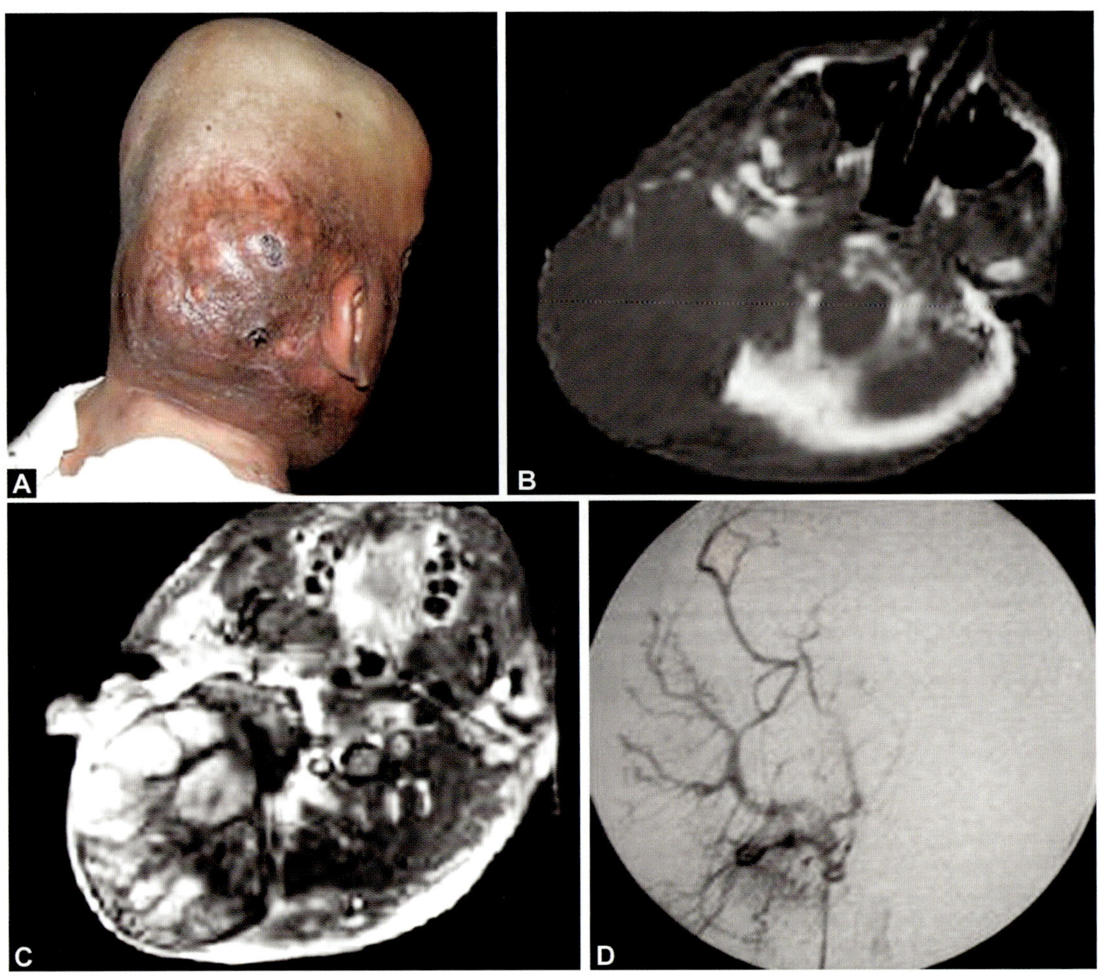

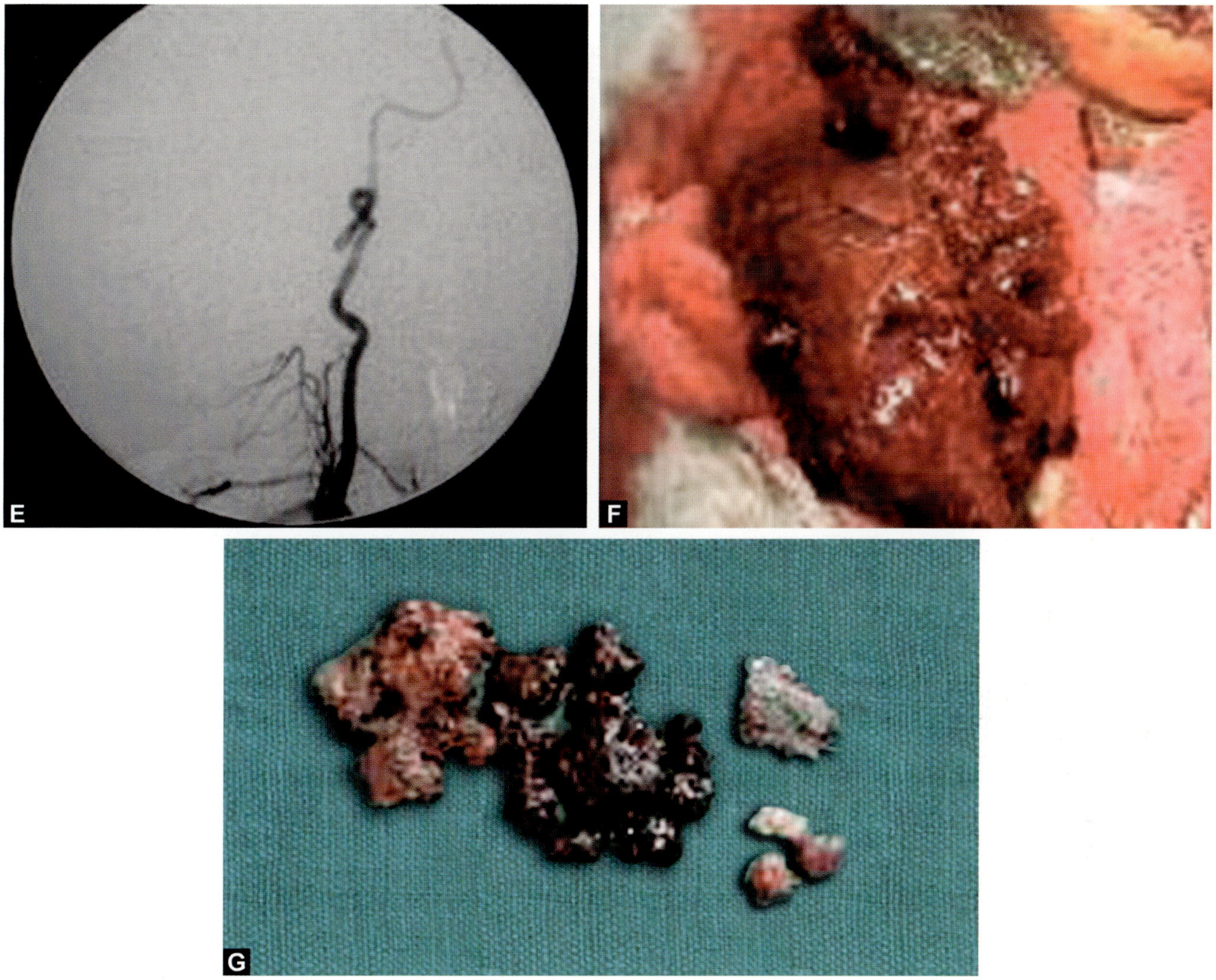

FIGURES 8.9A to G

Large occipital cavernous hemangioma: (A) Clinical photograph; (B) CT Scan showing skull defect in occipital bone and petrous temporal bone; (C) MRI showing the large variegated appearance of the lesion; (D and E) DSA showing avsacular lesion; (F) Surgical exposure; (G) Piecemeal radical excision

Vascular tumors of the maxillofacial bones in adults account for less than 1 percent of all osseous neoplasms (Dorfman 1971). In the jaw, they behave like slowly growing benign tumors and usually occur in females (female : male = 2:1) in the second decade of life (two-thirds of the patients reported by Batsakis 1979). Bone hemangiomas are extremely rare in the pediatric population.

BIBLIOGRAPHY

1. Al-Mefty O, Jinkins JR, Fox JL. Extensive dural arterio-venous malformation. J Neurosurg 1986;65:417-20.
2. Aminoff MJ. Vascular anomalies in intracranial duramater Brain 1973;96:601-12.

3. Barkovich AJ. Abnormal vascular drainage in anomalies of neuronal migration. AJNR 1988;9:939-42.
4. Barnwell SL, Halbach VV, Dowd CF. Multiple dural arteriovenous fistulas of the cranium and spine. AJNR 1991a;12:441-5.
5. Batjer HH, Devous MD Sr, Meyer YJ, Purdy PD, Samson DS. Cerebrovascular hemodynamics in arteriovenous malformation complicated by normal perfusion pressure breakthrough. Neurosurgery 1988;22:503-9.
6. Batjer HH. Treatment decision in brain AVMs: The case for and against surgery. Clin Neurosurg 2000;46:319-25.
7. Beers GJ, Carter AP, Ordia JI, Shapiro M. Sinus pericranii with dural venous lakes. AJNR 1984;5:629-31.
8. Benndorf G, Bender A, Lehmann R. Transvenous occlusion of dural cavernous sinus fistulas through thrombosed inferior petrosal sinus: Report of four cases and review of the literature. Surg Neurol 2000;54:42-54.
9. Berman MF, Sciacca RR, Pile-Spellman J, et al. The epidemiology of brain arteriovenous malformations. Neurosurgery 2000;47:389-96.
10. Bhattachaya JJ, Luo CB, Suh DC. Wyburn-Mason or Bonnet-Dechume-Blanc as cerebrofacial arteriovenous metameric syndromes (CAMS): A new concept and new classification. Interventional Neuroradiology 2001;7:5-17.
11. Biondi A, Le Jean L, Capelle L, et al. Fatal hemorrhagic complication following endovascular treatment of cerebral arteriovenous malformation. J Neuradiol 2006;33:96-104.
12. Bitoh S, Sasakis. Spontaneous cure of dural arteriovenous malformation in the posterior fossa. Surg Neurol 1979;12:111-4.
13. Boet RS, Poon WS, Chan MY. Childhood posterior fossa pial-dural arteriovenous fistula treated by endovascular occlusion. Childs Nerv Syst 2001;17:681-4.
14. Bouchacourt E, Carpena JP, Bories J, Koussa A, Chiras J. Ischemic accident caused by thrombosis of a venous angioma. Radiology 1986;67:631-5.
15. Bristot R, Santoro A, Fantozzi L, Delfini R. Cavernoma of the cavernous sinus: Case report. Surgical neurology 1997;48:160-63.
16. Brown RD, Wiebers DO, Forbes GS. The natural history of unruptured intracranial arteriovenous malformations. J Neurosurg 1988;68:352-7.
17. Brunon J, Nuti C. Natural history of cavernomas of the central nervous system. Neurochirugie 2007;53:122-30.
18. Bun YY, Ming CK, Ming CH, Lnig CY, Ming CC. Endovascular treatment of a neonate with dural arteriovenous fistula and other features suggestive of cerebrofacial arteriovenous metameric syndromes. Child Nerv Syst 2009;25:383-7.
19. Cabanes J, Blasco R, Garcia M, Tamarit L. Cerebral venous angioma. Surg Neurol 1979;11:385-89.
20. Campeau NG, Lane JL. De novo development of a lesion with the appearance of a cavernous malformation adjacent to an existing developmental venous anomaly. AJNR 2005;26:156-9.
21. Chaudhary MY, Sachdev VP, Cho SH. Dural arteriovenous malformation of the major venous sinuses: An acquired lesion AJNR 1982;3:13-9.
22. Chen JW, Kerber C, Hoi Sanf U. Spontaneous regression of large bilateral basal ganglia arteriovenous malformation. AJNR 1991;12:835-7.
23. Cognard C, Casasco A, Toevi M. Dural arteriovenous fistulas as a cause of intracranial hypertension due to impairment of cranial venous outflow. J Neurol Neurosurg Psychiatry 1998;65:308-16.
24. Davies M, Saleh J, Ter Brugge K. The natural history and management of dural arterio-venous fistulae Part 1. Benign lesions. Intervent Neuroradio 1997a;3:295-302.

25. Davies M, Ter Brugge K, Willinsky R. The natural history and management of dural arterio-venous fistulae Part 2. Aggressive lesions. Intervent Neuroradio 1997a;3:303-11.
26. Duffau H, Lopes M, Janosevic V, et al. Early rebleeeding from intracranial dural arteriovenous fistulas: Report of 20 cases and review of the literature. J Neurosurg 1999;90:78-84.
27. Enchev YP, Popov RV, Romansky KV, Marinov MB, Bussaraky VA. Neuronavigated surgery of intracranial cavernomas — Enthusiasm for high technologis or a golden standard. Folia Med (Plovdiv) 2008;50:11-7.
28. Garcia-Munoz L, Velasco-Camposb F, Lujan-Castilla P, Enriquez-Barrera M, Cervantes-Martinez A, Carrillo-Ruiz J. Radiosurgery in the treatment of brain cavernomas. Experience with 17 lesions treated in 15 patients. Neurochirurgie 2007;53:243-50.
29. Garner TB, Del Curling O Jr, Kelly DL Jr, Lester DW. The natural history of intracranial venous angiomas. J Neurosurg 1991;75:715-22.
30. Goel A, Muzumdar D, Sharma P. Extradural approach for cavernous hemangioma of the cavernous sinus: Experience with 13 cases. Neurol Med Chir (Tokyo) 2003;43:112-8.
31. Graf CJ, Perret GE, Torner JC. Bleeding from cerebral arteriovenous malformations as part of their natural history. J Neurosurg 1983;58:331-7.
32. Hamada Y, Goto K, Inoue T. Histopathological aspects of dural arteriovenous fistulas in the transverse-sigmoid region in 9 patients. Neurosurgery 1997;40:452-6.
33. Hamilton MG, Spetzler RF. The prospective application of of a grading system for arteriovenous malformations. Neurosurgery 1994;34:2-7.
34. Hartmann A, Mast H, Mohr JP. Morbidity of intracranial hemorrhage in patients with cerebral arteriovenous malformations. Stroke 1998;31:2361.
35. Hasegawa S, Hamada JI, Moriaki M, et al. Multiple cerebral arteriovenous malformations (AVMS) associated with spinal AVM. Acta Neurochir (Wien) 1999;141:315-9.
36. Hasegawa T, McInerney J, Kondziolka D, Lee JYK, Flickinger JC, Lunsford LD. Long term result after stereotactic radiosurgery for patients with cavernous malformations. Neurosurgery 2002;50:1190-98.
37. Hashimoto N, Nozali K, Takagi Y, et al. Surgery of cerebral arteriovenous malformations. Neurosurgery 2007;61:375-87.
38. Ishikawa T, Houkin K, Tokuda K, Kawaguchi S, Kashiwaba T. Development of anterior cranial fossa dural arteriovenous malformation following head trauma. Case report. J Neurosurg 1997;86:291-3.
39. Jones J, Jang J, Getcg CC, et al. Advances in the radiosurgical treatment of large inoperable arteriovenous malformations. Neurosurg Focus 2007;23:E7.
40. Kagawa K, Nishimura S, Seki K. Cavernous sinus dural arteriovenous fistula presenting with subarachnoid hemorrhage and subdural hematoma: A case report. No Shinkei Geka 2001;29:457-63.
41. Kaptain GJ, Lanzino G, Do HM, et al. Posterior inferior cerebellar artery aneurysms associated with posterior fossa arteriovenous malformation: Report of 5 cases and literature review. Surg. Neurol 1999;51:146-52.
42. Karlsson B, Kihlstroem L, Lindquist C, Ericson K, Steiner L. Radiosurgery for cavernous malformations. J Neurosurg 1998;88:293-97.
43. Kayali H, Sait S, Serdar K, Kaan O, Iker S, Erdener T. Intracranial cavernomas: Analysis of 37 cases and literature review. Neurol India 2004;52:439-42.
44. Kim DG, Park YG, Chung SS, Lee KC. An analysis of the natural history of cavernous malformations. Surg Neurol 1997;48:9-18.
45. Kim H, Marchuk DA, Pawlikowska L, et al. Genetic consideration relevant to intracranial hemorrhage and brain arteriovenous malformations. Acta Neurochi Suppl 2008;105:199-206.

46. King WA, Martin NA. Intracerebral hemorrhage due to dural arteriovenous malformations and fistulae. Neurosurg Clin N Am 1992;3:577-90.
47. Komiyama M, Yamanaka K, Iwai Y, Yasui T. Venous angiomas with arterio-venous shunts: Report of 3 cases and review of the literature. Neurosurgery 1999;44:1328-34.
48. Korinth MC, Moller-Hartmann W, Gilbasch JM. Microvascular decompression of a developmental venous anomaly in the cerebellopontine angle causing trigeminal neuralgia. Br J Neurosurg 2002;16:52-5.
49. Kuker W, Nacimiento W, Block F, Thron A. Presumed capillary telangiectasia of the pons.: MRI and Follow-up. Eur Radiol 2000;10:945-50.
50. Kurata A, Miyasaka Y, Oka H. Spontaneous carotid cavernous fistula with special reference to the influence of estradiol decrease. Neurol Res 1999;21:631-9.
51. Lasjaunias P, Chiu M, Ter Brugge K. Neurological manifestations of intracranial dural arterio-venous malformations. J Neurosurg 1986;64:724-3720.
52. Lasjaunias P, Terbrugge KG, Berenstein A. Chapter 11: Hemangiomas, In Lasjaunias p, Terbrugge KG, Berenstein A (Eds): Surgical Neuroangiography 3 clinical and interventional aspects in children. Springer-Verlag Berlin Heidelberg, 2nd edn 2006;595.
53. Lasjaunias P, Terbrugge KG, Berenstein A. Chapter 6: Craniofacial Arteriovenous Metameric Syndrome, In Lasjaunias P, Terbrugge KG and Berenstein A (Eds): Surgical Neuroangiography 3 clinical and interventional aspects in children. Springer-Verlag Berlin Heidelberg, 2nd edn 2006;359-64.
54. Lawton MT, Jacobowitz R, Spetzler R. Redefined role of angiogenesis in the pathogenesis of dural arterio-venous malformations. J Neurosurg 1997;87:267-74.
55. Lewis AI, Tomsick TA, Tew JM Jr. Management of tentorial dural arteriovenous malformations: Transarterial embolization combined with stereotactic radiation or surgery. J Neurosurg 1994;81:851-9.
56. Liebig T, Henkes H, Brew S. Reconstructive treatment of dural arterio-venous fistulas of the transverse and sigmoid sinus: Transvenous angioplasty and stent deployment. Neuroradiology 2005;47:543-51.
57. Maher CO, Piepgras DG, Brown JA, Friedman JA, Pollock BE. Cerebrovascular malformations in 321 cases of hereditary hemorrhagic telangiectasia. Stroke 2001;32:877-82.
58. Maiuri F, Iaconetta G, Sardo L, Briganti F. Dural arteriovenous malformation associated with recurrent subdural hematoma and intracranial hypertension. Br J Neurosurg 2001;15:173-276.
59. Mayberg MR, Zimmerman C. Vein of Galen aneurysm associated with dural AVM and straight sinsus thrombosis. Case report. J Neurosurg 1988;68:288-91.
60. Meyer B, Stangl AP, Schramm J. Association of venous and true arteriovenous malformation: A rare entity among mixed vascular malformations of the brain. J Neurosurg 1983:141-144, 1995.
61. Miller NR, Monsein LH, Debrun GM. Treatment of carotid cavernous fistulas using a superior ophthalmic vein approach. J Neurosurg 1995;83:838-42.
62. Naama O, Gazzaz M, Akhaddar A, Belhachmi A, Asri A, Elmostarchid B, Elbouzidi A, Kadiri B, Boucetta M. Cavernous hemangioma of the skull: 3 case reports. Surg Neurol 2008;70(6):654-9.9;43(2):75-81.
63. Ozawa T, Miyasaka Y, Tanaka R, Kurata A, Fujii K. Dural-pial arterio-venous malformation after sinsus thrombosis. Stroke 1998;29:1721-24.
64. Panciani PP, Fontanella M, Carlino C, et al. Progressive spontaneous occlusion of a cerebellar AVM: Pathogenetic hypothesis and review of the literature. Clin Neurol Neurosurg 2008;110:502-10.
65. Paolini S, Lanzino G, Colonnese C, Venditti E, et al. Three dimensional computed tomography in presurgical planning for treatment of infratentorial and dural arteriovenous fistulas. J Neurosurg 2009;110:85-9.

66. Pllock B. Stereotactic radiosurgery for arteriovenous malformations. Neurosurg Clin of North Am 1999;10:281-90.
67. Porter RW, Detwiler PW, Spetzler RF, Lawton MT, Baskin JJ, Derksen PT. Cavernous malformations of the brain stem: Experience with 100 patients. J Neurosurg 1999;90:50-8.
68. Pritz MB, Pribram HF. Spontaneous closure of high-risk dural arterio-venous malformation of the transverse sinus. Surg. Neurol 1991;36:226-8.
69. Richling B, Killer M, Al-Schameri AR, et al. Therapy of brain arteriovenous malformations: Multimodality treatment from a balanced standpoint. Neurosurgery 2006;59: Suppl 148-57.
70. Riel-Romero RM, Mattingly M. Developmental venous anomaly in association with neuromigrational anomalies. Pediatr Neurol 2005;32:53-5.
71. Roy D, Raymond J. The role of transvenous embolization in the treatment of intracranial dural arteriovenous fistulas. Neurosurgery 1997;40:1133-41.
72. Russell DS, Rubinstein LJ. Tumours and hamartomas of the blood vessels. In: The Pathology of tumours of the central nervous system. 5th edn 1989;727-90.
73. Sasaki T, Marimoto T, Nakase H, et al. Dural arteriovenous fistula of the posterior fossa developing after surgical occlusion of the sigmoid sinus: Report of 5 cases. J Neurosurg 1996;84:113-8.
74. Satoh K, Ohtsuka T, Abe T, Yokota K, Kunii K. Haemangioma of the forehead: Radiographic diagnosis and definitive surgical treatment in a Japanese series. Scand J plast Reinstr Surg Hand Surg 2009;43(2):75-81.
75. Soderman M, Andersson T, Karlsson B, et al. Eur J Radiol 2003;46:195-205.
76. Soderman M, Edner G, Ericson K. Gamma knife radiosurgery for dural arteriovenous shunts: 25 years of experience. J Neurosurg 2006;10:867-75.
77. Stancanello J, Cavedon C, Francescon P, Causin F, et al. BOLD fMRI integration into radiosurgery treatment planning of cerebral vascular malformations. Med Phys 2007;34:1176-84.
78. Stapf C. The neurology of cerebral arterio-venous malformations. Revue Neurol. (Paris) 2006;162:1189-203.
79. Stapf C. Unruptured brain arteriovenous malformations. Revue Neurol (Paris) 2008;164:787-92.
80. Sundt TM Jr, Piepgras DG. The surgical approach to arteriovenous malformations of the transverse and sigmoid sinuses. J Neurosurg 1983;59:32-9.
81. Suzuki S, Tanaka R, Miyasaka Y, et al. Dural arteriovenous malformations associated with cerebral aneurysms. J Clin Neurosci. 2000;7 (suppl 1):36-8.
82. Wilkins RH. Natural history of intracranial vascular malformations. Neurosurgery 1985;16:421-30.

9 ARTERIAL AND ARTERIOVENOUS MALFORMATIONS (AVMs)

CHARACTERIZED BY LARGE CHANNEL HIGH FLOW VASCULAR MALFORMATIONS

KS Goleria

Arterial malformations and arteriovenous malformations constitute this group. First described by Bell in 1816 and termed 'aneurysm by anasatomosis' it has been feared and recognized by various names such as, pulsating angioma, racemose aneurysm, cirsoid aneurysm and others over the last two centuries. Virchow in his monumental treatise on blood vessels (1863) devotes a lot of attention to these lesions, particularly their intracranial manifestations (see Chapter 8). For centuries, these had been feared for their 'malignant behavior', being associated with ulceration, hemorrhage and rapid growth after attempted removal.

MANIFESTATION

The lesion is present at birth, and is usually first noticed in early childhood as a local, reddish, pulsatile enlargement, attention to which is not uncommonly drawn by a sudden bleeding. Growth is usually in harmony with the body growth and the lesion may pass unnoticed. Even in an early lesion, a bruit on auscultation and a palpable thrill, gives away the diagnosis.

These lesions are characterized by a warm pulsatile mass, fed by one or more prominent blood vessels. The arterial malformations are uncommon. They are characterized by random arteriovenous fistulae from large arterial branches to adjacent venules. A single arteriovenous fistula is usually traumatic.

The more common arteriovenous malformations (AVMs) are characterized by numerous tiny arteriovenous fistulae, conglomerated into an identity called 'the nidus'. In these conditions, the veins exposed to a high pressure circulation, are often arterialized. Shunting of blood by the arterio venous fistulae also appears to be the cause of skin ulceration, which often leads to hemorrhage.

BIOLOGICAL BEHAVIOR

Untreated, the lesion grows steadily and relentlessly, incorrectly treated by blocking the main blood supply without ablation of the nidus, it shows a more rapid and severe growth. Multiple new 'feeders' are now established and both, the embolization and ablation of the lesion becomes far more difficult, challenging and sometimes impossible. This deserves emphasis, for it can truly be said—'a wrong beginning can create a subsequent hell'.

Usually, years pass by, before a relatively small lesion grows to life-threatening proportions, locally by the possibility of a severe bleeding and systematically, by the massive shunting effect on the circulatory system, resulting in cardiopulmonary decompensation. Patients with craniocervical lesions may suffer from a distressing buzzing sound in the ear, that can disturb both concentration and sleep.

AVMs are 20 times more common in the intracerebral vasculature than in extracerebral sites. They may be associated with excessive bone formation as illustrated in Figures 9.1A to D or with bone destruction as seen in Figures 9.8A to C. Increased

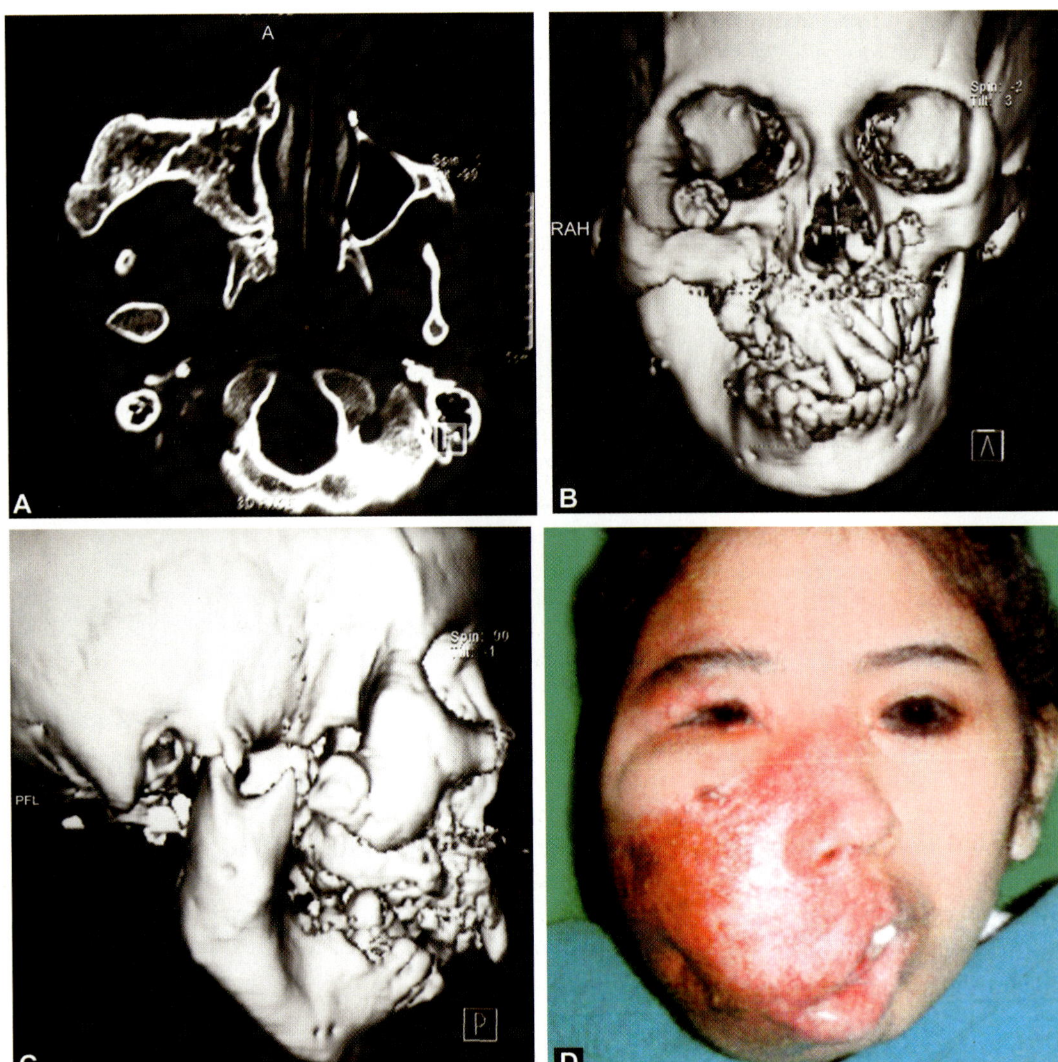

FIGURES 9.1A to D

Skeletal Hyperplasia in a longstanding AVM of the Face: (A) An axial section; (B and C) 3D reconstructions; (D) The clinical photograph bone formation, is attributed to increased vascularity and increased destruction, to bone proximity. In fact, increased bone destruction associated with new bone formation is a characteristic of an intraosseous AVM, e.g. those of the mandible. The lesions in the jaw may be asymptomatic—usually a swelling with a palpable pulsation. Occasionally, they are associated with pain, toothache, or hemorrhage. As in large venous malformations, here too, we can occasionally be faced with disseminated intravascular coagulopathy. Sometimes, longstanding AVMs of the face show new bone formation. An extreme form of hyper-circulation induced hypertrophy is shown in Figures 9.1A to D in a young lady aged 22 years, who has had multiple embolizations, two surgical interventions and a postoperative facial palsy. A craniofacial skeletal correction needs to be incorporated in her management plan.

MANAGEMENT

Wait and watch is never a good option because waiting can only aggravate the lesion. Before any intervention, a careful assessment of location, extent and approachability of the lesion is mandatory as is the necessity of planning, to minimize blood loss and to ensure its rapid substitution.

The key lies in the appropriate investigation and evaluation. The field is the best at the first attempt and a careful approach to evaluation, assessment, planning and the execution pays rich dividends.

Investigations

A contrast CT study or an MRI with appropriate reconstructions gives an insight into the location and extent of the lesion. However, it is the DSA which is invaluable in defining the feeding and the draining channels and planning the management. Usually a DSA has to be repeated for the preoperative embolization of the lesion.

Therapeutic Options

To treat these 'Large channel high flow lesions', the therapeutic options available are either a total obliteration by embolization of the feeders and the nidus and by a complete surgical ablation and frequently a combination of both these modalities. In fact, a close interaction between the interventional radiologist and the plastic surgeon is essential.

Embolization Alone—A Restricted Option

Embolization alone is usually restricted to a small lesion, with one or two feeders accessible to the embolizing catheter. The embolizing substance used for this type of intervention is non-absorbable. Quite often, this leaves behind a palpable and often visible nodule which is unpleasant, particularly if the lesion is superficial. Figures 9.2A to D shows a small pulsatile AVM treated by embolization and free from recurrence for over two years.

Embolization Followed by Surgery

For most of the larger lesions, embolization followed by surgery is a better option. To ensure an effective control of bleeding, the preparation begins prior to the surgical intervention. The help comes from the interventional radiologist by way of embolization of the nidus and all the major feeders.

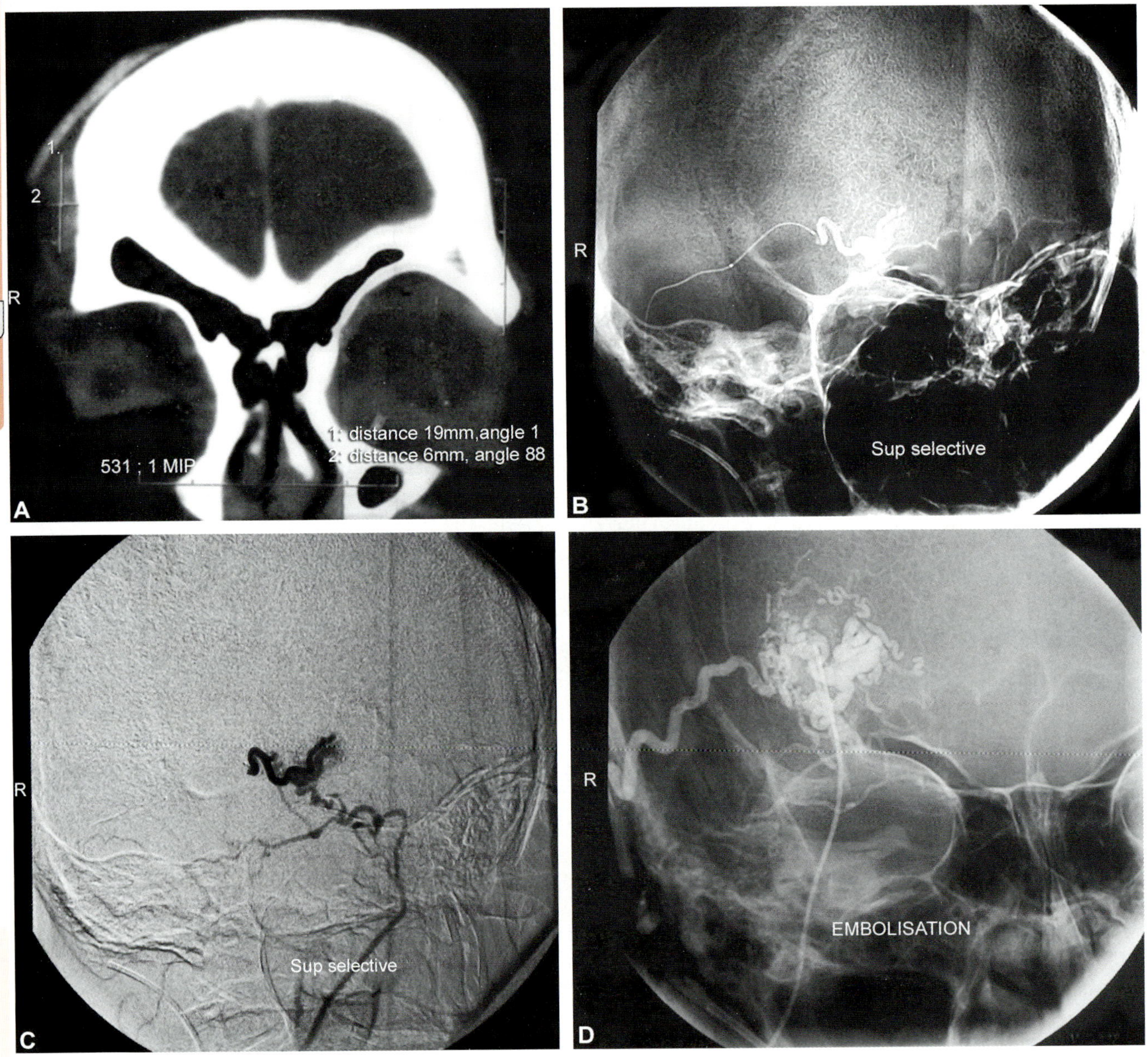

FIGURES 9.2A to D
A small AVM on the forehead: (A) A view of the lesion (in the CT section.); (B to D) Embolization

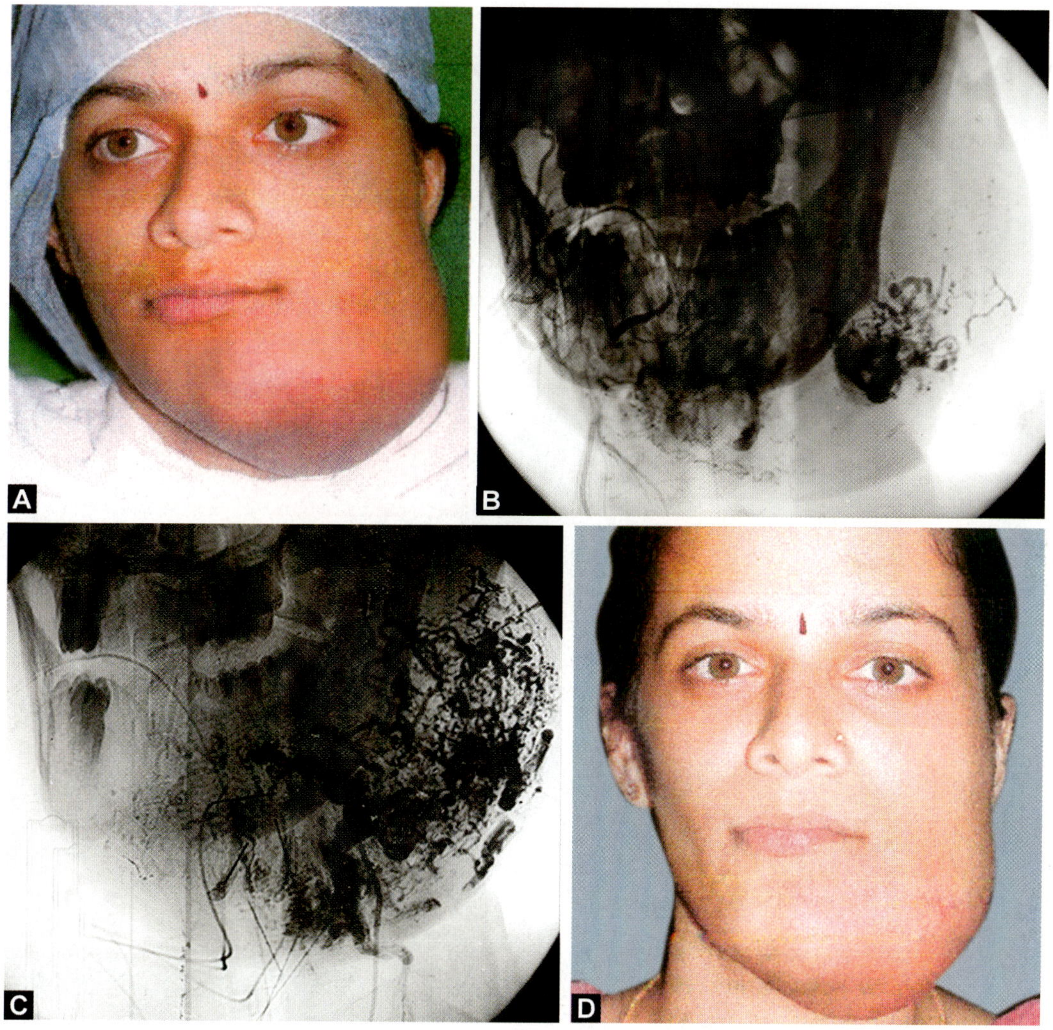

FIGURES 9.3A to D

Preoperative embolization with N-butyl 2- cyanoacrylate (NBCA) glue: (A) Postembolization clinical view; (B and C) Scans after embolization; (D) Preoperative view

For years, the choice for the presurgical embolizing agent was the gel-foam particles. The optimal control on surgical hemorrhage was available in the time window of 48 to 72 hours post embolization. A large time interval between this type of embolization and surgery compromises the benefit and defeats the objective of controlling the blood loss. Though gel-foam is still in use, the preferred embolizing agent is N-butyl 2-cyanoacrylate (NBCA) glue. This gives us more leeway between embolization and surgery (6 to 15 days) and facilitates surgery by a better localization, delineation and hemostasis (Figs 9.3A to D).

Any unembolized feeders must be recognized at the time of embolization and if possible, must be ligated as close to the nidus as possible, at the very start of the surgery. This objective of embolization can also be significantly achieved by ligation of all the major feeders at the commencement of surgery. However, it should be ensured that the ligation is carried out as close to the nidus as possible and the nidus is excised thereafter. A large distance between the ligature and the nidus (if not totally removed thereafter) leads to the development of the 'steal phenomenon' which has been dealt with, in Chapter 10.

The patient in Figures 9.4A to D had a large and longstanding AVM of the scalp at its vertex, fed by both the superficial temporal arteries and both the occipital arteries.

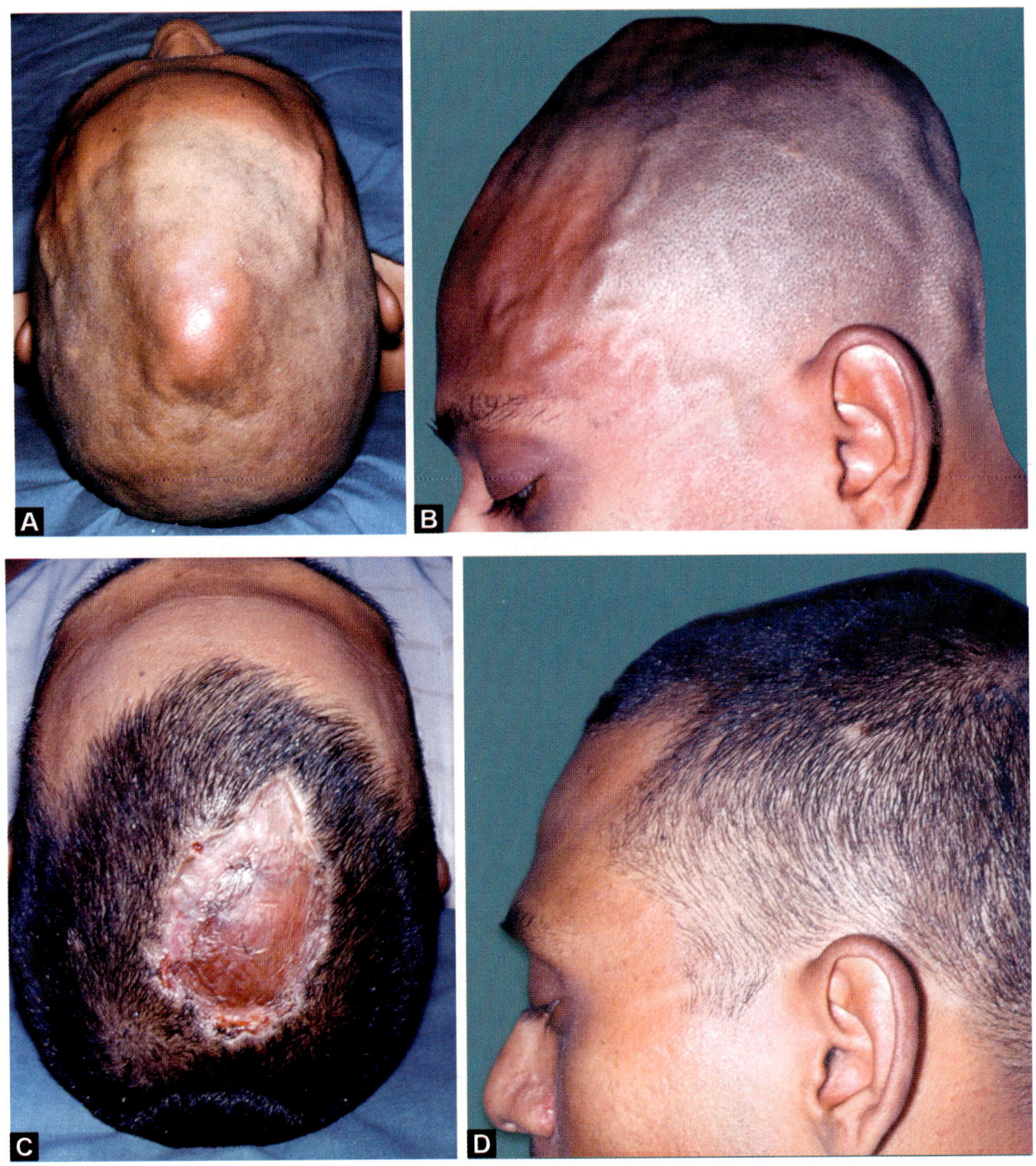

FIGURES 9.4A to D
(A and B) An AVM of the scalp with 4 main feeders; (C and D) show the postoperative status after gelfoam embolization of three feeders, immediate pre-ablation ligation close to the lesion of the fourth feeder, ablation and split skin graft

The right superficial temporal and both the occipital arteries were embolized with gelfoam. The left superficial temporal artery could not be embolized. The patient was operated two days later. The left superficial temporal artery was ligated near the nidus. The nidus was excised with its adherent skin cover and the raw surface grafted with a split skin graft. Of course the surgery must ensure a total excision of the nidus.

Any residual nidus should be recognized early, kept under observation and dealt with appropriately if growing (see Figs 10.7A).

AVM with Bone Destruction

Figures 9.5A to G illustrates an arteriovenous malformation (AVM) of the occipital and upper cervical region. The swelling in the retromastoid areas circled red, was present since birth. Swellings circled in blue have developed later. They are gradually increasing and are more prominent in sleep. The formation is fed by a branch of the vertebral artery.

Bone destruction is often associated with these lesions of the cranial skeleton. Figures 9.5D to G shows extensive resorption and bone destruction of the right occipital region of the skull upto the foramen magnum, with no evidence of intracranial communications.

These erosions are often associated with venous communication with the calvarial sinuses. After an adequate exposure, the malformation was stripped off the skull with control of bleeding with bone wax. Since bone destruction caused no significant problem, it was left alone. The patient has reportedly done well but unfortunately, a long term follow-up is not available.

The AMs, are uncommon compared to AVMs. However, their behavior pattern and their management are similar.

The Importance of Nidus Removal

The removal of a nidus after embolizing the lesion is essential to make the benefit lasting and reduce the chances of recurrence. Figure 9.6A shows an 18 years old patient

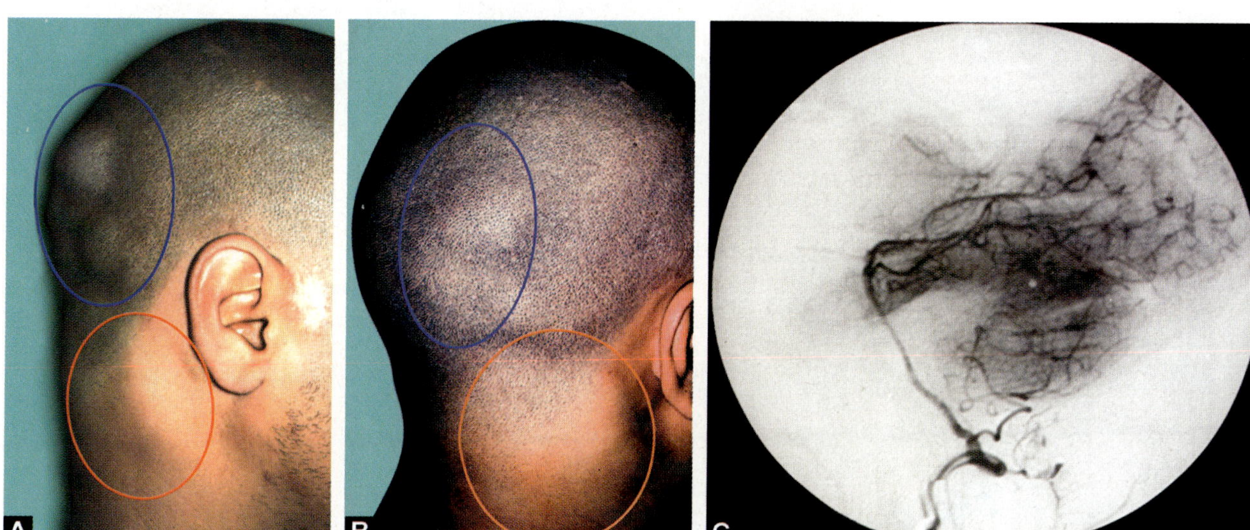

FIGURES 9.5A to C

AVM with bone destruction: (A and B) Upright and recumbent—note increased prominence in the recumbent position; (C) Fed by a branch of the vertebral artery—note a number of A-V fistulae with an AVM on the left side of the face. She was referred by an interventional radiology unit after four embolizations, the last, a few months earlier (Figs 9.6A and B). She gave history of a few injections, possibly sclerosants, prior to embolization.The lesion was still pulsatile with persistence of repeated episodes of bleeding.

It had been first noted at birth as a red spot which steadily and gradually increased. With the passage of time, the increase has been more rapid, with a significant swelling, changes in the skin surface, reddish and purplish discoloration, repeated bleeding episodes, redness and warmth. A surgical intervention, done on the ipsilateral side of the neck, at the age of seven years is said to be the cause of a hypoglossal nerve palsy on that side.

After discussion with the interventional radiologist, a fresh angiography and embolization was carried out. A few days later, followed a surgical intervention for the removal of the nidus and debulking. Care was taken to remain superficial to the facial muscles protecting deeper surface, where run the branches of the facial nerve.

Note the remarkable change in color, texture and form Figures 9.6L to N in just two months after surgery.

It must be emphasized that advances in interventional radiology have made many of the modern surgical interventions possible.

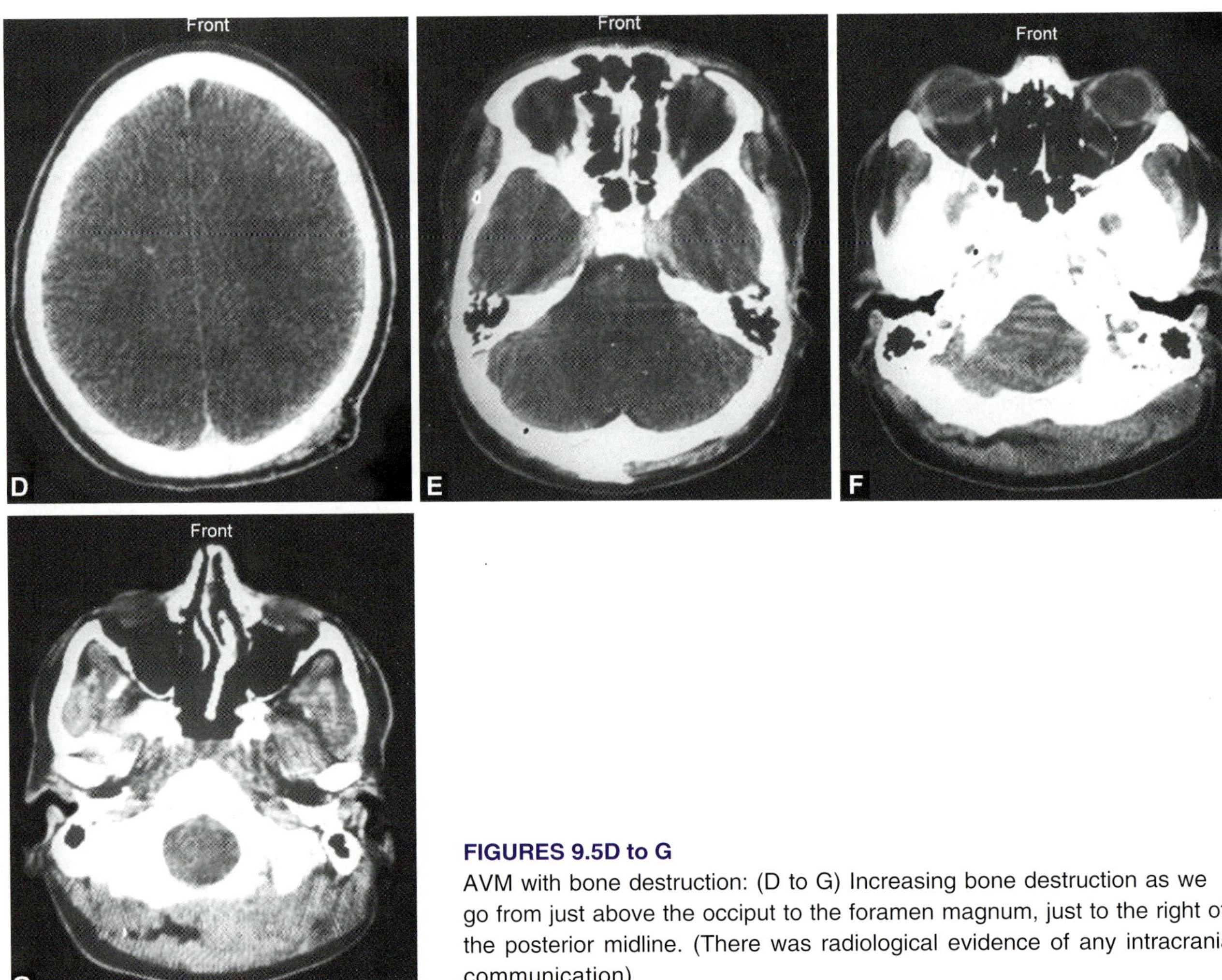

FIGURES 9.5D to G

AVM with bone destruction: (D to G) Increasing bone destruction as we go from just above the occiput to the foramen magnum, just to the right of the posterior midline. (There was radiological evidence of any intracranial communication)

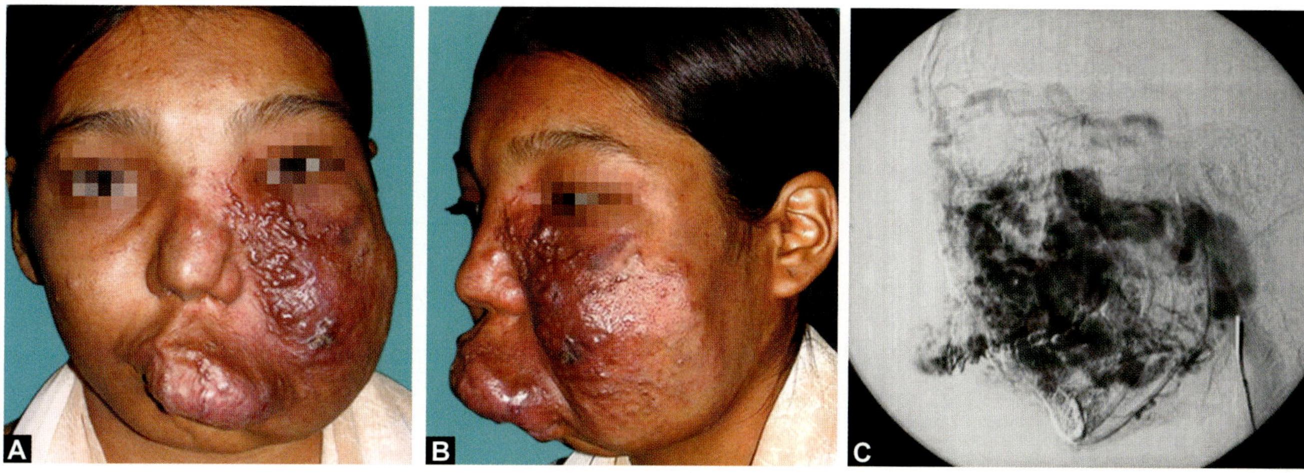

FIGURES 9.6A to C
(A and B) As first seen after four embolizations; (C) Nidus with numerous tiny arteriovenous fistulae

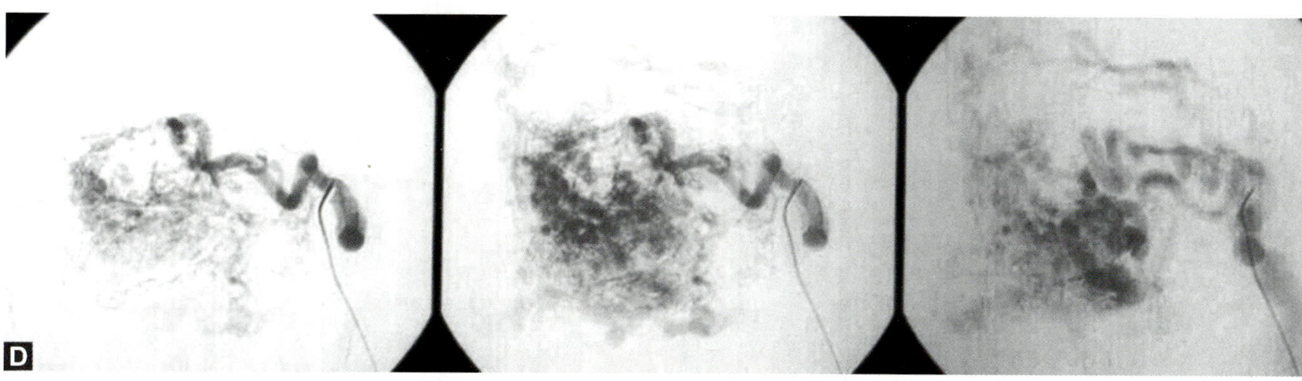

FIGURE 9.6D
(D) Angiogram—distal external carotid artery

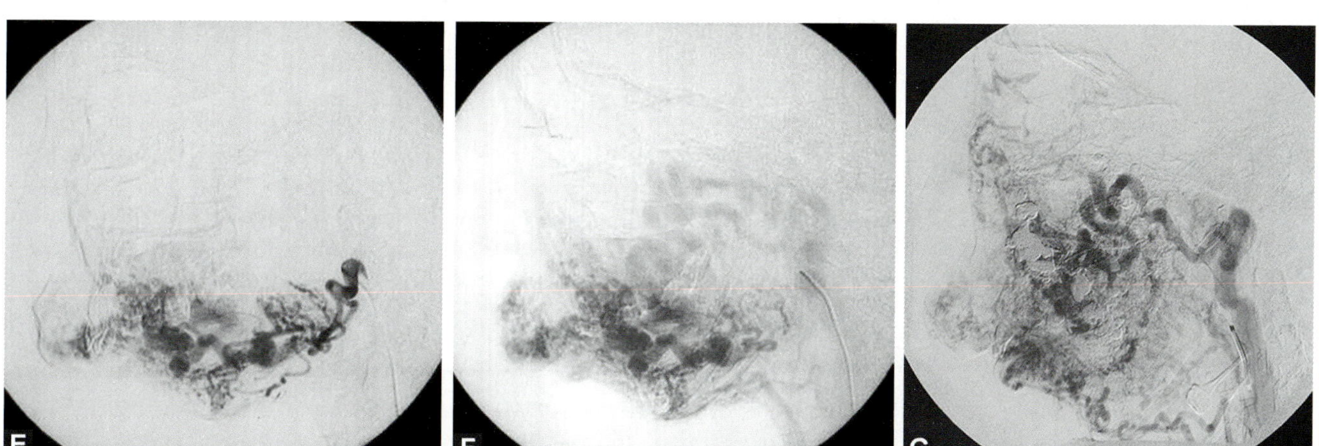

FIGURES 9.6E to G
(E) Angiogram—Selective left facial artery; (F and G) Pre and Postembolization of left facial artery

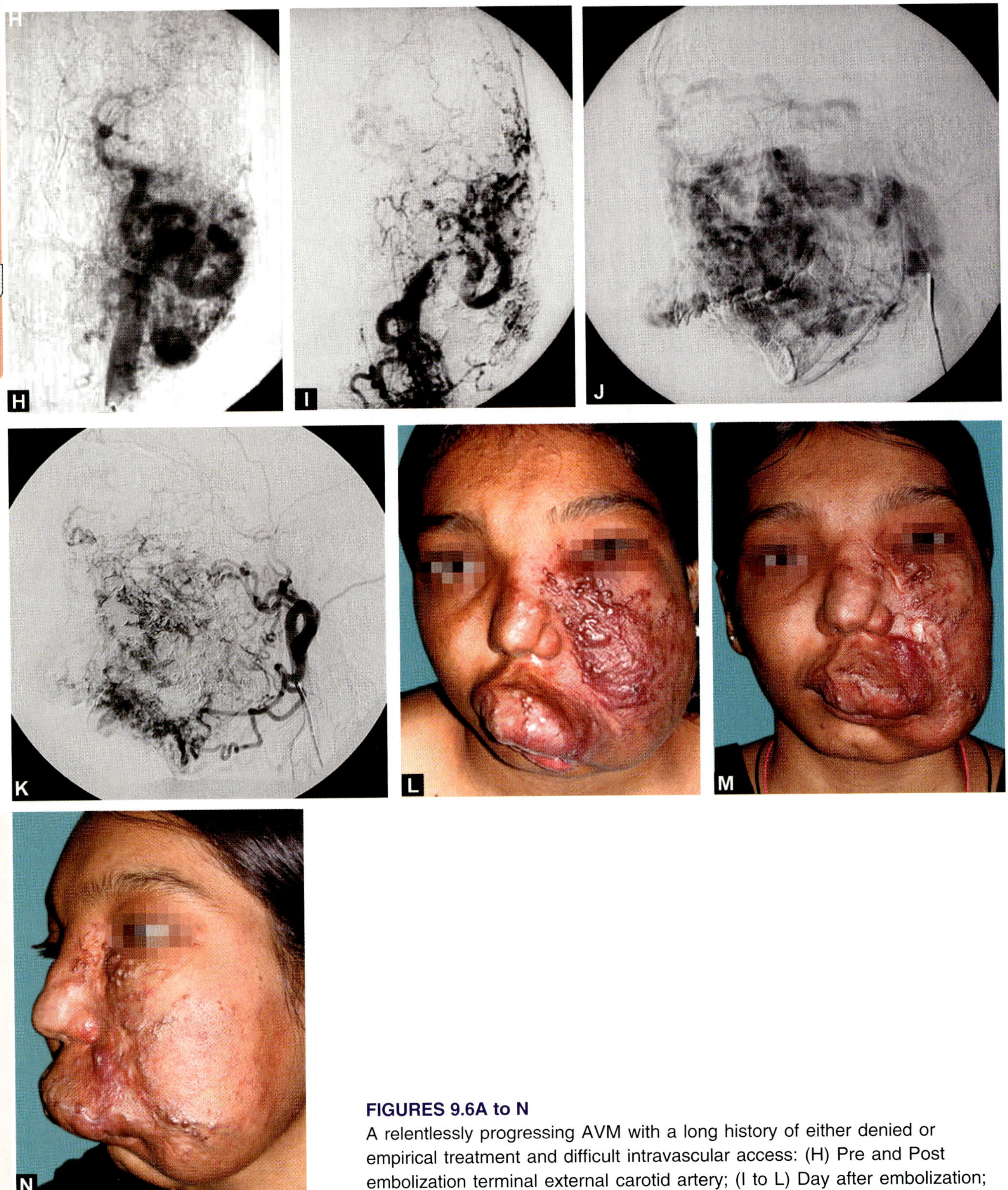

FIGURES 9.6A to N

A relentlessly progressing AVM with a long history of either denied or empirical treatment and difficult intravascular access: (H) Pre and Post embolization terminal external carotid artery; (I to L) Day after embolization; (M and N) 2 years after excision and shortly after 2 RF superpulse sessions

CASE STUDY

Importance of Early Eradication

The case study of a patient followed up for a long time has valuable lessons to offer.

The young man in Figure 9.7A, was referred to us by a colleague abroad for the treatment of an AVM in 1986.

He had a history of previous interventions since 1983.

The first surgery abroad in 1983, was a wedge excision from mucosal surface, an attempt to lower alar base and a ligature of the facial artery. A few months later, a small abscess at site of ligature had been drained. The second attempt, was made in India at another institution in 1985, involving an injection of boiling water and 'some surgery from inside and outside the mouth'. This was followed by episodes of severe bleeding from inside the mouth and an aggravation of facial deformity.

He came under our care in 1986. Angiography showed a number of feeders from facial artery and internal maxillary artery. The latter were embolized. We had no facilities to embolize the tiny feeders from the facial artery. The surgery was undertaken six days later. The nidus was excised and the vermillion readjusted. No blood transfusion was required and the recovery was uneventful (Figs. 9.7A to D).

Early recurrence a year later, was related to a branch of the maxillary artery. It was treated in the same way in 1987 (Figs. 9.7 E and F). A recurrence occurred again in three years (Fig. 9.7G). The treatment was delayed for two years because of educational considerations (Figs 9.7H and I). He was reoperated in 1992. By now we had better facilities and instrumentation. Again, the feeder was a branch of the maxillary artery which was embolized and the lesion resected (Fig. 9.7J). The patient has since done very well (Figs 9.7K and L) shows him 16 years later, lesion free and holding a very responsible position.

Relevant to this case, the question arises—*Why the recurrence twice?* The answer probably lies in the fact that the facial artery had been ligated at the first intervention, before he came under our care. The nidus had not been removed. Consequentially, feeders from maxillary artery had grown as a manifestation of the 'steal' phenomenon. Add to this the fact, that the embolizing armamentarium available to us at that time was poor.

Psychosocial Support

This patient's case history emphasizes that in dealing with these children, not only is a correct clinical evaluation relevant, but a careful emphasis on the need of follow-ups, and the possibility of multiple interventions.

Equally important is the incorporation of the needs of education, rehabilitation, psychological support and the cultivation of a positive attitude to life in the management plan. In most parts of the world, a strong psychosocial back-up is not available in the pediatric set-ups, and this role too, has to be effectively played by the clinicians.

AVM of the Jaws

AVMs of the jaws can present as a swelling or with a severe bleeding (usually at the time of a tooth extraction). These lesions of the facial skeleton have over the years,

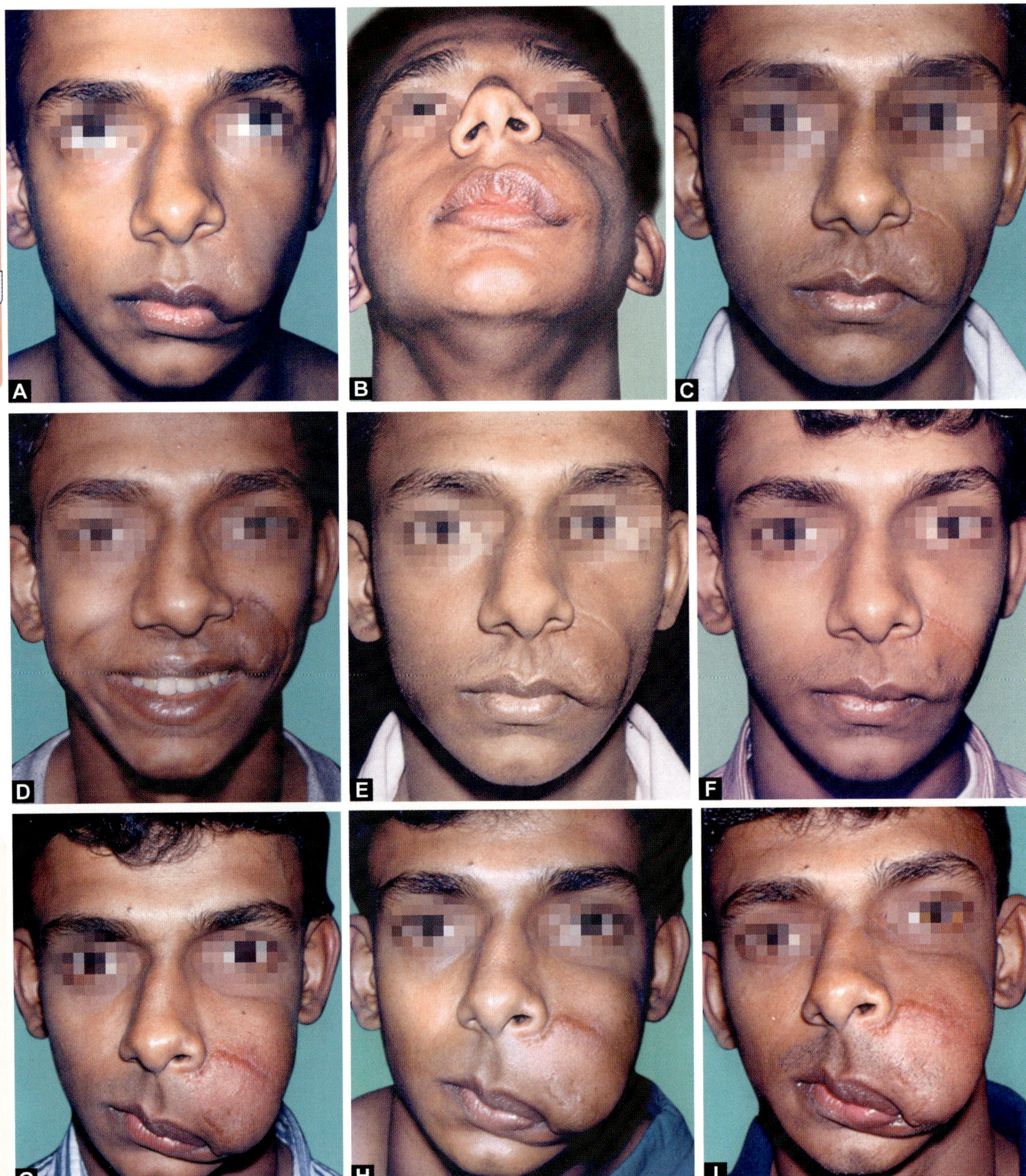
A
B
C
D
E
F
G
H
I

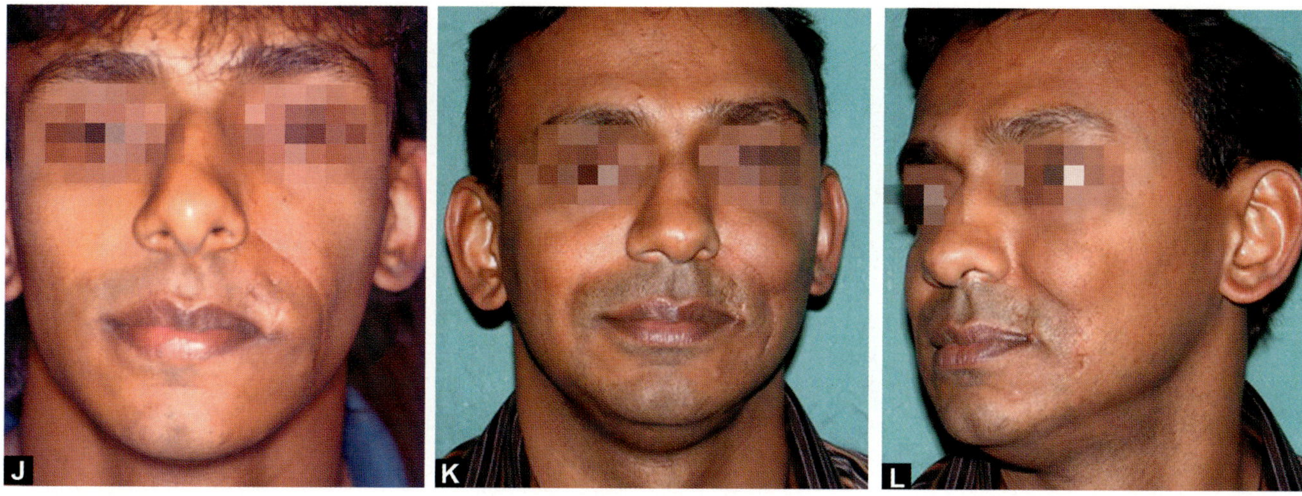

FIGURES 9.7A to L

A 16-year-old young boy presented with a swelling with recurrent hemorrhages, and two surgical interventions behind him: (A and B) Preoperative status, after embolization; (C and D) One month after the 1st surgical intervention; (E) Early recurrence 1 year later treated—embolization and surgery; (F) 2 months postoperative; (G) Recurrence after 3 years. Intervention delayed by 2 years for educational needs; (H and I) Note further yearly growth in a year; (I) As seen a year later. Maxillary artery perforators embolized and ablated; (J) The result; (K and L) 16 years later

posed special problems in management on two counts. The first, an access to the bleeders and the second, the preservation of the skeletal continuity, maintaining the shape and providing a bony platform to the bone graft. The management of both these problems has been facilitated by the development of interventional radiology.

A 24-year-old male, presented with a history of severe hemorrhage, following extraction of a left lower molar (Fig. 9.8). In view of the severe bleeding, a vascular malformation was suspected. Before anything could be done a massive recurrence of the hemorrhage led to an emergency angiography to locate and obliterate the bleeders.

The Figure 9.8A shows the bone defect in OPG and in (Fig. 9.8B) in the CT. The angiography (Fig. 9.8C) showed the lingual and facial arteries arising as a combined trunk from left external carotid artery. Arising from these, were multiple feeders leading to the malformation in the mandible.

Ablation of the nidus was carried out with absolute alcohol (ethanol) followed by an embolization and obliteration of these channels with cyanoacrylate glue (Figs 9.8D and E). The lesion was later curetted with the double objective of removing the nidus of the malformation and eliminating the chances of infection posed by the glue acting as a foreign body.

The patient had an uneventful recovery. No hemorrhagic episode occurred later. Bony remodeling was complete and the morphology of the mandible restored (Fig. 9.8F).

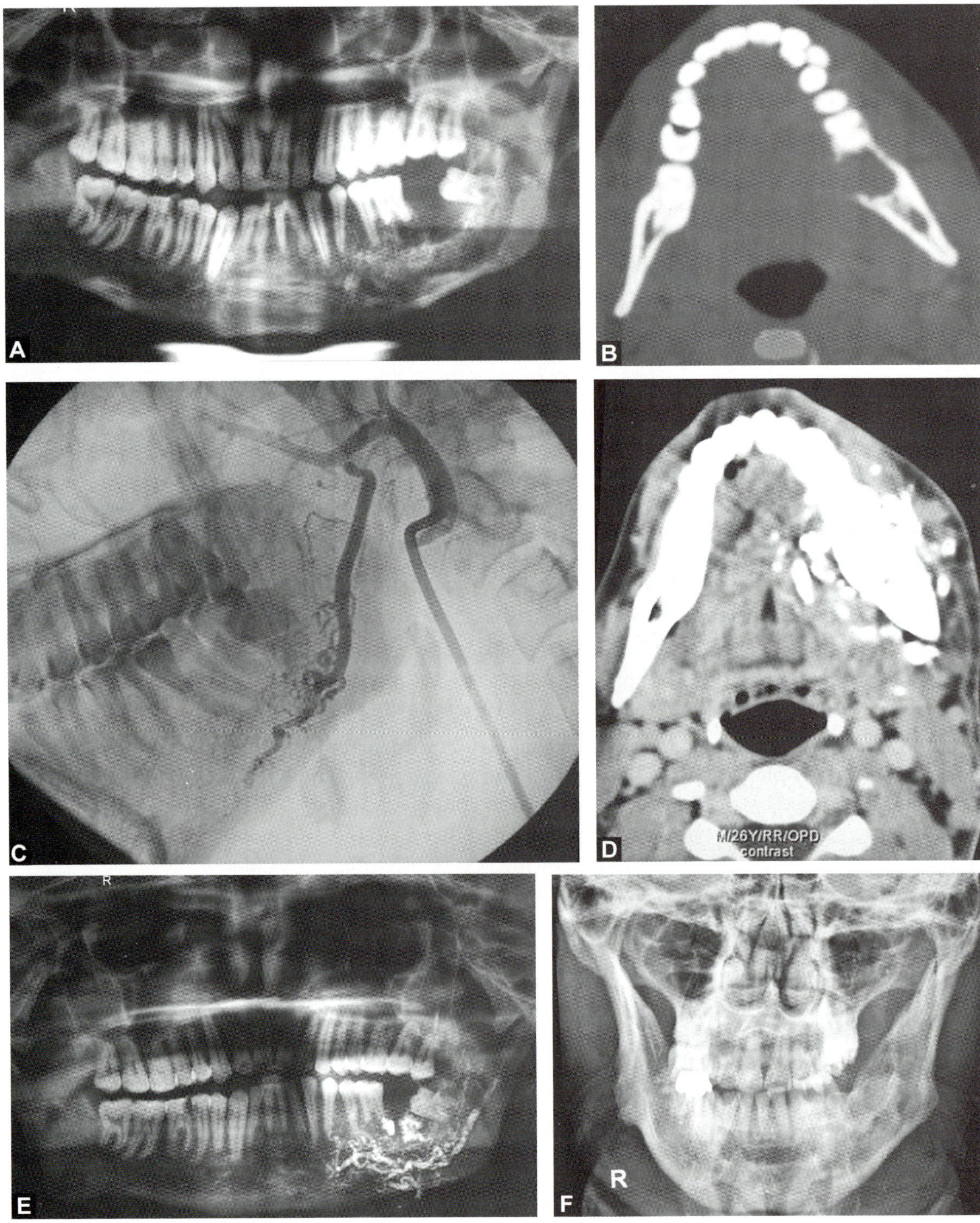

FIGURES 9.8A to F

Skeletal (Mandibular) AVM: (A and B) Pre-intervention view of the mandible; (C) Embolizing catheter in place showing the common origin of the ligual and facial arteries; (D) The embolized area of the malformation; (E) The embolized vessels in bone; (F) The remodeled skeleton. *Courtesy: Prof Dr Ashok V Dabir, MDS, Oral and Maxillofacial Surgeon*

SUMMARY

The AVMs, in the mandible can be life-threatening malformations and should be tackled early and effectively.

For localized lesions, which can be accessed by the embolizing catheter, total embolization using nonabsorbable particles is curative. However, if the lesion is on the surface, it can leave a small visible nodule.

For most lesions, the effective treatment is a total ablation of the nidus, preferably shortly after an effective embolization.

Reconstruction following ablation, whenever necessary, must conform to the principles and techniques of such reconstruction, taking into consideration the disturbance of the pattern of blood supply due to the malformation itself and following ablation.

To ensure minimum blood loss and a clean field for an effective ablation, needs a knowledge of the vascular supply and its pattern. To meet both these objectives, a close collaboration with an interventional radiologist is an absolute necessity.

All imaging modalities contribute to the preoperative assessment. However, a DSA study enables planning of the surgical approach and facilitates surgery by preoperative embolization.

Contrast CT and DSA, are invaluable in managing a recurrence, which is normally attributed to a part or the whole of the nidus escaping the ablative procedure. This recurrence draws its blood supply from the neighboring blood vessels—the 'steal phenomenon'—and if not recognized and dealt with early, becomes a formidable barrier to further management because of intense growth of the 'nidus', now fed by innumerable vessels making effective embolization impossible.

These large-lumen high flow malformations can be easily suspected because of their pulsatile nature, thrills and bruits. 'Fiddling' with them without careful evaluation and planning, is usually counter-productive. Ligations of main feeder trunks alone without removing the nidus can be disastrous.

Should the 'steal phenomenon' manifest itself, it should be tackled as soon as possible. Extensive steal phenomenon is a formidable problem which can be fatal. The principles of managing it are dealt with in the next chapter.

BIBLIOGRAPHY

1. Bryant WM, Maull KI. Arteriovenous malformations of the mandible. Graduated surgical management. Plast. Reconstr. Surg 1975;55:690.
2. Coleman CC Jr. Diagnosis and treatment of congenital arteriovenous fistulas of the head and neck. Am. J. Surg 1973;126:557.
3. Coleman CC Jr, Hoopes JE. Congenital arteriovenous anomalies of the head and neck. Plast. Reconstr. Surg 1971;47:354.
4. Cunningham DD, Paletta FX. Control of arteriovenous fistulae in massive facial hemangioma by muscle emboli. Plast. Reconstr. Surg 1970;46:305.
5. Engel JD, Supancic JS, Davis LF. Arteriovenous malformation of the mandible: Life-threatening complications during tooth extraction. J Am Dent Assoc 1995;126(2):237-42.
6. Gomes AS. Embolization therapy of congenital arteriovenous malformations: Use of alternate approaches. Radiology 1994;190:191-198 [Abstract/Free Full Text].
7. Noreau G, Landry Pierre-É, Morais D. Arteriovenous malformation of the Mandible: Review of Literature and Case History: J Can Dent Assoc 2001;67(11):646-651.

8. Haller JA Jr, Pickard LR, Kumar AJ, White RI Jr. A new percutaneous technique for occluding arterial flow to massive congenital A-V malformation to prevent major hemorrhage during resection. J. Pediatr. Surg 1980;15:523.
9. Jackson IT, Clifford RJ, Aycock B, Dubin B, Irons GB. The management of intraosseous arteriovenous malformations in the head and neck area. Plast Reconstr Surg 1989; 84(1):47-54.
10. Lamberg MA, Tasanen A, Jääskeläinen J. Fatality from central hemangioma of the mandible. J Oral Surg 1979; 37(8):578-84.
11. Olcott C, Newton TH, Stoney RJ, Ehrenfeld WK. Intra-arterial embolization in the management of arteriovenous malformations. Surgery 1976;79:3.
12. Shenoy SN, Raja A. Scalp arteriovenous malformations. Neurol India 2004;52:478-81.
13. Williams HB. Facial bone changes with vascular tumors in children. Plast. Reconstr. Surg 1979;63:309.

10

THE STEAL PHENOMENON AND ITS MANAGEMENT

KS Goleria

The 'steal phenomenon' deserves to be kept in mind when planning and managing the arteriovenous malformations (AVMs) which have been an enigma, since the times of Virchow, over one and half century ago. Keeping a postoperative eye for recurrence is an equally important part of the management. Recurrence too needs an early and effective management.

STEAL AND NIDUS

An arteriovenous malformation is distinguished by a direct communication between the arteries and the veins without the intervention of the capillary system. A single such communication is referred to as an arteriovenous fistula (AVF), and a conglomeration of such fistulae as an arteriovenous malformation (AVM). The AVMs are far more common. AVFs are usually post-traumatic and AVMs usually congenital.

When dealing with these lesion, the concept of 'nidus' and 'steal' needs to be elaborated. The 'nidus' is a fast flow system involving both the arteries and the veins. It is a high pressure system wherein, even the veins tend to be arterialized. Being a very high flow, low resistance system, it tends to suck in blood from the neighborhood. It was the intracranial AVMs which first drew attention of the surgical world to the associated neurological morbidity and deficits which were attributed to the steal phenomenon. The closure or ablation of the intracranial AVMs, in turn, is associated with hyperperfusion (Nakagawa, et al 2005)—the high input now has no quick, resistance free exit. In the closed space of the cranium, the effect of these changes on the brain is readily recognizable. It is of great concern and has received a lot of attention.

However, the AVMs on the more accessible areas also exhibit the effects of the 'steal' phenomenon. Here, the manifestation is dusky discoloration, congestion, stasis and poor oxygenation, often associated with ulceration and bleeds as seen in Figures 10.2A to C. The 'nidus' is the cause and the promoter of the 'steal', which in turn aggravates the 'nidus'. The changes are believed to be mediated by biological factors. The persistent hypoxia initiates the changes. The vascular endothelial growth factor (VEGF) and the basic fibroblast growth factors (bFGF) are supposed to play a part. The shunts that are created cause enlargement of the feeder arteries and then form a tangled nidus with enlarged draining veins and feeding arteries.

When the feeders are ligated leaving the nidus intact, the 'steal' takes on another form, viz. development of vascularization from the neighboring vascular systems (Fig. 10.4).

Thus the 'steal' phenomenon has two expressions. With the intact blood supply, the 'nidus' per se, steals blood from the neighboring tissues. When the main blood supply is blocked the nidus draws blood from the neighboring blood supply, creating a huge network of feeders and consequentially the draining veins.

The only effective solution to break this cycle and eliminate its consequences is the elimination of the nidus with embolization or ablation, preferably both sequentially.

Haphazard management can be disastrous. What follows is a case study which documents the genesis of a most aggressive steal phenomenon with a giant nidus and its hazardous management.

A CASE STUDY OF AN ARTERIOVENOUS MALFORMATION

This case study encompasses 16 years of interventional management with steady aggravation, before he was referred to us in a desperate state. The management thereafter, the rehabilitation and the team work involved are enumerated.

According to the history, the first manifestation of the problem, was a bleed from his right lower gum (during a religious ceremony) when he was about seven years old. Figure 10.1 shows the patient on the day of the first bleed. The picture clearly shows an enlarged right pinna and if one looks carefully, the right lower face shows a bulge.

PAST SURGICAL HISTORY

In 1987, the first angiography was done but no details are available. A short time later, in the same year an ***external carotid ligation above superior thyroid artery*** was performed and 6 months later a Hemimandibulectomy and a rib graft reconstruction was carried out. Apparently, this did not do well and in 1990, a titanium implant was substituted. In 1992, the patient had a partial excision of the lower lip.

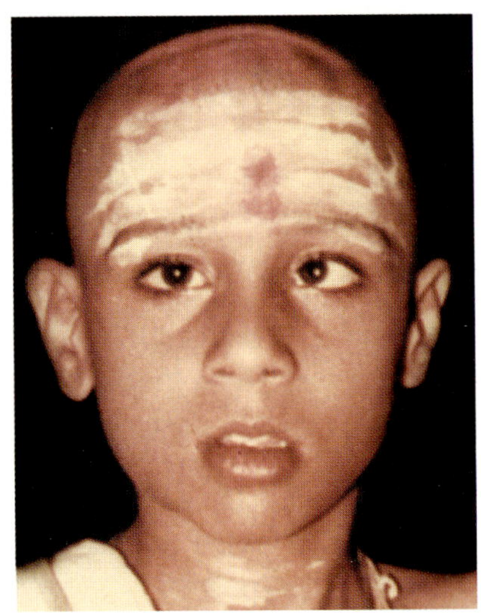

FIGURE 10.1
The patient on the day of the first bleed from the right lower gum. Note the enlarged right pinna and the slight bulge in the right lower face

In 1994, both the hospital and the surgeon were changed and the 'hemangioma' excised by a lip splitting incision. More interventions followed. In 1995, removal of the right ear was carried out and the ear cartilage banked on the trunk. In 1996, partial reconstruction of the right ear was carried out.

According to the patient, between 1992 and 1996 an angiography was carried out before every operative intervention but the documents were not made available to the patient.

Thereafter, the patients management mainly consisted of repeated sutures to arrest hemorrhages from the lip, as well inj. Setral and other sclerosants till 2003. Yet the AVM continued to grow aggressively.

MANAGEMENT

Evaluation

When first seen by us in 2003 *(16 years after the first bleed),* the patient was desparate, having had innumerable interventions, recurrent bleeds and severe disfigurement.

Figures 10.2A to C show the widespread vascular malformation, the dusky appearance and the extent of the physical disfigurement showing the engorgement, discoloration and deformity. The OPG and the radiograph of the face reveal that more than half of the mandible is missing with an implant, whose condylar head is far from the articular fossa (probably displaced downwards by the malformation) and the fixation of the medial end to the left mandible loose—the implant only a little short of freely floating (Figs 10.2D and E).

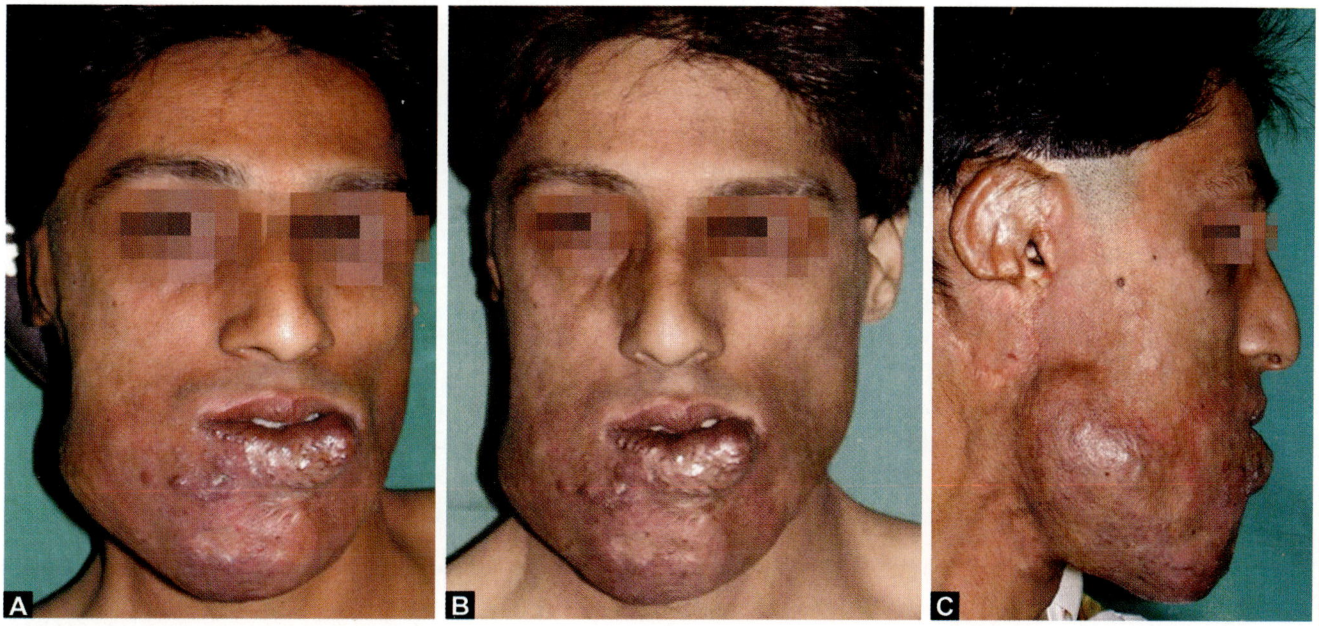

FIGURES 10.2A to C
The status on presentation: (A) Standing; (B) Recumbent showing increased engorgement; (C) Profile standing

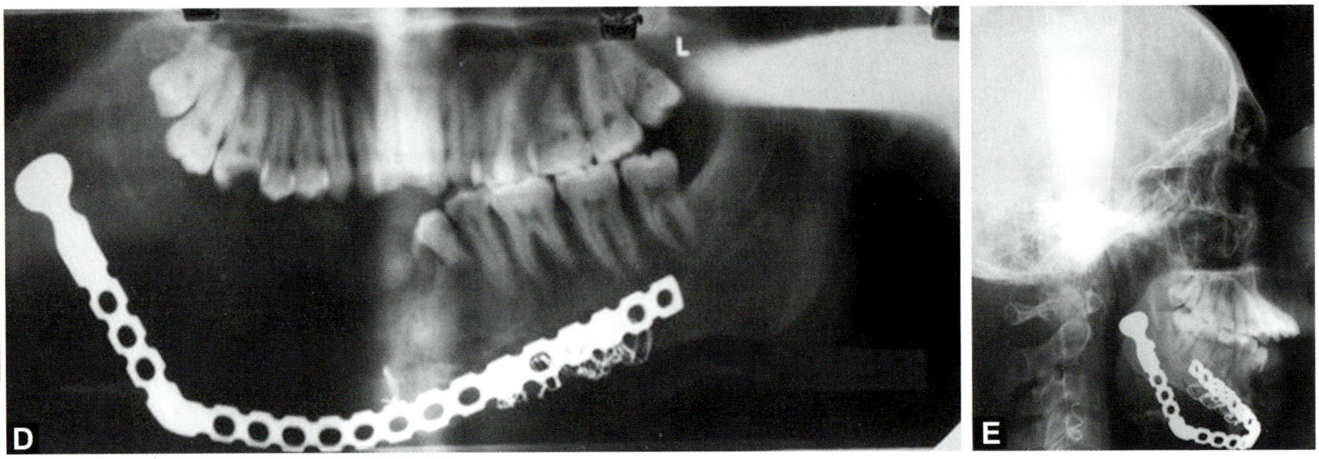

FIGURES 10.2D and E

(D and E) The OPG and the lateral cephalogram showing the extent of ablation and the almost floating implant

The CT studies (Figs 10.3A to C) show the widespread vascular malformation. These show the loss of over half of the mandible and the massive extent of the AV malformation and its nidus both within and outside the oral cavity.

With the history of the ligation of the right external carotid artery, distal to the origin of the superior thyroid artery and away from the nidus 16 years earlier, this was obviously an expression of 'the steal phenomenon'.

Our worst fears were confirmed by a DSA study as shown in Figure 10.4. The lesion is fed not only by the innumerable branches arising from the ligated right external carotid artery, but also by feeders arising from the opposite external carotid artery, both the internal carotid arteries and both the vertebral arteries.

There was no way that all these could be embolized near the massive nidus where the feeding vessels were innumerable.

The patient had suffered so much, that the he was willing to get rid of the lesion even if it meant the loss of the total lower face. In fact he felt that even death would be more welcome than the life he was leading.

After due deliberations among the team members and with the patient accepting the risks involved, it was decided to carry out an ablation of the total nidus and to follow it up with an immediate total reconstruction using a free microvascular latissimus dorsi muscle flap with an appropriate skin paddle.

Ablation and Disseminated Intravascular Coagulation (DIC)

Ablation was the only available solution. It involved the removal of the implant, the affected soft tissues, a significant part of the floor of the mouth and a massive blood loss. It took about 7 hours of surgery and 7 units of blood. After considerable hemostasis was achieved, a fresh increase in bleeding from the raw surface raised doubts of an early DIC. Appropriate measures were taken and it was decided to abandon reconstruction and do a wound closure (Figs 10.5A and B).

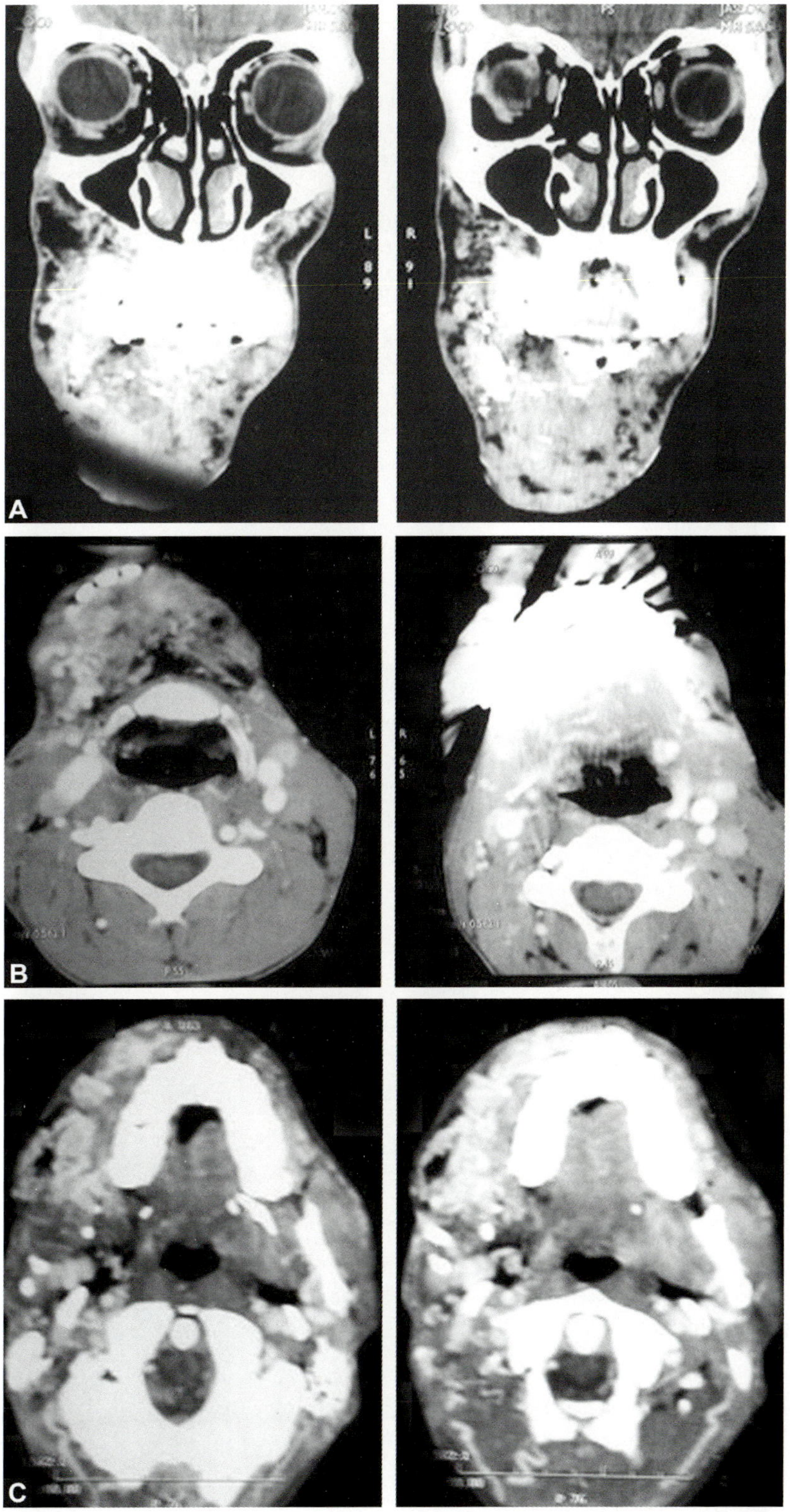

FIGURES 10.3A to C

The extent of the nidus — A CT study: (A) A couple of sections in the coronal plane; (B) Axial sections at the level of the mandible; (C) Axial sections at the level of the maxillary arch

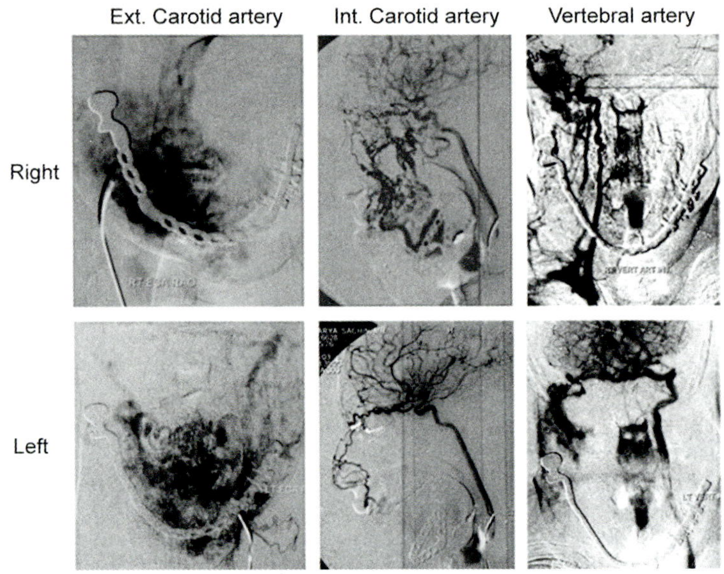

FIGURE 10.4
A DSA study of The 'steal' phenomenon. Note the feeders from both the external carotid arteries, both the internal carotid arteries and both the vertebral arteries

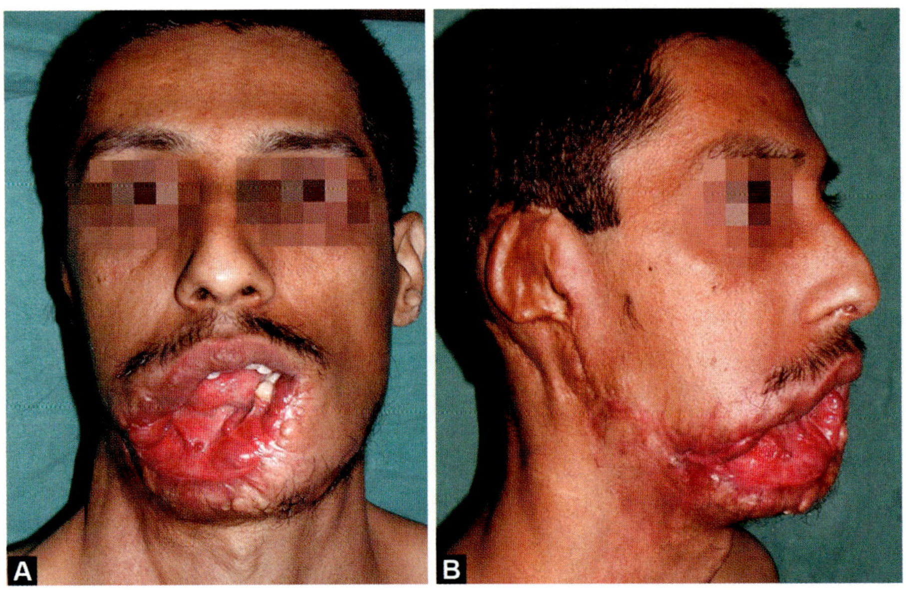

FIGURES 10.5A and B
Status after ablation and wound closure

The DIC was confirmed by the hematology department. The patient responded to the therapy and made a rapid recovery.

THE RECONSTRUCTION

He was taken up for repair 5 months later. Ipsilateral musculocutaneous latissimus dorsi muscle flap was planned to repair the defect. The design ensured that the free border of the muscle forms the free border of lower lip. A length of the nerve to latissimus dorsi muscle was harvested with the pedicle for anastamosis to the now spare lower division of the facial nerve. For saving costs, the removed implant duly sterilized was used for structural support.

However, when it came to ipsilateral vascular anastomosis, extensive vascularity of the region posed considerable problems. The result was excellent and remained so for the next 2 days. The disaster stuck on the 3rd day. Re-exploration showed that the block was on the donor side of the anastamosis and the intense vascularity made reanastomosis impossible. The flap had to be discarded and the wounds closed. The healing was uneventful.

Since, the tissues were clean and healthy, the patient fit and not merely willing but keen, the operating team after due deliberation decided to make the second attempt at reconstruction a week later, re-enacting the same plan, using the opposite, latissimus dorsi muscle, recipient vessels and the lower branch of the facial nerve with expected result (Figs 10.6A to D).

Figures 10.7A and B show a 30 months follow-up with a good muscle support of the reconstructed lower lip, restoration of continence to the right angle of the mouth. and an effective sphincteric action of the oral stoma. However, the small residual lesion on the upper lip had grown slightly (Figs 10.7C and D).

Removal of the residual lesion and the restoration of the sphincteric action to both the angles of the mouth has given a totally competent oral sphincter (Figs 10.8A to D).

There was no evidence of recurrence for over three years. The patient is happy, socially well adjusted, self-supporting and doing reasonably well.

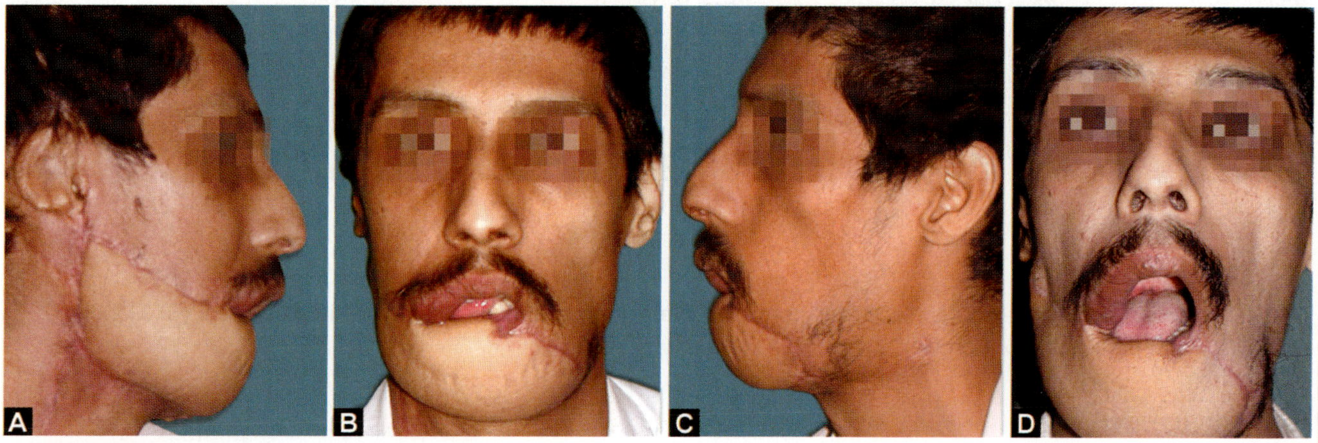

FIGURES 10.6A to D

Shape resonably restored. Muscle reintervention still to take place. Oral feeding possible with some oral incontinence. Note a small residual lesion. The postoperative result: (A) Left profile; (B) Front; (C) Right profile; (D) Mouth opening

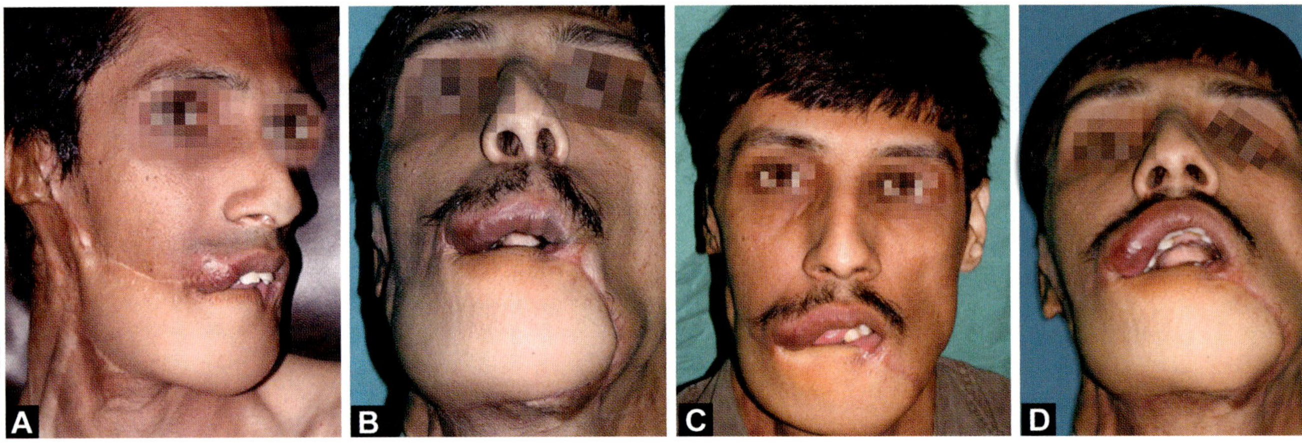

FIGURES 10.7A to D
A 30 month follow-up (A and B). Note the formation of the right angle of the mouth and the restoration of the sphincteric action; (C and D) The residual lesion of the upper lip shows a small growth

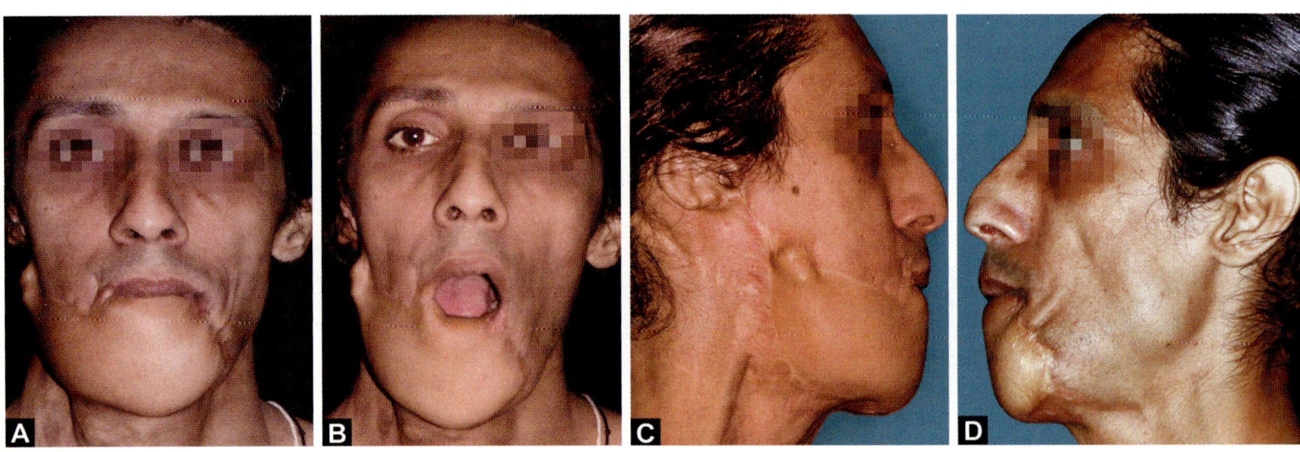

FIGURES 10.8A to D
The lesion is cleared and the oral sphincter fully restored. No evidence of recurrence. (A) Mouth closed; (B) Mouth open; (C) Right profile; (D) Left profile

SUMMARY

The 'steal' phenomenon is a deadly characteristic of arteriovenous malformation (AVMs). The basic pathological unit of this malformation is the arteriovenous fistula.

A conglomeration of the arteriovenous fistulae is its 'nidus'. An AVM, can have a number of 'nidi'. The fast flow that the 'nidus' generates, is the cause of the 'steal phenomenon' which expresses itself in different ways.

Untouched by direct interventional effort, when in the confines of the cranial cavity, it expresses itself as neurological deficits. In the more accessible areas, it is a pulsatile swelling with a dusky discoloration, poor oxygenation and with a tendency to ulcerate and bleed.

Following surgical intervention, when the feeders are ligated, the steal has a different face. The 'nidus' draws blood from the neighboring blood supply creating a huge network of feeders and draining veins.

The 'nidus' is the cause of the 'steal' which in turn promotes the 'nidus'. The only way to cure an AVM is to totally eliminate the nidus. Total ablation can at times produce hideous deformity which needs reconstruction.

Defining the limits of ablation and a prior thought for reconstruction, can make a profound difference. The choice of tissue to be preserved even temporarily, prior identification of a nerve here or a vessel there and the identification of the tissue to be brought in for repair are essential to an aesthetic and functionally adequate result.

Merely ligating the main feeding vessel, without total elimination of the 'nidus, can be disastrous.

As mentioned earlier "steal phenomenon" is confined to AVMs, and of AVMs it can truly be said, 'A wrong beginning by ligating the feeding vessels without ablation of the nidus can create a subsequent hell.'

ACKNOWLEDGMENT

The contributions of Dr Shaji Marar, MD, Interventional Radiologist and Dr Sameer Kumta, MS, MCh, Microvascular Plastic and Reconstructive Surgeon, Jaslok Hospital and Research Center, Mumbai, Maharashtra, India

BIBLIOGRAPHY

1. Ichiro N, Shoichiro K, Junichi I, Hidehiro H, Toshisuke S. Postoperative hyperperfusion associated with steal phenomenon caused by a small arteriovenous malformation. Neurologia medico-chirurgica 2005;45:363-6.
2. Moussa, Ronad F, Wong, John H. Chapter on Pathology and Genetic Factors, pg 22. in Intracranial Arteriovenous Malformations By Philip E Stieg, H Hunt Batjer, Duke Samson. Google Books.

APPENDIX: EXISTING NOMENCLATURE OF HEMANGIOMAS AND VASCULAR MALFORMATIONS

A SOURCE OF CONFUSION

VASCULAR TUMORS OF INFANCY AND CHILDHOOD

Capillary hemangioma of infancy
- Syn. Infantile hemangioma
  - Common hemangioma of infancy

Congenital hemangioma
Miliary hemangiomatosis of infancy
Tufted angioma
- Syn. Angioblastoma

Kaposiform hemangioendothelioma
Kasabach-Merritt phenomenon
- Syn. Hemangioma — hemorrhage syndrome

Verrucous hemangioma
Digital verrucous fibroangioma
Hemangiopericytoma
Glomangiomas
- Syn. Multiple glomus tumors
  - Glomangiomatosis
  - Disseminated multiple glomangiomas
  - Localized multiple glomangiomas
  - Congenital plague-like glomangiomas

VASCULAR MALFORMATIONS

Capillary vascular malformations
- Syn. Telangiectatic nevi
  - Vascular stains

Salmon patch
- Syn. Nevus simplex
  - Erythema nuchae

Unna's nevus
Stork bite
Angel's kiss
Port-wine stain
Syn. Nevus flammeus
The Sturge-Weber syndrome
Syn: Encephalofacial angiomatosis
Encephalotrigeminal angiomatosis
Proteus syndrome
Craniofacio cutaneous syndrome
Nevus anemicus
Nevus oligaemicus
Roberts' syndrome
Syn: Hypomelia-hypotrichosis-facial hemangioma syndrome
Thrombocytopenia-absent radii syndrome
Wyburn-Mason syndrome
Syn: Bonnet-Dechaume-Blanc syndrome
Beckwith-Wiedemann syndrome
Syn: Exomphalos-macroglossia-gigantism syndrome

MIXED VASCULAR MALFORMATIONS

Macrocephaly cutis marmorata telangiectatica congenita
Syn: Macrocephaly with cutis marmorata
Hemangioma and syndactyly syndrome
Macrocephaly, cutis marmorata, midline telangiectatic nevus and syndactyly syndrome
Cutis marmorata telangiectatica congenita
Syn. Reticulate vascular nevus
Divry-van Bogaert syndrome
Syn. Corticomeningeal angiomatosis
Recticulate vascular nevus
Klippel-trenaunay syndrome

OTHER MULTIPLE VASCULAR MALFORMATION SYNDROMES

Bannayan-Riley-Ruvalcaba syndrome
Syn. Bannyan Zonnana syndrome
Riley Smith syndrome
Hereditary neurocutaneous vascular malformations
Syn. Hereditary neurocutaneous angiomas
Hereditary hemorrhagic telangiectasia
Syn. Osler-Weber-Rendu disease

ANGIOKERATOMAS

Angiokeratoma circumscriptum
    Syn. Angiokeratoma corporis cicumscriptum neviforme
Angikeratoma of Mibelli
Solitary papular angiokeratoma
Angiokeratomas of the scrotum and vulva
Angiokeratoma corporis diffusion universale
Angiokeratoma fucocidosis
Angiokeratoma of fordyce

LYMPHATIC MALFORMATIONS

Microcystic lymphatic malformation
Small channel lymphatic malformation
Lymphangioma
Large channel lymphatic malformation
Cystic hygroma
Macrocystic lymphatic malformation

VENOUS MALFORMATIONS

Blue rubber bleb nevus syndrome
Maffucci's syndrome
    Syn. Dyschondroplasia with hemangiomas
        Unilateral dermatomal hemangiomatosis
Zosteriform venous malformations
Gortham's disease
    Syn: Hemangiomas with osteolysis
        Disappearing bone disease
        Osteovascular dysplasia
Other multiple dysplasia syndromes

ARTERIAL AND ARTERIOVENOUS MALFORMATIONS

Arteriovenous fistula —AVF
Arteriovenous malformation—AVM, with aneurysm

Index

Page numbers followed by *f* refer to figures and *t* refer to tables